Topics in Cardiology

Guest Editor

JONATHAN A. ABBOTT, DVM

VETERINARY CLINICS
OF NORTH AMERICA:
SMALL ANIMAL PRACTICE

www.vetsmall.theclinics.com

July 2010 • Volume 40 • Number 4

SAUNDERS an imprint of ELSEVIER, Inc.

W.B. SAUNDERS COMPANY
A Division of Elsevier Inc.

1600 John F. Kennedy Blvd. • Suite 1800 • Philadelphia, PA 19103-2899
http://www.vetsmall.theclinics.com

VETERINARY CLINICS OF NORTH AMERICA: SMALL ANIMAL PRACTICE Volume 40, Number 4
July 2010 ISSN 0195-5616, ISBN-13: 978-1-4377-2506-3

Editor: John Vassallo; j.vassallo@elsevier.com

Veterinary Clinics of North America: Small Animal Practice (ISSN 0195-5616) is published bimonthly (For Post Office use only: volume 40 issue 4 of 6) by Elsevier Inc., 360 Park Avenue South, New York, NY 10010-1710. Months of issue are January, March, May, July, September, and November. Business and Editorial Offices: 1600 John F. Kennedy Blvd., Ste. 1800, Philadelphia, PA 19103-2899. Customer Service Office: 3251 Riverport Lane, Maryland Heights, MO 63043. Periodicals postage paid at New York, NY and additional mailing offices. Subscription prices are $245.00 per year (domestic individuals), $388.00 per year (domestic institutions), $122.00 per year (domestic students/residents), $324.00 per year (Canadian individuals), $477.00 per year (Canadian institutions), $360.00 per year (international individuals), $477.00 per year (international institutions), and $177.00 per year (international and Canadian students/residents). To receive student/resident rate, orders must be accompanied by name of affiliated institution, date of term, and the *signature* of program/residency coordinator on institution letterhead. Orders will be billed at individual rate until proof of status is received. Foreign air speed delivery is included in all *Clinics* subscription prices. All prices are subject to change without notice. **POSTMASTER:** Send address changes to *Veterinary Clinics of North America: Small Animal Practice*, Elsevier Health Sciences Division, Subscription Customer Service, 3251 Riverport Lane, Maryland Heights, MO 63043. Customer Service (orders, claims, online, change of address): Elsevier Periodicals Customer Service, Elsevier Health Sciences Division Subscription Customer Service 3251 Riverport Lane Maryland Heights, MO 63043. Tel: 1-800-654-2452 (U.S. and Canada); 314-447-8871 (outside U.S. and Canada). Fax: 314-447-8029. E-mail: journalscustomerservice-usa@elsevier.com (for print support); journalsonlinesupport-usa@elsevier.com (for online support).

Reprints. For copies of 100 or more of articles in this publication, please contact the Commercial Reprints Department, Elsevier Inc., 360 Park Avenue South, New York, NY 10010-1710. Tel.: 212-633-3812; Fax: 212-462-1935; E-mail: reprints@elsevier.com.

Veterinary Clinics of North America: Small Animal Practice is also published in Japanese by Inter Zoo Publishing Co., Ltd., Aoyama Crystal-Bldg 5F, 3-5-12 Kitaaoyama, Minato-ku, Tokyo 107-0061, Japan.

Veterinary Clinics of North America: Small Animal Practice is covered in *Current Contents/Agriculture, Biology and Environmental Sciences, Science Citation Index, ASCA, MEDLINE/PubMed (Index Medicus), Excerpta Medica,* and *BIOSIS.*

Printed and bound by CPI Group (UK) Ltd, Croydon, CR0 4YY

Transferred to Digital Print 2011

Contributors

GUEST EDITOR

JONATHAN A. ABBOTT, DVM
Diplomate, American College of Veterinary Internal Medicine (Cardiology); Associate
Professor of Cardiology, Department of Small Animal Clinical Sciences, Virginia-Maryland
Regional College of Veterinary Medicine, Virginia Polytechnic Institute and State
University, Blacksburg, Virginia

AUTHORS

JONATHAN A. ABBOTT, DVM
Diplomate, American College of Veterinary Internal Medicine (Cardiology); Associate
Professor of Cardiology, Department of Small Animal Clinical Sciences, Virginia-Maryland
Regional College of Veterinary Medicine, Virginia Polytechnic Institute and State
University, Blacksburg, Virginia

LAWRENCE T. BISH, PhD
Department of Physiology, University of Pennsylvania School of Medicine, Philadelphia,
Pennsylvania

MICHELE BORGARELLI, DMV, PhD
Diplomate, European College of Veterinary Internal Medicine (Cardiology); Associate
Professor of Cardiology, Department of Clinical Sciences, Kansas State University College
of Veterinary Medicine, Manhattan, Kansas

ADRIAN BOSWOOD, MA, VetMB, DVC, MRCVS
Diplomate, European College of Veterinary Internal Medicine-Companion Animals
(Cardiology); Professor of Veterinary Cardiology, Department of Veterinary Clinical
Sciences, The Royal Veterinary College, North Mymms, Hatfield, Hertfordshire,
United Kingdom

VALÉRIE CHETBOUL, DVM, PhD
Diplomate, European College of Veterinary Internal Medicine - Companion Animals
(Cardiology); Professor of Veterinary Cardiology and Internal Medicine, Unité de
Cardiologie d'Alfort, UMR INSERM-ENVA U955, Ecole Nationale Vétérinaire d'Alfort,
Maisons-Alfort Cedex, France

DAVID J. CONNOLLY, BSc, BVetMed, PhD, CertSAM, CertVC
Diplomate, European College of Veterinary Internal Medicine-Companion Animals;
Department of Veterinary Clinical Sciences, Royal Veterinary College, Hatfield,
Hertfordshire, United Kingdom

ETIENNE CÔTÉ, DVM
Diplomate, American College of Veterinary Internal Medicine (Cardiology, SAIM);
Associate Professor, Department of Companion Animals, Atlantic Veterinary College,
University of Prince Edward Island, Charlottetown, Prince Edward Island, Canada

LEIGH G. GRIFFITHS, VetMB, MRCVS, PhD
Assistant Professor, Department of Veterinary Medicine and Epidemiology, University of California, Davis, California

JENS HAGGSTROM, DVM, PhD
Diplomate, European College Veterinary Internal Medicine (Cardiology); Professor of Internal Medicine, Department of Clinical Sciences, Swedish University of Agricultural Sciences, Uppsala, Sweden

HEIDI B. KELLIHAN, DVM
Clinical Assistant Professor-Cardiology, Department of Medical Sciences, School of Veterinary Medicine, University of Wisconsin, Madison, Wisconsin

KRISTIN MACDONALD, DVM, PhD
Diplomate, American College of Veterinary Internal Medicine (Cardiology); VCA-The Animal Care Center of Sonoma, Rohnert Park, California

KATHRYN M. MEURS, DVM, PhD
Professor, Department of Veterinary Clinical Sciences, Washington State University College of Veterinary Medicine, Pullman, Washington

MARK A. OYAMA, DVM
Diplomate, American College of Veterinary Internal Medicine - Cardiology; Associate Professor, Department of Clinical Studies-Philadelphia, Matthew J. Ryan Veterinary Hospital, University of Pennsylvania, Philadelphia, Pennsylvania

GRETCHEN E. SINGLETARY, DVM
Resident Cardiology, Department of Clinical Studies-Philadelphia, Matthew J. Ryan Veterinary Hospital, University of Pennsylvania, Philadelphia, Pennsylvania

MEG M. SLEEPER, VMD
Associate Professor of Cardiology, Section of Cardiology, Department of Clinical Studies, University of Pennsylvania Veterinary School, Philadelphia, Pennsylvania

CHRISTOPHER D. STAUTHAMMER, DVM
Diplomate, American College of Veterinary Internal Medicine (Cardiology); Assistant Clinical Professor of Cardiology, Veterinary Clinical Sciences Department, College of Veterinary Medicine, University of Minnesota, St Paul, Minnesota

REBECCA L. STEPIEN, DVM, MS
Clinical Professor-Cardiology, Department of Medical Sciences, School of Veterinary Medicine, University of Wisconsin, Madison, Wisconsin

H. LEE SWEENEY, PhD
Chairman of Physiology, Department of Physiology, University of Pennsylvania School of Medicine, Philadelphia, Pennsylvania

ANTHONY H. TOBIAS, BVSc, PhD
Diplomate, American College of Veterinary Internal Medicine (Cardiology); Associate Professor and Section Chief of Cardiology, Veterinary Clinical Sciences Department, College of Veterinary Medicine, University of Minnesota, St Paul, Minnesota

Contents

Advanced Techniques in Echocardiography in Small Animals 529

Valérie Chetboul

Transthoracic echocardiography has become a major imaging tool for the diagnosis and management of canine and feline cardiovascular diseases. During the last decade, more recent advances in ultrasound technology with the introduction of newer imaging modalities, such as tissue Doppler imaging, strain and strain rate imaging, and 2-dimensional speckle tracking echocardiography, have provided new parameters to assess myocardial performance, including regional myocardial velocities and deformation, ventricular twist, and mechanical synchrony. An outline of these 4 recent ultrasound techniques, their impact on the understanding of right and left ventricular function in small animals, and their application in research and clinical settings are given in this article.

The Use of NT-proBNP Assay in the Management of Canine Patients with Heart Disease 545

Mark A. Oyama and Gretchen E. Singletary

The diagnosis and management of canine heart disease could be facilitated by a highly sensitive and specific laboratory test that predicts risk of morbidity and mortality, is helpful in directing therapy, easy to perform, inexpensive, and widely available. This article details if, how, and when the cardiac biomarker, N-terminal fragment of the prohormone B-type natriuretic peptide (NT-proBNP), helps in the diagnosis and management of canine heart disease. Veterinary cardiac biomarkers, specifically NT-proBNP, hold great promise. The incorporation of NT-proBNP assay into successful clinical practice requires an understanding of the science behind the technology, as well as the clinical data available to date.

Natriuretic Peptides: The Feline Experience 559

David J. Connolly

In feline medicine natriuretic peptides (NP), particularly NT-proBNP, have emerged as biomarkers with significant potential. Since the introduction of the commercial ELISA that enabled the convenient and accurate measurement of circulating N terminal ANP and BNP fragments research examining the utility of these peptides as an aid to the diagnosis of feline cardiovascular disease has accelerated. This article describes the results of these studies and tries to put them in the context of clinical practice by exploring the areas of agreement and controversy and explaining the influence of confounding factors on the interpretation of NP concentrations. Considerable further work is needed to fully evaluate the clinical utility of NP regarding their potential for diagnosis, prognosis, and guidance of treatment.

Pimobendan is a drug with both inotropic and vasodilatory properties and is widely used for the treatment of heart failure in dogs. The best evidence regarding its efficacy is derived from several clinical studies of dogs with the two most common conditions that result in heart failure: dilated cardiomyopathy (DCM) and degenerative mitral valve disease (DMVD). The main studies addressing the effectiveness of pimobendan in dogs with DCM and DVMD are discussed in this article.

With ever-increasing sophistication of veterinary cardiology, minimally invasive per-catheter occlusion and dilation procedures for the treatment of various congenital cardiovascular abnormalities in dogs have become not only available, but mainstream. Much new information about minimally invasive per-catheter patent ductus arteriosus occlusion has been published and presented during the past few years. Consequently, patent ductus arteriosus occlusion is the primary focus of this article. Occlusion of other less common congenital cardiac defects is also briefly reviewed. Balloon dilation of pulmonic stenosis, as well as other congenital obstructive cardiovascular abnormalities is discussed in the latter part of the article.

The feasibility of surgical correction for almost all canine congenital or acquired cardiac diseases has been demonstrated. Current surgical success rates are remarkably high considering the infrequency with which such procedures are performed. Such results are a testament to the dedication and skill of the various cardiac surgical teams offering these procedures worldwide. However, experience from the medical field indicates that the only way to increase success rates above those presently achieved will be to dramatically increase the frequency with which cardiac surgical teams perform these procedures. Fortunately, lack of case load does not appear to be the limiting factor to such efforts. Rather, lacks of infrastructure and manpower are the major obstacles for expansion of cardiac surgical programs.

Pulmonary hypertension (PH) has been recognized as a clinical syndrome for many years in veterinary medicine, but routine accurate clinical diagnosis in dogs was greatly enhanced by widespread use of echocardiography and Doppler echocardiography. Most cases of PH in veterinary medicine can be categorized as precapillary or postcapillary. These subsets of patients often differ with regard to clinical presentation, response to therapy, and prognosis. Effective medical therapy is now available to treat this often-devastating clinical complication of common chronic diseases, making accurate diagnosis even more important to patient longevity and quality of life.

In the cat, electrocardiography is indicated for assessing the rhythm of the heartbeat and identifying and monitoring the effect of certain systemic disorders on the heart. Basic information regarding feline electrocardiography is contained in several textbooks, and the reader is referred to these sources for background reading. This article describes selected clinical advances in feline cardiac arrhythmias and electrocardiography from the past decade.

Myxomatous mitral valve disease is a common condition in geriatric dogs. Most dogs affected are clinically asymptomatic for a long time. However, about 30% of these animals present a progression to heart failure and eventually die as a consequence of the disease. Left atrial enlargement, and particularly a change in left atrial size, seems to be the most reliable predictor of progression in some studies, however further studies are needed to clarify how to recognize asymptomatic patients at higher risk of developing heart failure. According to the published data on the natural history of the disease and the results of published studies evaluating the effect of early therapy on delaying the progression of the disease, it seems that no currently available treatment delays the onset of clinical signs of congestive heart failure (CHF). Although the ideal treatment of more severely affected dogs is probably surgical mitral valve repair or mitral valve replacement, this is not a currently available option. The results of several clinical trials together with clinical experience suggest that dogs with overt CHF can be managed with acceptable quality of life for a relatively long time period with medical treatment including furosemide, an angiotensin-converting enzyme inhibitor, pimobendan, and spironolactone.

Infective endocarditis (IE) is the invasion of a heart valve or endocardium by a microbe. Difficulty in diagnosis and underreporting of IE in dogs contribute

RELATED INTEREST

Veterinary Clinics of North America: Exotic Animal Practice
January 2009 (Vol. 12, No. 1)
Cardiology
J. Jill Heatley, DVM, MS, Dipl. ABVP—Avian, Dipl. ACZM, *Guest Editor*

THE CLINICS ARE NOW AVAILABLE ONLINE!

Access your subscription at:
www.theclinics.com

Erratum

The editor of *Veterinary Clinics of North America: Small Animal Practice* would like to confirm the retraction of "Idiopathic Granulomatous and Necrotizing Inflammatory Disorders of the Canine Central Nervous System," by Scott J. Schatzberg from the January 2010 issue (Vol. 40(1): 101-120) at the request of the editor and author. This article was a duplication of a paper that had already appeared in the *Journal of Small Animal Practice*, Published Online: October 8, 2009 9:28AM; DOI: 10.1111/j.1748-5827.2009.00823.x. The author would like to apologize for this administrative error.

Vet Clin Small Anim 40 (2010) xi
doi:10.1016/j.cvsm.2010.04.006
0195-5616/10/$ – see front matter © 2010 Elsevier Inc. All rights reserved.

Preface
Topics in Cardiology

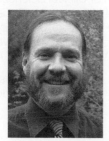

Jonathan A. Abbott, DVM
Guest Editor

Six years ago, it was my privilege to provide guest editorial direction when an issue of the *Veterinary Clinics of North America: Small Animal Practice* addressed topics in cardiology. There have been notable advances since I last contributed to this series: the practice of veterinary echocardiography has continued to evolve; we are beginning to realize the diagnostic potential of biomarkers, such as the natriuretic peptides; recent discoveries have improved understanding of recognized diseases; and new therapeutic approaches have been developed.

As in 2004, this issue addresses a broad range of subjects in an attempt to provide an overview of current topics in veterinary cardiology. The initial articles outline progress in cardiovascular diagnosis. The current role of the natriuretic peptides is assessed and recent advances in the practice of echocardiography are reviewed. Subsequent articles address current issues in cardiovascular therapy: recent clinical data regarding the use of the pimobendan are reviewed; the growing field of interventional catheterization is addressed as is the role of surgical techniques in the management of small animal cardiovascular disease. In a series of updates, current issues in the diagnostic and therapeutic management of specific disorders and syndromes are addressed. Finally, the subject of genetics is addressed in two separate reviews that relate, respectively, to heritability of disease and therapy.

I was fortunate that talented clinical scientists generously provided their expertise— I wish to acknowledge these authors and express sincere thanks for their willingness to contribute to this issue. I am certain, however, that it is the readership that will be the

Vet Clin Small Anim 40 (2010) xiii–xiv
doi:10.1016/j.cvsm.2010.04.005
0195-5616/10/$ – see front matter © 2010 Elsevier Inc. All rights reserved.

vetsmall.theclinics.com

true beneficiary of their efforts. Readers are fortunate that prominent experts were willing to share their views on such vital and exciting topics in veterinary cardiology.

Jonathan A. Abbott, DVM
Department of Small Animal Clinical Sciences
Virginia-Maryland Regional College of Veterinary Medicine
Virginia Polytechnic Institute and State University
Duck Pond Drive
Blacksburg, VA 24061-0442, USA

E-mail address:
abbottj@vt.edu

Advanced Techniques in Echocardiography in Small Animals

Valérie Chetboul, DVM, PhD

KEYWORDS

- Tissue Doppler • Speckle tracking • Strain • Strain rate
- Tissue tracking

Over the last 30 years, standard transthoracic echocardiography has become a major imaging tool for the diagnosis and management of canine and feline cardiovascular diseases. In the late 1980s miniaturization of transducer components allowed the development of transesophageal echocardiography, which is used for analyzing specific abnormalities (congenital heart diseases, thrombosis, cardiac tumors) and for monitoring surgical and interventional procedures.[1–3] During the last decade, more recent advances in ultrasound technology with the introduction of newer imaging modalities, such as tissue Doppler imaging (TDI), strain (St) and strain rate (SR) imaging, and 2-dimensional (2D) speckle tracking echocardiography (STE), have provided new parameters to assess myocardial performance, including regional myocardial velocities and deformation, ventricular twist, and mechanical synchrony. An outline of these 4 recent ultrasound techniques, their impact on the understanding of right and left ventricular function in small animals, and their application in research and clinical settings are given in this article.

TISSUE DOPPLER IMAGING

TDI is a recently developed echocardiographic technique that enables global and regional myocardial function to be quantified from measurements of myocardial velocities in real time.[4]

Isaaz and colleagues[5] were the first (in 1989) to record the left ventricular free wall (LVFW) velocities in human patients using the pulsed-wave Doppler mode of standard ultrasound equipment. The wall filter was set at 100 Hz to record the low myocardial velocities (<10 cm/s). Several years later, the first software was developed for quantifying myocardial velocities using color Doppler imaging.[6] Since then, TDI has been more and more investigated in human and veterinary cardiology, providing information on myocardial function, and also improving our understanding of cardiac physiopathology.

Unité de Cardiologie d'Alfort, UMR INSERM-ENVA U955, Ecole Nationale Vétérinaire d'Alfort, 7 Avenue du Général de Gaulle, 94704 Maisons-Alfort Cedex, France
E-mail address: vchetboul@vet-alfort.fr

Vet Clin Small Anim 40 (2010) 529–543
doi:10.1016/j.cvsm.2010.03.007
0195-5616/10/$ – see front matter © 2010 Elsevier Inc. All rights reserved.

Technical Characteristics

Standard spectral and color Doppler instrumentation detects high-frequency, low-amplitude Doppler signals reflected from rapidly moving red blood cells, and filters out low-frequency, high-amplitude Doppler signals that arise from the myocardium. With the TDI technique, modifications of high-pass frequency and amplitude filter settings are needed to allow Doppler signals from myocardial motion to be processed and displayed.[7]

Three TDI modes are available.[4,7] The pulsed-wave TDI mode provides information on myocardial movements through a single sample volume, which is placed within

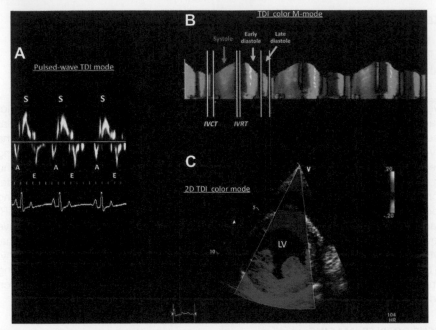

Fig. 1. The 3 TDI modes. (*A*) The pulsed-wave TDI mode provides information on myocardial movements through a single sample volume, which is placed within the myocardial wall thickness (here in the left ventricular free wall [LVFW], using the right parasternal transventricular short-axis view). When the myocardium moves toward the transducer, myocardial velocities are positive (above the baseline), and when it moves away from the transducer, myocardial velocities are negative (below the baseline). S, E, A: peak systolic, early diastolic, and late diastolic velocities, respectively. (*B*) This color M-mode TDI tracing of the LVFW (radial motion) obtained in a healthy dog shows on the same image colored systolic and diastolic velocities within the entire wall thickness. Myocardial velocities toward the transducer are encoded in red, and those away from the transducer in blue. Using specific software, the mean myocardial velocity (defined as the average of velocity values measured along each M-mode scan line throughout the entire myocardial wall thickness) may then be calculated during the whole cardiac cycle. The mean myocardial velocity in the 2 layers of the LVFW, that is, subendocardial and subepicardial layers, may also be assessed. IVCT, isovolumic contraction time; IVRT, isovolumic relaxation time. (*C*) Using the 2D color mode, myocardial velocities are superimposed on 2D mode images (here right parasternal transventricular short-axis view). Velocities toward the transducer are colored in red whereas those away from the transducer are colored in blue. In this view taken at end systole, the LVFW is depicted in red while the interventricular septum, which moves in the opposite direction, is depicted in blue. Using specific software, myocardial velocities may then be analyzed in 1 or several segments (see **Fig. 2**). LV, left ventricle.

the myocardial wall (**Fig 1**A). With color M-mode TDI (**Fig. 1**B), myocardial velocities are analyzed along a selected single scan line, which is directed by the operator in the same manner as for conventional transventricular M-mode; this method is used to analyze the radial motion of the interventricular septum (IVS) or the LVFW. Using 2D color TDI mode (**Fig. 1**C), real-time color Doppler is superimposed on the gray-scale of 2D mode images. Specific software is then used to quantify velocities throughout the cardiac cycle in myocardial segments of various sizes (**Fig. 2**). One of the main advantages of 2D color TDI mode over the 2 others is its ability to simultaneously quantify velocities in several segments within 1, 2, or 3 myocardial walls, thereby allowing assessment of intra- and interventricular synchrony (see **Fig. 2**; **Figs. 3** and **4**).[8]

Normal TDI Myocardial Velocity Profiles

Radial and longitudinal LVFW velocities, as well as longitudinal right ventricular myocardial velocities, may be quantified using 2D color TDI with adequate to good repeatability and reproducibility for a trained observer in awake cats and dogs.[9–11] For example, using 2D color TDI in the cat, the lowest coefficients of variation were observed in endocardial segments (8.2% and 6.5% for systole [S] and early diastole [E], respectively) and for E at the base (5.5%).[9] By contrast, with the pulsed-wave

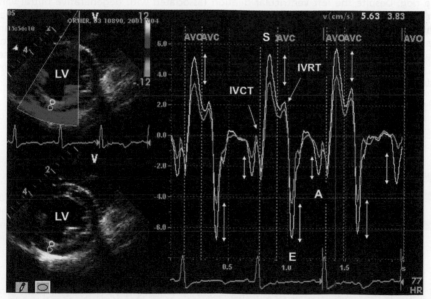

Fig. 2. An example of normal radial velocity profiles recorded within 2 segments of the left ventricular free wall using the 2D color TDI mode in a dog (right parasternal transventricular short-axis view). This simultaneous recording of myocardial velocities in a subendocardial (*yellow*) and subepicardial (*green*) segment confirms myocardial synchrony and indicates that the subendocardium is moving more rapidly than the subepicardium in systole and also in diastole, thus defining systolic and diastolic myocardial velocity gradients (*white double arrows*). As with the pulsed wave TDI mode, myocardial velocities are positive when the myocardium moves toward the transducer whereas they are negative when it moves away from the transducer. The color display of velocity is superimposed on the right parasternal transventricular short-axis view (*left upper panel*). A, peak myocardial velocity during late diastole; AVC, aortic valve closure; AVO, aortic valve opening; E, peak myocardial velocity during early diastole; IVCT, isovolumic contraction time; IVRT, isovolumic relaxation time; LV, left ventricle; S, peak myocardial velocity during systole.

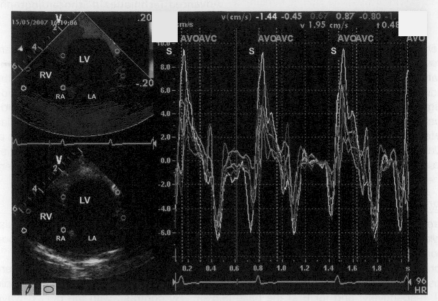

Fig. 3. An example of normal interventricular synchrony assessed by the 2D color TDI mode in a dog. Despite the left ventricular dilation (associated with degenerative mitral valve disease), all peak systolic velocities (S) assessed in 6 myocardial segments from the left ventricular free wall (*red and green*), the interventricular septum (*blue and orange*), and the right myocardial wall (*yellow and pink*) occur almost simultaneously at early systole between aortic valve opening and closure. The color display of velocity is superimposed on the left apical 4-chamber view (*left upper panel*). S, peak myocardial velocity during systole; LA, left atrium; LV, left ventricle; RA, right atrium; RV, right ventricle.

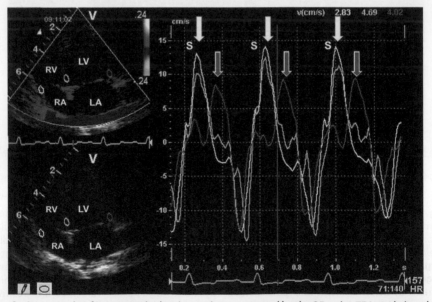

Fig. 4. An example of interventricular dyssynchrony assessed by the 2D color TDI mode in a dog with degenerative mitral valve disease. Unlike the dog from **Fig. 3**, the longitudinal velocity profiles obtained from 3 basal segments of the left ventricular free wall (LVFW, *red*), the interventricular septum (*green*), and the right myocardial wall (*yellow*) show a delayed peak systolic LVFW velocity (*red arrows*) compared with the 2 others (*yellow arrows*). The color display of velocity is superimposed on the left apical 4-chamber view (*left upper panel*). S, peak myocardial velocity during systole; LA, left atrium; LV, left ventricle; RA, right atrium; RV, right ventricle.

TDI mode, velocities recorded during the isovolumic phases or within the IVS may have coefficients of variation of more than 20%, and should therefore be interpreted with caution.[12]

Whatever the TDI mode used, all myocardial velocity profiles include, after a short isovolumic contraction phase, one positive systolic wave (S), and after a short isovolumic relaxation phase, 2 diastolic negative waves (E and A, respectively, in early and late diastole, with E/A ratio >1, see **Fig. 2; Fig. 5**).[9–18] Fusion of the 2 negative diastolic waves E and A into one negative diastolic wave EA is often observed in the cat owing to high heart rate. This phenomenon may represent a limitation of the TDI technique for the accurate assessment of diastolic myocardial function in this species.[16,17]

As shown in **Fig. 2**, normal radial LVFW motion is heterogeneous, with myocardial layers moving more rapidly in the subendocardium than in the subepicardium, thus creating a radial intramyocardial velocity gradient (MVG) in both systole and diastole.[9,10,15,16] Normal right and left longitudinal myocardial motion is also characterized by nonuniformity, with myocardial velocities decreasing from the base to the apex, thus producing a longitudinal MVG (see **Fig. 5**).[9–11,15,16] Moreover, right ventricular myocardial velocities have been shown to be higher than LVFW velocities.[11]

Main Applications

The most important TDI applications in humans are the assessment of diastolic function and myocardial synchrony, the early detection of myocardial dysfunction, and

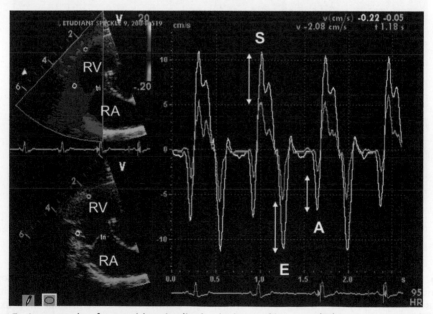

Fig. 5. An example of normal longitudinal velocity profiles recorded in 2 segments of the right ventricular myocardial wall using the 2D color TDI mode in a dog (left apical 4-chamber view). This simultaneous recording of myocardial velocities in a basal (*yellow*) and apical (*green*) segment indicates that the base is moving more rapidly than the apex in systole and also in diastole, thus defining systolic and diastolic myocardial velocity gradients (*double arrows*) during the whole cardiac cycle. The color display of velocity is superimposed on the left apical 4-chamber view (*left upper panel*). A, peak myocardial velocity during late diastole; E, peak myocardial velocity during early diastole; RA, right atrium; RV, right ventricle; S, peak myocardial velocity during systole; tri, tricuspid valve.

quantification of the myocardial functional reserve during stress echocardiography, enabling an accurate diagnosis of coronary diseases.[7,19]

The high sensitivity of the TDI technique compared with conventional ultrasound imaging in detecting regional myocardial abnormalities has also been demonstrated in small animals. The author's group first demonstrated that TDI allowed early detection of systolic as well as diastolic myocardial dysfunction in a dystrophin-deficient Golden Retriever Muscular Dystrophy (GRMD) model of dilated cardiomyopathy (DCM; **Figs. 6** and **7A**).[20,21] These regional TDI myocardial alterations including decreased radial and longitudinal systolic and early diastolic MVGs could be detected during the preclinical phase of the disease, before occurrence of left ventricular dilation and overt myocardial dysfunction.[20,21] In a dystrophin-deficient hypertrophic feline muscular dystrophy (HFMD) model of hypertrophic cardiomyopathy (HCM), TDI has also been shown to consistently detect LVFW dysfunction despite the absence of myocardial hypertrophy in all mutated animals.[22] Compared with healthy controls, HFMD cats without LVFW hypertrophy showed higher longitudinal TDI isovolumic relaxation times, longitudinal TDI E/A ratio less than 1 at the base and, for some of them, radial TDI E/A ratio less than 1 in the subendocardium and subepicardium as well as decreased systolic longitudinal myocardial velocities at the base and the apex. Similarly, in hypertensive cats or cats affected by spontaneous HCM, and in Maine Coon cats heterozygous for the A31P

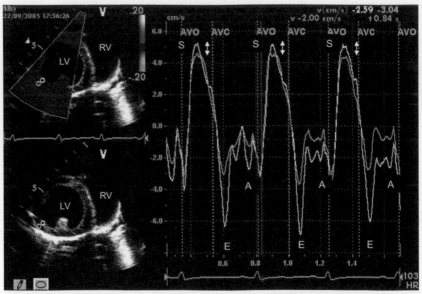

Fig. 6. An example of abnormal radial velocity profiles recorded in 2 segments of the left ventricular free wall using the 2D color TDI mode in a young Golden Retriever dog with muscular dystrophy (GRMD dog, 7 month-old; right parasternal transventricular short-axis view). The subendocardial (*yellow*) and subepicardial (*green*) velocity profiles are nearly superimposed in systole, thus indicating a very low systolic myocardial velocity gradient (*double arrows*, for comparison see normal radial velocity profiles in **Fig. 2**). This TDI systolic dysfunction was not detected using conventional echocardiography (fractional shortening of 38%, ie, within the normal ranges). The color display of velocity is superimposed on the right parasternal transventricular short-axis view (*left upper panel*). A, peak myocardial velocity during late diastole; AVC, aortic valve closure; AVO, aortic valve opening; E, peak myocardial velocity during early diastole; LV, left ventricle; RV, right ventricle; S, peak myocardial velocity during systole.

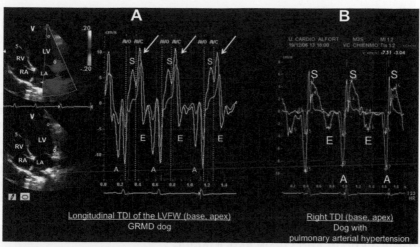

Fig. 7. Examples of abnormal left (*A*) and right (*B*) longitudinal velocity profiles recorded in 2 myocardial segments using the 2D color TDI mode (left apical 4-chamber views). (*A*) Young Golden Retriever dog with muscular dystrophy (GRMD dog, 6 month-old). Although no abnormality was detected on conventional echo-Doppler examination, the longitudinal velocity profiles recorded simultaneously in 2 segments of the left ventricular free wall at the base (*yellow*) and at the apex (*green*) show 2 myocardial alterations: first, E is lower than A, thus confirming diastolic dysfunction. Second, both curves show postsystolic contraction waves (*white arrows*), occurring after S waves (and after aortic valve closure) and greater than the latter. This marked postsystolic motion was confirmed using strain imaging (data not shown). (*B*) Cavalier King Charles Spaniel (9 year-old) with mild systolic pulmonary arterial hypertension (35 mmHg) secondary to degenerative mitral valve disease. Pulmonary arterial hypertension is associated with systolic and diastolic right myocardial dysfunction, with an inverted E/A ratio and decreased peak systolic velocities (mean S wave of 4.8 cm/s) compared with reference ranges (7.7–18.5 cm/s).[11] A, peak myocardial velocity during late diastole; AVC, aortic valve closure; AVO, aortic valve opening; E, peak myocardial velocity during early diastole; LA, left atrium; LV, left ventricle; RA, right atrium; RV, right ventricle; S, peak myocardial velocity during systole.

mutation in the myosin-binding protein C gene, TDI detected segmental functional changes in nonhypertrophied myocardial wall segments.[23,24] Lastly, in a recent study comparing the diagnostic value of echo-Doppler and TDI in dogs with pulmonary arterial hypertension, conventional echo-Doppler variables were less discriminating than TDI indices for predicting increased systolic pulmonary arterial pressure (SPAP).[25] The TDI technique also demonstrated that alterations in right-sided systolic and diastolic myocardial function could occur with mild increases in SPAP (**Fig. 7**B).[25] Compared with dogs with normal SPAP, dogs with mild pulmonary arterial hypertension (between 30 and 41 mmHg) showed a significant decrease in right longitudinal systolic velocities and E/A ratio at the base.[25]

TDI has contributed to a better understanding of the nature of myocardial dysfunction that is associated with several heart diseases, thus providing new insights into their physiopathology and suggesting the possibility of new therapeutic approaches. For example, using the 2D color TDI mode and the color M-mode, feline HCM was recently shown to be associated not only with diastolic myocardial dysfunction but also systolic myocardial alteration, particularly regarding the longitudinal LVFW motion.[23,26] Similarly, not only systolic but also diastolic myocardial function has been shown to be impaired in dogs with DCM.[27]

Another important TDI application is the accurate assessment of a treatment effect on myocardial function. For example, the author's group has recently used the TDI technique to demonstrate the beneficial regional systolic myocardial effect of muscle cell transplantation in an animal model of DCM.[28]

Limitations

One limitation of the TDI technique is angle dependency. A perfect alignment of the Doppler beam with the direction of the myocardial wall motion must always be obtained. Imperfect alignment leads to an underestimation of assessed myocardial velocities. Moreover, several TDI variables may be affected by breed, heart rate, and age.[9,10,13,15,16] Lastly, myocardial velocities assessed by TDI do not discriminate between actively contracting myocardium and passive motion due to translational movement of the heart within the ultrasound beam and tethering effects. This limitation may be overcome by measuring MVGs (which reflect the rate of myocardial deformation, see **Figs. 2, 5** and **6**) or by using St and SR imaging.

TDI-DERIVED STRAIN AND STRAIN RATE IMAGING
Definitions and Normal Aspect

Strain is defined as the deformation of a material that results from a force or stress. In the context of echocardiography, strain refers to the decrease or increase in length of a myocardial segment; it is a dimensionless quantity expressed as a proportion of initial segment length. Echocardiographic St and SR provide measurements of 1-dimensional myocardial segmental deformation (contraction or stretching) and rate of deformation, respectively.[29,30] St and SR initially were derived from TDI data, but these quantities can also be obtained from STE. Myocardial St represents the deformation of a myocardial segment over a period of time and is expressed as the percent change from its original dimension (**Fig. 8**). Myocardial SR (expressed in s^{-1}) is the

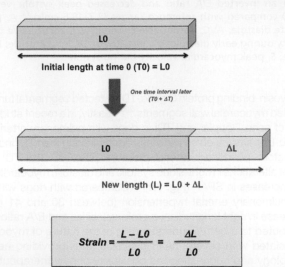

Fig. 8. Calculation of deformation (strain) and rate of deformation (strain rate). The initial myocardial length (at T0) is L0 (*gray bar*). One time interval (ΔT) later (at T0 + ΔT), the myocardial length increased from L0 to L0 + ΔL (*gray bar added to red bar*). The strain (St, expressed in %) undergone by the myocardial segment is ΔL/L0 and is positive. Rate at which length changes occur is strain rate (St/ΔT, expressed in s^{-1}).

temporal derivative of St, and therefore describes the rate of myocardial deformation (ie, how quickly a myocardial segment shortens or lengthens).[29,30] SR is also equivalent to the deformation velocity per myocardial segment length (or the myocardial velocity gradient normalized by the distance).[31] In practice, TDI-derived SR data are obtained through computer analysis of the TDI myocardial velocity gradient. From this comes a graphical representation of the relationship between time and SR. The integral of this curve describes temporal variation in St.

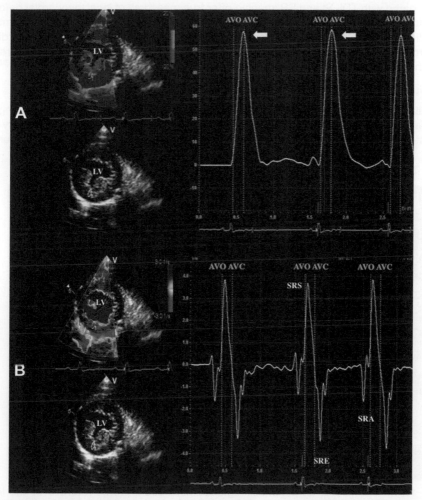

Fig. 9. Examples of normal regional radial strain (A) and strain rate (B) profiles recorded within the left ventricular free wall in a healthy dog (right parasternal transventricular short-axis view). (A) The radial strain profile (expressed in %) is positive and maximal in end systole (arrows) reflecting regional systolic thickening of the left ventricular free wall. (B) The strain rate profile (expressed in s⁻¹) is positive during systole (SRS), indicating regional thickening, then features 2 negative diastolic peaks during early filling and atrial contraction (SRE and SRA) corresponding to a biphasic thinning phase. The color displays of strain and strain rate are superimposed on the right parasternal transventricular short-axis views (left upper panels). Strain length = 12 mm. Region of interest size = 6/3 mm. AVC, aortic valve closure; AVO, aortic valve opening; LV, left ventricle.

The normal ranges of regional systolic St and SR values have already been determined in the awake dog for the radial and longitudinal motions of the LVFW, and for the longitudinal motion of the IVS and the right ventricular myocardial wall.[30] Moreover, when assessed by a trained observer, systolic St and SR values have been shown to be repeatable and reproducible in this species.[30] Examples of normal St and SR curves are presented in **Fig. 9**.

Advantages

Compared with TDI, St and SR imaging offer true measures of local myocardial deformation, thereby separating active from passive myocardial motion.[29–31] Experimental studies and clinical studies performed in human patients with DCM and myocardial infarction have shown that these "deformation imaging techniques" were accurate methods for quantifying regional myocardial function and synchrony (**Fig. 10**).[8,32–34]

Limitations

Similar to the TDI technique, one of the disadvantages of St and SR imaging is angle dependency. St and SR imaging present other limitations including a high variability of diastolic SR variables, a high signal to noise ratio (particularly for SR imaging), and

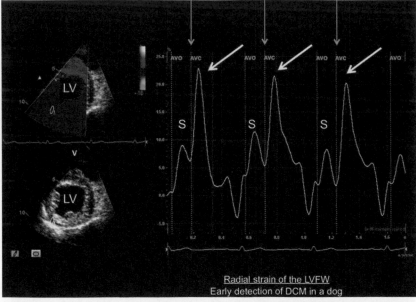

Fig. 10. An example of an abnormal regional radial strain profile recorded in the left ventricular free wall (LVFW) in a dog with occult dilated cardiomyopathy (DCM; right parasternal transventricular short-axis view). The radial strain profile is positive, thus confirming a regional expansion during systole, which is normal. However, the maximal strain values are measured after the T wave on the ECG tracing (or after aortic valve closure, *green arrows*). These postsystolic contraction waves (*yellow arrows*) confirm a marked left myocardial systolic dysfunction. This systolic dysfunction is also characterized by a peak systolic strain (S, between the 2 aortic time events) that is lower (9.7%) than the published reference ranges (45%–87%).[30] The color display of velocity is superimposed on the right parasternal transventricular short-axis view (*left upper panel*). Region of interest size = 6/3 mm. AVC, aortic valve closure; AVO, aortic valve opening; LV, left ventricle.

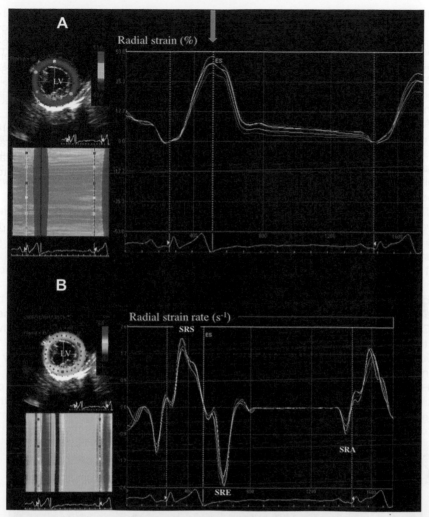

Fig. 11. Examples of normal left ventricular (LV) radial strain (*A*) and strain rate (*B*) profiles recorded in 6 myocardial segments using 2D STE in a dog (right parasternal transventricular short-axis view). The software algorithm has automatically defined 6 equidistant myocardial segments within the interventricular septum and the LV free wall. (*A*) The 6 corresponding LV radial strain versus time curves are shown on the right. All 6 LV segments undergo a homogeneous and coordinated systolic myocardial thickening during systole (positive strain, maximal at end systole [ES], *pink arrow*); this may also be observed on the 2D and M-curves color-coded views (*left*) showing a positive strain during systole (*red*). (*B*) The 6 LV radial strain rate versus time curves, including a positive systolic wave (SRS) and 2 diastolic negative waves (SRE and SRA), are shown on the right; this may also be observed on the M-curves color-coded views (*left*) showing a positive strain rate during systole (*red*) and negative strain rate during diastole (*green and blue*). LV, left ventricle.

many types of artifacts due to stationary reverberations, drop-out zones, and low lateral resolution.[29–33] These artifacts may create false regional myocardial akinesia or dyskinesia. However, some of the aforementioned limitations may, at least in part, be overcome by non-Doppler–based methods such as 2D STE.

TWO-DIMENSIONAL SPECKLE TRACKING ECHOCARDIOGRAPHY

2D STE is the most recent ultrasound tool allowing assessment of regional myocardial function.[35–38] This imaging technique is based on the tracking of speckle patterns created by interference between the ultrasound beam and the myocardium on gray-scale 2D echocardiographic images. These speckles appear as small and bright elements within the myocardium and represent natural acoustic tissue markers that can be tracked from frame to frame throughout the cardiac cycle.

As the tracking is based on routine 2D echocardiographic images, 2D STE allows a non-Doppler assessment of regional myocardial motion by filtering out random speckles, and then performing autocorrelations to evaluate the motion of stable structures (**Fig. 11**).[35–38] Therefore, compared with the Doppler-based techniques such as TDI or TDI-derived techniques, 2D STE is independent of both cardiac translation and insonation angle.

Two-dimensional STE can be used to assess the complex pattern of regional myocardial motion concomitantly in several segments, providing similar indices to the TDI (velocity) and TDI-derived techniques (St and SR), and also new indices of systolic LV function (such as systolic rotation or circumferential St).[35–40]

Two-dimensional STE has been shown to be a repeatable and reproducible method for assessing the systolic LV wringing motion and for analyzing systolic radial LV St and SR in the awake normal dog, with a good correlation with values obtained by the TDI-based techniques.[39,40] As in human patients with various heart diseases (DCM and myocardial infarction), systolic LV torsion, defined as apical rotation relative to the base, has been shown to be altered in dogs with hypokinesia using 2D STE.[40] Two-dimensional STE can also be used to accurately assess myocardial synchrony in humans and in small animals (**Fig. 12**).[37,39]

However, 2D STE has known technical limitations, including its dependence on frame rate and image resolution, and potential out-of-plane movements of the speckles, decreasing the reliability of the speckle tracking process.[37] Lastly, there is

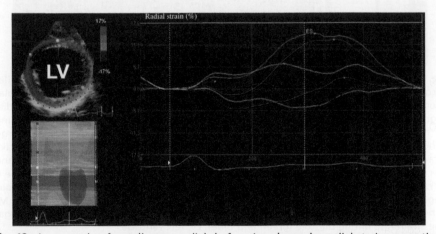

Fig. 12. An example of systolic myocardial dysfunction shown by radial strain versus time curves using 2D STE in a dog with dilated cardiomyopathy. The maximal positive strain values for the green and blue segments are obtained after the T wave (ie, in diastole), and not at end systole (for comparison see normal radial profiles in **Fig. 2**A). Note also the dyskinesia of 3 myocardial segments (*pink, red* and *green curves*) characterized by an abnormal negative strain during systole. ES, end systole; LV, left ventricle.

still limited experience regarding its prognostic and diagnostic abilities as well as its use in veterinary cardiology as compared with the TDI and TDI-based techniques. Further studies are therefore required in large populations of diseased animals to determine the comparative clinical and research relevance of 2D STE and the 3 other imaging techniques.

SUMMARY

TDI and its derived modalities, St and SR imaging, are newly developed ultrasound techniques permitting quantitative assessment of myocardial function by calculating regional myocardial velocities in real time and by measuring myocardial segmental deformation and rate of deformation, respectively. STE is an even more recent ultrasound modality, based on 2D gray-scale echocardiographic images, allowing a non-Doppler assessment of regional myocardial motion.

REFERENCES

1. Quintavalla C, Pradelli D, Domenech O, et al. Transesophageal echocardiography of the left ventricular outflow tract, aortic valve and ascending aorta in Boxer dogs with heart murmurs. Vet Radiol Ultrasound 2006;47(3):307–12.
2. Borenstein N, Daniel P, Behr L, et al. Successful surgical treatment of mitral valve stenosis in a dog. Vet Surg 2004;33(2):138–45.
3. Chetboul V, Tessier D, Borenstein N, et al. Familial aortic aneurysm in Leonberg dogs. J Am Vet Med Assoc 2003;223(8):1159–62.
4. Chetboul V. Tissue Doppler imaging: a promising technique for quantifying regional myocardial function. J Vet Cardiol 2002;4(2):7–12.
5. Isaaz K, Thompson A, Ethevenot G, et al. Doppler echocardiographic measurement of low velocity motion of the left ventricular posterior wall. Am J Cardiol 1989;64(1):66–75.
6. McDicken WN, Sutherland GR, Moran CM, et al. Colour Doppler velocity imaging of the myocardium. Ultrasound Med Biol 1992;18(6–7):651–4.
7. Brodin LA. Tissue Doppler, a fundamental tool for parametric imaging. Clin Physiol Funct Imaging 2004,24(3):147–55.
8. Estrada A, Chetboul V. Tissue Doppler evaluation of ventricular synchrony. J Vet Cardiol 2006;8(2):129–37.
9. Chetboul V, Athanassiadis N, Carlos Sampedrano C, et al. Quantification, repeatability, and reproducibility of feline radial and longitudinal left ventricular velocities by tissue Doppler imaging. Am J Vet Res 2004;65(5):566–72.
10. Chetboul V, Athanassiadis N, Carlos Sampedrano C, et al. Assessment of repeatability, reproducibility, and effect of anesthesia on determination of radial and longitudinal left ventricular velocities via tissue Doppler imaging in dogs. Am J Vet Res 2004;65(7):909–15.
11. Chetboul V, Carlos Sampedrano C, Gouni V, et al. Quantitative assessment of regional right ventricular myocardial velocities in awake dogs by Doppler tissue imaging: repeatability, reproducibility, effect of body weight and breed, and comparison with left ventricular myocardial velocities. J Vet Intern Med 2005; 19(6):837–44.
12. Simpson KE, Devine BC, Gunn-Moore DA, et al. Assessment of the repeatability of feline echocardiography using conventional echocardiography and spectral pulse-wave Doppler tissue imaging techniques. Vet Radiol Ultrasound 2007; 48(1):58–68.

13. Koffas H, Dukes-McEwan J, Corcoran BM, et al. Peak mean myocardial velocities and velocity gradients measured by color M-mode tissue Doppler imaging in healthy cats. J Vet Intern Med 2003;17(4):510–24.

14. Gavaghan BJ, Kittleson MD, Fisher KJ, et al. Quantification of left ventricular diastolic wall motion by Doppler tissue imaging in healthy cats and cats with cardiomyopathy. Am J Vet Res 1999;60(12):1478–86.

15. Chetboul V, Carlos Sampedrano C, Concordet D, et al. Use of quantitative two-dimensional color tissue Doppler imaging for assessment of left ventricular radial and longitudinal myocardial velocities in dogs. Am J Vet Res 2005; 66(6):953–61.

16. Chetboul V, Carlos Sampedrano C, Tissier R, et al. Quantitative assessment of velocities of the annulus of the left atrioventricular valve and left ventricular free wall in healthy cats by use of two-dimensional color tissue Doppler imaging. Am J Vet Res 2006;67(2):250–8.

17. MacDonald KA, Kittleson MD, Kass PH, et al. Tissue Doppler imaging in Maine Coon cats with a mutation of myosin binding protein C with or without hypertrophy. J Vet Intern Med 2007;21(2):232–7.

18. Koffas H, Dukes-McEwan J, Corcoran BM, et al. Pulsed tissue Doppler imaging in normal cats and cats with hypertrophic cardiomyopathy. J Vet Intern Med 2006; 20(1):65–77.

19. Naqvi TZ. Recent advances in echocardiography. Expert Rev Cardiovasc Ther 2004;2(1):89–96.

20. Chetboul V, Escriou C, Tessier D, et al. Tissue Doppler imaging detects early asymptomatic myocardial abnormalities in a dog model of Duchenne's cardiomyopathy. Eur Heart J 2004;25(21):1934–9.

21. Chetboul V, Carlos C, Blot S, et al. Tissue Doppler assessment of diastolic and systolic alterations of radial and longitudinal left ventricular motions in Golden Retrievers during the preclinical phase of cardiomyopathy associated with muscular dystrophy. Am J Vet Res 2004;65(10):1335–41.

22. Chetboul V, Blot S, Carlos Sampedrano C, et al. Tissue Doppler imaging for detection of radial and longitudinal myocardial dysfunction in a family of cats affected by dystrophin-deficient hypertrophic muscular dystrophy. J Vet Intern Med 2006;20(3):640–7.

23. Carlos Sampedrano C, Chetboul V, Gouni V, et al. Systolic and diastolic myocardial dysfunction in cats with hypertrophic cardiomyopathy or systemic hypertension. J Vet Intern Med 2006;20(5):1106–15.

24. Carlos Sampedrano C, Chetboul V, Mary J, et al. Prospective echocardiographic and tissue Doppler imaging screening of a population of Maine Coon cats tested for the A31P mutation in the myosin-binding protein C gene: a specific analysis of the heterozygous status. J Vet Intern Med 2009;23(1):91–9.

25. Serres F, Chetboul V, Gouni V, et al. Diagnostic value of echo-Doppler and tissue Doppler imaging in dogs with pulmonary arterial hypertension. J Vet Intern Med 2007;21(6):1280–9.

26. Koffas H, Dukes-McEwan J, Corcoran BM, et al. Colour M-mode tissue Doppler imaging in healthy cats and cats with hypertrophic cardiomyopathy. J Small Anim Pract 2008;49(7):330–8.

27. Chetboul V, Gouni V, Carlos Sampedrano C, et al. Assessment of regional systolic and diastolic myocardial function using tissue Doppler and strain imaging in dogs with dilated cardiomyopathy. J Vet Intern Med 2007;21(4): 719–30.

28. Borenstein N, Chetboul V, Bruneval P, et al. Non-cultured cell transplantation in an ovine model of non-ischemic heart failure. Eur J Cardiothorac Surg 2007;31(3): 444–51.
29. D'hooge J, Heimdal A, Jamal F, et al. Regional strain and strain rate measurements by cardiac ultrasound: principles, implementation and limitations. Eur J Echocardiogr 2000;1(3):154–70.
30. Chetboul V, Carlos Sampedrano C, Gouni V, et al. Ultrasonographic assessment of regional radial and longitudinal systolic function in healthy awake dogs. J Vet Intern Med 2006;20(4):885–93.
31. Urheim S, Edvardsen T, Torp H, et al. Validation of a new method to quantify regional myocardial function. Myocardial strain by Doppler echocardiography. Circulation 2000;102:1158–64.
32. Thibault H, Derumeaux G. Assessment of myocardial ischemia and viability using tissue Doppler and deformation imaging: the lessons from the experimental studies. Arch Cardiovasc Dis 2008;101(1):61–8.
33. Yip G, Abraham T, Belohlavek M, et al. Clinical applications of strain rate imaging. J Am Soc Echocardiogr 2003;16(12):1334–42.
34. Nesbitt GC, Mankad S. Strain and strain rate imaging in cardiomyopathy. Echocardiography 2009;26(3):337–44.
35. Perk G, Tunick PA, Kronzon I. Non-Doppler two-dimensional strain imaging by echocardiography-from technical considerations to clinical applications. J Am Soc Echocardiogr 2007;20(3):234–43.
36. Helle-Valle T, Crosby J, Edvardsen T, et al. New noninvasive method for assessment of left ventricular rotation: speckle tracking echocardiography. Circulation 2005;112(20):3149–56.
37. Nesser HJ, Winter S. Speckle tracking in the evaluation of left ventricular dyssynchrony. Echocardiography 2009;26(3):324–36.
38. Artis NJ, Oxborough DL, Williams G, et al. Two-dimensional strain imaging: a new echocardiographic advance with research and clinical applications. Int J Cardiol 2008;123(3):240–8.
39. Chetboul V, Serres F, Gouni V, et al. Radial strain and strain rate by two-dimensional speckle tracking echocardiography and the tissue velocity based technique in the dog. J Vet Cardiol 2007;9(2):69–81.
40. Chetboul V, Serres F, Gouni V, et al. Non-invasive assessment of systolic left ventricular torsion by 2-dimensional speckle tracking imaging in the awake dog: repeatability, reproducibility, and comparison with tissue Doppler imaging variables. J Vet Intern Med 2008;22(2):342–50.

The Use of NT-proBNP Assay in the Management of Canine Patients with Heart Disease

Mark A. Oyama, DVM*, Gretchen E. Singletary, DVM

KEYWORDS

• Biomarkers • Natriuretic peptides • Mitral valve disease
• Dilated cardiomyopathy

The diagnosis and management of canine heart disease could be facilitated by a highly sensitive and specific laboratory test that predicts risk of morbidity and mortality, is helpful in directing therapy, easy to perform, inexpensive, and widely available. This article details if, how, and when the cardiac biomarker, N-terminal fragment of the prohormone B-type natriuretic peptide (NT-proBNP), helps in the diagnosis and management of canine heart disease. Veterinary cardiac biomarkers, specifically NT-proBNP, hold great promise; however, NT-proBNP should be considered as work in progress. Until ongoing clinical studies are completed, there remain substantial gaps in existing knowledge on how recommendations for this technology are formulated for everyday patients, which require a slow and cautious approach. Thus, the incorporation of NT-proBNP assay or any diagnostic test into successful clinical practice requires an understanding of the science behind the technology, as well as the clinical data available to date. These aspects of NT-proBNP testing and their contribution to clinical management of canine heart disease are discussed.

THE BIOLOGY OF NT-proBNP

NT-proBNP belongs to the family of natriuretic peptides and regulates fluid homeostasis. Six different natriuretic peptides have been described, and along with atrial

Disclosure: One of the authors (M.A.O.) consults for IDEXX Laboratories and IDEXX Telemedicine, Westbrook, ME, and both authors have received funding for clinical studies from IDEXX Laboratories.
Department of Clinical Studies-Philadelphia, Matthew J. Ryan Veterinary Hospital, University of Pennsylvania, 3900 Delancey Street, Philadelphia, PA 19104, USA
* Corresponding author.
E-mail address: maoyama@vet.upenn.edu

natriuretic peptide (ANP), B-type natriuretic peptide (BNP) is the predominant cardiac natriuretic peptide in dogs and cats.[1] BNP and ANP are produced by cardiac muscle tissue and released in response to a variety of stimuli, including volume overload, hypertrophy, and hypoxia. They are can also be secreted in conjunction with the release of other neurohormonal peptides such as norepinephrine and angiotensin II.[2] The natriuretic peptides are produced in the myocardium as preprohormones, which are subsequently cleaved first into prohormones (eg, proBNP, proANP) and then into a mature, active hormone. Thus, proANP and proBNP are ultimately split by specific serum and myocardial proteases into an active carboxy-terminal fragment (C-ANP, C-BNP) and an inactive N-terminal byproduct (NT-proANP, NT-proBNP). C-ANP or C-BNP binds to 2 main natriuretic peptide receptors, which are predominantly found in the kidney, lungs, vasculature, and adrenal glands. Activation of these receptors elicits natriuresis and vasodilation and also results in antihypertrophic and antifibrotic effects. Thus, the natriuretic system counteracts the vasoconstrictive and sodium-retaining effects of the renin-angiotensin-aldosterone system. The relative balance between these 2 systems contributes to the development of congestive heart failure.[2,3] As the heart disease worsens, the activities of both systems increase. However, the net effect favors vasoconstriction as well as fluid and sodium retention, because the efficacy of the natriuretic peptide system is diminished and overwhelmed in the later stages of heart disease.

From a diagnostic perspective, human ANP and BNP serve as markers of underlying cardiac function and are used to diagnose congestive heart failure, differentiate etiologies of respiratory signs, and provide information regarding risk of morbidity and mortality.[4,5] BNP assays are available for the detection of C-BNP and NT-proBNP, and, in general, the diagnostic utilities of the tests are similar.[4] In dogs, a commercial test specifically detects NT-proBNP, for which the most recent clinical trial data are available. Interest in BNP in veterinary patients stems from the recognition of how and when BNP tests are used in human patients. Thus, it is helpful to briefly review the corresponding guidelines and recommendations regarding BNP and NT-proBNP tests in this population.

HOW BNP TESTING IS USED IN HUMAN MEDICINE

The strongest indication for BNP or NT-proBNP testing is to help rule out or confirm a diagnosis of congestive heart failure.[4,6] The usefulness of the test is greatest in the cases of patients with ambiguous respiratory signs and symptoms. The usefulness of the test declines with the increase in the clinical suspicion of heart failure based on conventional modalities such as history taking, physical examination, radiography, and echocardiography.[7] This relationship makes sense, considering that an additional test provides little diagnostic value in patients already having clear evidence of heart failure using conventional diagnostics. In contrast, in cases where traditional testing is ambiguous or confusing, the addition of NT-proBNP assay to the clinical assessment improves the accuracy of diagnosis.[8,9] BNP or NT-proBNP assay combined with clinical assessment was superior to clinical assessment alone in identifying the cause of acute respiratory distress, shortening hospitalization time, and reducing cost of treatment.[10]

Another indication for testing is identification of patients with asymptomatic (occult) left ventricular dysfunction. The diagnostic utility and cost-effectiveness of screening increase with the increase in the prevalence of the disease.[11] Thus, screening is best performed in a patient population thought to be at a high risk for the disease (ie, patients with a family history of the disease, with previous infarction, and so forth), whereas routine screening of large community populations is not recommended at present.[12]

A third indication for BNP or NT-proBNP testing is to stratify a patient's risk of morbidity and mortality. Practice guidelines indicate that either one-time or serial testing can be used to assess risk level or to track a patient's clinical status.[12] In humans, the risk of death increases by 35% for every 100-ng/L increase in BNP level above the reference range.[13] Serial measurements that detect an increase greater than 85% or a decrease greater than 46% of either BNP or NT-proBNP concentration are associated with a subsequent worsening or improvement in clinical status and risk level, respectively.[14,15] In human patients with early primary mitral valve disease, elevated BNP concentration was associated with a 4.7-times higher risk for eventual congestive heart failure or death compared with patients with lower values.[16] BNP assay provides prognostic information independent of information gathered from conventional diagnostics, such as clinical signs, echocardiographic severity of mitral regurgitation, and heart size.[16–18]

A final indication for BNP or NT-proBNP testing is to help in guiding therapy.[19] When the most recent guidelines were published (in 2007),[12] routine testing was not recommended to help guide specific therapeutic decisions (ie, if diuretics should be increased, if additional cardiac medications should be started, and so forth). Since then, a large meta-analysis[20] of more than 1600 human patients reported that the risk of mortality was decreased 31% when using biomarker-guided strategies, and in no instance was this practice associated with an increase in adverse events. The indications for BNP and NT-proBNP testing in humans are summarized in **Table 1**. If and how these recommendations are applicable in the cases of dogs with heart failure is the subject of the remainder of this article.

NT-proBNP TESTING IN DOGS WITH RESPIRATORY SIGNS

Perhaps the best supported veterinary indication for NT-proBNP assay is in dogs with respiratory signs of unknown cause.[21–24] Often, data gathered from the medical history, clinical signs, and conventional diagnostics fail to clearly indicate either primary respiratory disease or congestive heart failure as the most likely cause. Concomitant respiratory and mitral valve diseases are common in geriatric dogs,

Table 1
Potential indications for BNP or NT-proBNP testing in humans and dogs

Indication	Evidence in Humans[4,6]	Evidence in Dogs
Diagnosis of heart failure	Strong	Moderately strong[21–24]
Patients with ambiguous signs	Strong	Moderately strong
Patients with suspicious signs	Moderately strong	Moderately strong
Patients with obvious heart failure signs	Not useful	Not useful
Detection of occult left ventricular dysfunction	Moderate	
High-risk populations	Moderate	Moderate[30–32]
General population screening	Not useful	Likely not useful
Risk stratification and prognostication	Strong	Moderately strong[37–39]
Biomarker-guided therapy	Unknown	Few data available[40]

and the presence of a heart murmur may subvert recognition of respiratory disease as the primary cause of signs. Two veterinary studies specifically support the use of NT-proBNP assay in ruling in or ruling out the presence of congestive heart failure in dogs with respiratory signs. Fine and colleagues[21] examined 46 dogs with respiratory distress or coughing and found that median NT-proBNP concentration was significantly higher in dogs with heart failure than in dogs with respiratory diseases such as chronic bronchitis, infection, or neoplasia. In each of the 21 dogs with respiratory disease, NT-proBNP concentration was less than 800 pmol/L, conferring 100% specificity for pulmonary disease to this value. In 23 of the 25 (92%) dogs with heart failure, NT-proBNP concentration was greater than 1400 pmol/L. In another study,[24] NT-proBNP concentration greater than 1158 pmol/L differentiated dogs with respiratory disease from dogs with congestive heart failure with a relatively high accuracy (in terms of percentage of correct diagnoses) of 83.6%. This study included a subset of dogs with concurrent primary respiratory disease and asymptomatic mitral valve disease (**Fig. 1**). Studies such as these seek to dichotomize a patient's clinical status (ie, evaluate a state with only 2 options; in heart failure or not in heart failure) using a continuous variable (ie, concentration of NT-proBNP). By doing so, it should be recognized that NT-proBNP values close to the proposed cutoff (1158 pmol/L) have less predictive power than values on either extreme of the assay's diagnostic range. Thus, a slightly more sophisticated interpretation of results[24] is that values approximately less than 900 pmol/L are highly specific for respiratory disease, and values approximately greater than 1800 pmol/L are highly specific for congestive heart failure, whereas values intermediate to these (ie, between 900 and 1800 pmol/L) have less clinical value and should be interpreted more cautiously. Thus, results

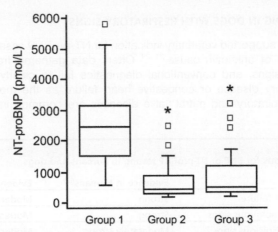

Fig. 1. Box and whisker plot of serum NT-proBNP concentration in dogs, in which the cause of respiratory signs is congestive heart failure (group 1, n = 62), primary respiratory tract disease (group 2, n = 21), or respiratory tract disease with concurrent heart disease (group 3, n = 27). For each plot, the box represents the interquartile range (IQR), the horizontal line in the middle of the box represents the median, and the whiskers denote the range extending to 1.5 times the IQR from the upper and lower quartiles. Outlier values between 1.5 and 3 times the IQR are denoted as open squares. Asterisks in groups 2 and 3 denote values significantly (P<.005) different from value for group 1 dogs. (*From* Oyama MA, Rush JE, Rozanski EA, et al. Assessment of serum N-terminal pro-B-type natriuretic peptide concentration for differentiation of congestive heart failure from primary respiratory tract disease as the cause of respiratory signs in dogs. J Am Vet Med Assoc 2009;235:1319–25; with permission.)

from veterinary studies closely mimic those in human studies, wherein the likelihood ratio of heart failure versus respiratory disease is very low when NT-proBNP concentration is low, whereas the likelihood of heart failure is very high when NT-proBNP concentration is high.[7]

In such clinical studies[21–24] and others,[9,10] the gold standard for the diagnosis of either congestive heart failure or respiratory disease is the review of case material (ie, history, clinical signs, radiographs, echocardiographs, electrocardiograms, and so forth) by one or more specialists. It is this "expert opinion" against which the clinical utility of the NT-proBNP assay is evaluated. This study design emphasizes an important aspect of biomarker testing; that is, as an individual's proficiency in assessing the conventional diagnostic studies increases, the value of or need for biomarker testing likely decreases. As stated earlier, the greatest value of NT-proBNP assay is in those patients whose diagnostic results are ambiguous.[7] Thus, depending on the individual examiner's experience, the value of NT-proBNP testing is likely variable. For instance, a specialist who routinely examines patients with cardiac diseases may not rely on NT-proBNP assay as much as a general practitioner. In humans, the accuracy of heart failure diagnosis by emergency physicians is typically less than 80% and can be as low as 60%,[25–27] leading to improper treatment in as many as a third of patients, resulting in a subsequent doubling of mortality.[8,25] In a study involving more than 1500 human patients with congestive heart failure admitted to the emergency room, the accuracy of the primary physician rose from 74% to 81.5% when NT-proBNP results were used in conjunction with conventional diagnostics.[28] Although, to the authors' knowledge, the accuracy of heart failure diagnosis by veterinarians has not been studied, it is likely similar to that by physicians, suggesting that NT-proBNP assay can be useful. The cause and clinical presentation of dogs with respiratory signs is extremely heterogeneous, and no one test is likely to provide 100% accuracy. Even in human medicine, there is no broad consensus over what NT-proBNP cutoff value yields the best diagnostic utility.[29] Hence, NT-proBNP values should be interpreted in the context of the entire clinical picture, realizing that the lower the NT-proBNP value, the less likely is the chance of congestive heart failure.

NT-proBNP TESTING IN DOGS SUSPECTED TO HAVE HEART DISEASE

A potential indication for NT-proBNP testing is detection of asymptomatic or occult heart disease. During this stage, early diagnosis is required to monitor progression and, possibly, to intervene before the onset of clinical signs. In achieving a diagnosis of degenerative mitral valve disease, NT-proBNP assay (or any biochemical testing) plays no role. Auscultation represents an easy, inexpensive, and highly sensitive and specific screening method.

What about the use of biomarker assay for other types of canine heart disease? In the case of occult dilated cardiomyopathy (DCM), NT-proBNP assay may have value in that characteristic physical examination findings, such as diastolic gallops or heart murmurs, may be subtle or absent. Moreover, the diagnostic gold standard for occult cardiomyopathy, which involves electrocardiographic (ECG) and echocardiographic examinations, is relatively expensive and requires additional expertise and equipment. Studies suggest that BNP or NT-proBNP may have a limited role in the detection of occult cardiomyopathy. In Doberman pinschers, BNP testing possesses a relatively high sensitivity (95.2%) but low specificity (61.9%) for detection of occult disease.[30] Thus, many false-positive results would be expected, limiting the test utility. Wess and colleagues[31] examined 324 Doberman pinschers and found that NT-proBNP assay possessed relatively low sensitivity and specificity (76.1% and 76.9%, respectively) in detecting dogs with either echocardiographic or ECG abnormalities. However, in the subset of dogs limited to those with abnormal echocardiographic findings, sensitivity rose to 90%. In another study[32] of 71 Doberman pinschers, the combination of NT-proBNP assay and 24-hour ambulatory ECG (Holter) monitoring was 100% sensitive, 93.2% specific, and 94.4% accurate in detecting a subset of 19 affected dogs. Thus, it is possible that NT-proBNP testing together with Holter monitoring is a useful diagnostic combination. The cost-effectiveness of screening assays increases with increase in the prevalence of disease within the screened population.[11] The prevalence of occult DCM in adult Doberman pinschers may be as high as 40%[33]; however, the routine screening of dogs for occult cardiomyopathy is not recommended until additional studies are conducted. NT-proBNP testing reveals information specific to a single point in time, and a normal value does not exclude the possibility of disease in the future. A normal NT-proBNP value in a young dog does not guarantee fitness for breeding programs, because DCM is a late-onset disease. In the case of widespread screening of young healthy dogs for acquired diseases such as DCM, identification of and testing for specific genetic mutations remains the gold standard. Thus, in the case of occult DCM detection, NT-proBNP may play a role in the initial testing of individual animals in adult high-risk populations.

NT-proBNP TESTING TO STRATIFY RISK

Clinicians possess a limited ability to predict risk of future morbidity and mortality in dogs with heart disease. In dogs with mitral valve disease, the ratio of left atrial diameter to that of aortic root (LA/Ao) is a variable shown to be significantly and independently associated with outcome, but even this variable tends not to change dramatically until heart failure is imminent.[34] Other studies[35] indicate that natriuretic peptide concentration increases with increasing disease severity among dogs with and without history of clinical signs.[36] Thus, it is possible that biomarkers such as NT-proBNP could accurately predict when heart failure or mortality is expected. In a prospective study[37] of 72 dogs with asymptomatic mitral valve disease, NT-proBNP was 1 of 8 variables, including LA/Ao ratio, that were predictive of death or onset of congestive heart failure during the subsequent 12 months after their initial examination. Similarly, in a separate population of 100 dogs with mitral valve disease, only 2 variables—normalized left ventricular diameter and NT-proBNP concentration— were found to be predictive of all-cause and cardiac mortality over a 3-year study period.[38] For every 100-pmol/L increase in NT-proBNP concentration, the risk of death from all causes increased by 7%. The median survival time in dogs with NT-proBNP concentration greater than 738.5 pmol/L was 318 days versus 786 days in dogs with NT-proBNP concentration between 391.1 and 738.5 pmol/L ($P = .001$). In the subpopulation of dogs dying specifically of cardiac causes, median survival time in dogs with NT-proBNP concentration greater than 738.5 pmol/L was 351 days. Median survival time in dogs with NT-proBNP concentration less than or equal to 738.5 pmol/L could not be calculated because more than half of these dogs were still alive at the end of study duration, suggesting that NT-proBNP was specifically predictive of risk of cardiac mortality (**Fig. 2**).

Serres and colleagues[39] reported that NT-proBNP concentration was closely correlated with clinical severity of mitral valve disease in dogs with congestive heart failure. These investigators also reported that that NT-proBNP assay yielded a sensitivity of 80% and specificity of 73% in predicting mortality over the subsequent 6 months, with NT-proBNP concentration greater than 1500 pmol/L, conferring a worse prognosis (**Fig. 3**). These studies provide a glimpse of how biomarker testing can provide

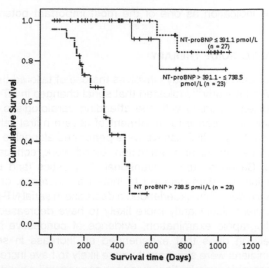

Fig. 2. Survival curves for 73 dogs with mitral valve disease based on NT-proBNP assay with cardiac mortality as the end point. Median survival of dogs with NT-proBNP values in the highest tercile (NT-proBNP concentration >738.5 pmol/L) was significantly shorter than dogs in the middle or lowest tercile (*P* = .001). (*From* Moonarmart W, Boswood A, Luis-Fuentes V, et al. N-terminal proBNP and left ventricular diameter independently predict mortality in dogs with mitral valve disease. J Small Anim Pract 2010;51:84–96; with permission.)

clinically important information regarding risk stratification. Additional studies are needed to better define the diagnostic cut points and target patient populations, but clearly the prediction of outcome and risk in dogs with mitral valve disease has great potential impact, especially if it can be demonstrated that after the identification of high-risk patients, intervention can favorably alter the natural history of disease. The

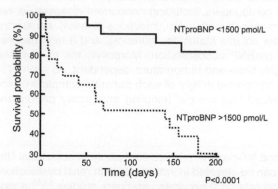

Fig. 3. Survival curves of dogs with mitral valve disease according to NT-proBNP concentration less than 1500 pmol/L (n = 23, *solid line*) and greater than 1500 pmol/L (n = 23, *dashed line*) on initial presentation. Survival probability is significantly greater in dogs with NT-proBNP concentration less than 1500 pmol/L. (*Adapted from* Serres F, Pouchelon JL, Poujol L, et al. Plasma N-terminal pro-B-type natriuretic peptide concentration helps to predict survival in dogs with symptomatic degenerative mitral valve disease regardless of and in combination with the initial clinical status at admission. J Vet Cardiol 2009;11:103–21; with permission.)

authors regard this indication as one of the most important potential uses of NT-proBNP assay.

NT-proBNP TESTING TO GUIDE THERAPY

A final indication for biomarker assays involves the use of tailored therapy guided by biomarker levels. A pilot study[40] indicated that serial changes in NT-proBNP in dogs with mitral valve disease agreed with the attending cardiologist's clinical decision making. Dogs receiving diuretics for treatment of severe mitral valve disease were monitored, and serial NT-proBNP assays were performed alongside the conventional workup, which included physical examination, blood work, echocardiography, and chest radiographs. Based on the conventional diagnostics (and blind to the NT-proBNP results), clinicians then decided to increase, decrease, or not change the diuretic dose. In those dogs that experienced a decrease in serial NT-proBNP concentrations, clinicians were significantly more likely to have decreased the furosemide dose, and on radiographic examination, evidence of congestive heart failure was unlikely. Conversely, in dogs that experienced an increase in serial NT-proBNP concentrations, clinicians were significantly more likely to have increased furosemide dose, and on radiographic examination, evidence of congestive heart failure was more likely. These results, although preliminary, suggest that NT-proBNP concentrations track changes in clinical status and may help clinicians determine need for treatment. In the authors' experience successful resolution of congestive heart failure usually decreases NT-proBNP concentrations, but not to the normal reference range. Whether more aggressive therapy to further decrease NT-proBNP concentrations would change progression of disease or recurrence of heart failure is unknown. As discussed earlier, studies of biomarker-directed therapy in humans have yielded positive[16,19,20] and negative[41] results, and until more data are available, routine testing to guide therapy in dogs is not recommended.

PRACTICALITIES AND LIMITATIONS OF NT-proBNP TESTING

As with all diagnostic tests, NT-proBNP assay is not without certain limitations. Multiple potential confounders, including concurrent diseases (ie, renal dysfunction, systemic and pulmonary hypertension, infectious disease), administration of medications that may alter volume status (ie, diuretics), and a high degree of weekly variability, affect NT-proBNP concentration. Moreover, the ex vivo stability of canine NT-proBNP is highly time- and temperature-dependent. As such, NT-proBNP values must be carefully interpreted in light of each patient's complete clinical picture, and it should be recognized that sample handling and assay performance could affect results.

Renal Function

In humans, BNP and NT-proBNP are excreted partly through renal filtration; therefore, circulating levels can be elevated in individuals with renal dysfunction and decreased glomerular filtration rate. In 2 separate veterinary studies,[42,43] a significantly higher mean NT-proBNP concentration was documented in azotemic dogs as compared with healthy controls. The difference in NT-proBNP concentration between these groups ranged from 2.4 to 4.7 times higher in the dogs with renal disease. In both studies, the presence of azotemia often was enough to increase the NT-proBNP concentration above the normal reference range, thus producing dogs with a false-positive result. This confounding effect can be partially mitigated by using values corrected for azotemia (ie, a NT-proBNP/creatinine ratio) (**Fig. 4**).[42] In patients with renal

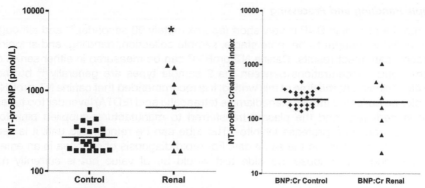

Fig. 4. (*Left panel*) Scatterplot of serum NT-proBNP concentration in 23 healthy control dogs and 8 dogs with renal disease. Asterisk indicates that value of geometric mean is significantly (*P*<.05) different from value for control dogs. (*Right panel*) Scatterplot of NT-proBNP/creatinine ratio in 23 healthy dogs and 8 dogs with renal disease. The median value is not significantly different between the groups. (*Adapted from* Schmidt MK, Reynolds CA, Estrada AH, et al. Effect of azotemia on serum N-terminal proBNP concentration in dogs with normal cardiac function: a pilot study. J Vet Cardiol 2009;11(Suppl 1):S81–6; with permission.)

disease or systemic or pulmonary hypertension, it is likely that elevated NT-proBNP concentrations are not solely the result of decreased renal filtration. Increased release of BNP in chronic renal disease could occur secondary to either diastolic dysfunction or expanded plasma volume, leading to increased myocardial stretch. Systemic and/or pulmonary hypertension is a frequent sequela of extracardiac disease, and both are associated with elevations in NT-proBNP in dogs.[24,44] Elevations in natriuretic peptides may reflect the so-called cardiorenal syndrome,[45] a complex clinical entity characterized by concurrent cardiac and renal dysfunction that results from pathophysiologic interactions of the cardiovascular system and kidneys. In dogs,[43] the lack of[42] or weak[30] correlation between NT-proBNP and serum creatinine supports the theory that NT-proBNP is not simply the result of decreased glomerular filtration. Thus, in dogs with renal disease, elevated BNP or NT-proBNP may still convey important prognostic information. In human patients, BNP or NT-proBNP concentrations have been convincingly and repeatedly shown to be predictors of morbidity and mortality independent of renal function, echocardiographic heart size, and results of other conventional testing.[46–51] This finding suggests that natriuretic peptides add unique information to the clinical assessment rather than just acting as a surrogate measure of other parameters.

Biologic Variability

Unlike ANP, little BNP is stored before release. Secretion of BNP is modulated by an increase in transcription, requiring a sufficiently long period (generally 1–3 hours) between the initial stimulus for release and the elevation in circulating peptide.[3] Biologic variation in NT-proBNP concentration exists on a day-to-day level and may affect assay results, leading to false positives or false negatives.[52] Fluctuations in human patients can affect assay interpretation, and substantial week-to-week variation has been demonstrated in healthy dogs.[53] These fluctuations can result from a variation in production because of circadian rhythm or may be related to daily variation in volume status resulting from changes in diet, water intake, exercise, or neurohormonal peptide clearance.[14,52]

Sample Handling and Processing

The half-life of canine BNP is very short (approximately 90 seconds),[54] and although NT-proBNP is thought to be more stable, sample collection, handling, and shipping protocols can affect results. Canine NT-proBNP can be measured in either serum or plasma, and concentrations between the 2 sample types are generally,[55] but not entirely,[53] similar. At the time of this writing, it is recommended that canine NT-proBNP samples be collected into ethylenediamine tetraacetic acid (EDTA) lavender top tubes, spun immediately, and the plasma transferred to manufacturer-supplied pink top tubes that contain a protease inhibitor. The tube can be refrigerated until it is sent to a central laboratory on the same day. For rapid diagnosis of dyspnea in an emergency setting, an in-house, pet-side test would be of value but is currently not available.

Assay Variability

The canine BNP assay has evolved from a time-consuming and highly variable C-BNP radioimmunoassay to a first-generation C-BNP enzyme-linked immunosorbent assay (ELISA), several iterations of a veterinary NT-proBNP assay, and finally to the currently available canine- and feline-specific NT-proBNP ELISA.[56] Widespread adoption of NT-proBNP assay into clinical practice requires results from well-designed clinical trials, as well as an assay platform that is stable and consistently performing. Since its introduction, the reference values associated with the canine NT-proBNP assay have undergone several changes, leading to confusion in the usage and interpretation of the assay. Changes in assay performance and sample handling have likely contributed to important differences in reference ranges and diagnostic cut points reported across clinical studies. Going forward, assay consistency at the level of the manufacturer is critical in establishing consistent reference ranges and in knowing how to best use NT-proBNP results in everyday clinical practice.

THE FUTURE OF NATRIURETIC PEPTIDE TESTING

BNP and NT-proBNP tests have become widely accepted as diagnostic tools in human medicine, and their application in canine patients holds great promise. In the authors' estimation, NT-proBNP assay is useful for the differentiation of respiratory distress in dogs and is likely to be especially useful in instances where the conventional diagnostic results are ambiguous. For veterinarians who are experienced in interpreting cardiac diagnostics, the value of the test lies not with its diagnostic utility but with its potential for either one-time or serial NT-proBNP measurements to provide risk stratification and prognosis. Ideally, risk stratification would be accompanied by interventions proved to delay or alter the natural progression of disease at various stages of disease. Whether NT-proBNP has a role in the screening of high-risk populations for occult canine cardiomyopathy requires additional study, but it is unlikely that NT-proBNP assay alone can be used. The use of NT-proBNP–directed therapy is an intriguing and attractive possibility, but it requires longitudinal studies with careful planning and execution.

Regardless of the final role that NT-proBNP assumes in the diagnosis and management of canine heart disease, proper use of the test is almost certainly as a complement and not as a replacement for conventional diagnostics. It is unlikely and, in fact, not particularly helpful for any biomarker assay to perfectly mirror the results of conventional diagnostics. To realize its maximal promise, NT-proBNP would add unique data to the clinical assessment, which cannot be gathered from currently existing means, and the combination of biomarker testing with conventional diagnostics would lead to outcomes superior to that of conventional means alone.

REFERENCES

1. van Kimmenade RR, Januzzi JL Jr. The evolution of the natriuretic peptides—current applications in human and animal medicine. J Vet Cardiol 2009;11(Suppl 1): S9–21.
2. Potter LR, Yoder AR, Flora DR, et al. Natriuretic peptides: their structures, receptors, physiologic functions and therapeutic applications. Handb Exp Pharmacol 2009;191:341–66.
3. Mair J. Biochemistry of B-type natriuretic peptide—where are we now? Clin Chem Lab Med 2008;46:1507–14.
4. Tang WH, Francis GS, Morrow DA, et al. National Academy of Clinical Biochemistry Laboratory Medicine Practice Guidelines: clinical utilization of cardiac biomarker testing in heart failure. Clin Biochem 2008;41:210–21.
5. Rehman SU, Januzzi JL Jr. Natriuretic peptide testing in clinical medicine. Cardiol Rev 2008;16:240–9.
6. Beilby J. National Academy of Clinical Biochemistry (NACB) laboratory medicine guidelines on the clinical utilization and analytical issues for cardiac biomarker testing in heart failure. Clin Biochem Rev 2008;29:107–11.
7. Steinhart B, Thorpe KE, Bayoumi AM, et al. Improving the diagnosis of acute heart failure using a validated prediction model. J Am Coll Cardiol 2009;54: 1515–21.
8. Mueller C, Scholer A, Laule-Kilian K, et al. Use of B-type natriuretic peptide in the evaluation and management of acute dyspnea. N Engl J Med 2004;350: 647–54.
9. Januzzi JL Jr, Camargo CA, Anwaruddin S, et al. The N-terminal Pro-BNP investigation of dyspnea in the emergency department (PRIDE) study. Am J Cardiol 2005;95:948–54.
10. Maisel AS, Krishnaswamy P, Nowak RM, et al. Rapid measurement of B-type natriuretic peptide in the emergency diagnosis of heart failure. N Engl J Med 2002;347:161–7.
11. Heidenreich PA, Gubens MA, Fonarow GC, et al. Cost-effectiveness of screening with B-type natriuretic peptide to identify patients with reduced left ventricular ejection fraction. J Am Coll Cardiol 2004;43:1019–26.
12. Tang WH, Francis GS, Morrow DA, et al. National Academy of Clinical Biochemistry Laboratory Medicine practice guidelines: clinical utilization of cardiac biomarker testing in heart failure. Circulation 2007;116:e99–109.
13. Doust JA, Pietrzak E, Dobson A, et al. How well does B-type natriuretic peptide predict death and cardiac events in patients with heart failure: systematic review. BMJ 2005;330:625–34.
14. O'Hanlon R, O'Shea P, Ledwidge M, et al. The biologic variability of B-type natriuretic peptide and N-terminal pro-B-type natriuretic peptide in stable heart failure patients. J Card Fail 2007;13:50–5.
15. Wu AH, Smith A, Wieczorek S, et al. Biological variation for N-terminal pro- and B-type natriuretic peptides and implications for therapeutic monitoring of patients with congestive heart failure. Am J Cardiol 2003;92:628–31.
16. Pizarro R, Bazzino OO, Oberti PF, et al. Prospective validation of the prognostic usefulness of brain natriuretic peptide in asymptomatic patients with chronic severe mitral regurgitation. J Am Coll Cardiol 2009;54:1099–106.

17. Detaint D, Messika-Zeitoun D, Avierinos JF, et al. B-type natriuretic peptide in organic mitral regurgitation: determinants and impact on outcome. Circulation 2005;111:2391–7.
18. Detaint D, Messika-Zeitoun D, Chen HH, et al. Association of B-type natriuretic peptide activation to left ventricular end-systolic remodeling in organic and functional mitral regurgitation. Am J Cardiol 2006;97:1029–34.
19. Jourdain P, Jondeau G, Funck F, et al. Plasma brain natriuretic peptide-guided therapy to improve outcome in heart failure: the STARS-BNP Multicenter Study. J Am Coll Cardiol 2007;49:1733–9.
20. Felker GM, Hasselblad V, Hernandez AF, et al. Biomarker-guided therapy in chronic heart failure: a meta-analysis of randomized controlled trials. Am Heart J 2009;158:422–30.
21. Fine DM, Declue AE, Reinero CR. Evaluation of circulating amino terminal-pro-B-type natriuretic peptide concentration in dogs with respiratory distress attributable to congestive heart failure or primary pulmonary disease. J Am Vet Med Assoc 2008;232:1674–9.
22. Prosek R, Sisson DD, Oyama MA, et al. Distinguishing cardiac and noncardiac dyspnea in 48 dogs using plasma atrial natriuretic factor, B-type natriuretic factor, endothelin, and cardiac troponin-I. J Vet Intern Med 2007;21:238–42.
23. DeFrancesco TC, Rush JE, Rozanski EA, et al. Prospective clinical evaluation of an ELISA B-type natriuretic peptide assay in the diagnosis of congestive heart failure in dogs presenting with cough or dyspnea. J Vet Intern Med 2007;21:243–50.
24. Oyama MA, Rush JE, Rozanski EA, et al. Differentiation of congestive heart failure versus respiratory disease in dogs with respiratory signs using NT-proBNP assay. J Am Vet Med Assoc 2009;235:1319–25.
25. Ray P, Birolleau S, Lefort Y, et al. Acute respiratory failure in the elderly: etiology, emergency diagnosis and prognosis. Crit Care 2006;10:R82.
26. Mueller C, Frana B, Rodriguez D, et al. Emergency diagnosis of congestive heart failure: impact of signs and symptoms. Can J Cardiol 2005;21:921–4.
27. Ray P, Delerme S, Jourdain P, et al. Differential diagnosis of acute dyspnea: the value of B natriuretic peptides in the emergency department. QJM 2008;101:831–43.
28. McCullough PA, Nowak RM, McCord J, et al. B-type natriuretic peptide and clinical judgment in emergency diagnosis of heart failure: analysis from Breathing Not Properly (BNP) Multinational Study. Circulation 2002;106:416–22.
29. Worster A, Balion CM, Hill SA, et al. Diagnostic accuracy of BNP and NT-proBNP in patients presenting to acute care settings with dyspnea: a systematic review. Clin Biochem 2008;41:250–9.
30. Oyama MA, Sisson DD, Solter PF. Prospective screening for occult cardiomyopathy in dogs by measurement of plasma atrial natriuretic peptide, B-type natriuretic peptide, and cardiac troponin-I concentrations. Am J Vet Res 2007;68:42–7.
31. Wess G, Butz V, Killich K, et al. Evaluation of NT-proBNP in the diagnosis of various stages of dilated cardiomyopathy in Doberman pinschers [abstract]. J Vet Intern Med 2009;23:686.
32. Morris N, Oyama MA, O'Sullivan ML, et al. Utility of NT-proBNP assay to detect occult dilated cardiomyopathy in Doberman pinschers [abstract]. J Vet Intern Med 2009;23:686.
33. O'Grady MR, O'Sullivan ML. Dilated cardiomyopathy: an update. Vet Clin North Am Small Anim Pract 2004;34:1187–207.

34. Haggstrom J, Hoglund K, Borgarelli M. An update on treatment and prognostic indicators in canine myxomatous mitral valve disease. J Small Anim Pract 2009;50(Suppl 1):25–33.

35. Tarnow I, Olsen LH, Kvart C, et al. Predictive value of natriuretic peptides in dogs with mitral valve disease. Vet J 2009;180:195–201.

36. Oyama MA, Fox PR, Rush JE, et al. Clinical utility of serum N-terminal pro-B-type natriuretic peptide concentration for identifying cardiac disease in dogs and assessing disease severity. J Am Vet Med Assoc 2008;232:1496–503.

37. Chetboul V, Serres F, Tissier R, et al. Association of plasma N-terminal pro-B-type natriuretic peptide concentration with mitral regurgitation severity and outcome in dogs with asymptomatic degenerative mitral valve disease. J Vet Intern Med 2009;23:984–94.

38. Moonarmart W, Boswood A, Luis-Fuentes V, et al. N-terminal proBNP and left ventricular diameter independently predict mortality in dogs with mitral valve disease. J Small Anim Pract 2010;51:84–96.

39. Serres F, Pouchelon JL, Poujol L, et al. Plasma N-terminal pro-B-type natriuretic peptide concentration helps to predict survival in dogs with symptomatic degenerative mitral valve disease regardless of and in combination with the initial clinical status at admission. J Vet Cardiol 2009;11:103–21.

40. Achen SE, Gordon SG, Roland RM, et al. Serial evaluation of NT-proBNP in dogs with CHF predicts clinical score and the presence or absence of radiographic pulmonary edema [abstract]. J Vet Intern Med 2009;23:687.

41. Pfisterer M, Buser P, Rickli H, et al. BNP-guided vs symptom-guided heart failure therapy: the Trial of Intensified vs Standard Medical Therapy in Elderly Patients with Congestive Heart Failure (TIME-CHF) randomized trial. JAMA 2009;301: 383–92.

42. Schmidt MK, Reynolds CA, Estrada AH, et al. Effect of azotemia on serum N-terminal proBNP concentration in dogs with normal cardiac function: a pilot study. J Vet Cardiol 2009;11(Suppl 1):S81–6.

43. Raffan E, Loureiro J, Dukes-McEwan J, et al. The cardiac biomarker NT-proBNP is increased in dogs with azotemia. J Vet Intern Med 2009;23:1184–9.

44. Atkinson KJ, Fine DM, Thombs LA, et al. Evaluation of pimobendan and N-terminal probrain natriuretic peptide in the treatment of pulmonary hypertension secondary to degenerative mitral valve disease in dogs. J Vet Intern Med 2009;23:1190–6.

45. Ronco C, Haapio M, House AA, et al. Cardiorenal syndrome. J Am Coll Cardiol 2008;52:1527–39.

46. Paniagua R, Ventura MD, Avila-Diaz M, et al. NT-proBNP, fluid volume overload and dialysis modality are independent predictors of mortality in ESRD patients. Nephrol Dial Transplant 2009. DOI:10.1093/ndt/gfp395.

47. Maisel AS. Cardiovascular and renal surrogate markers in the clinical management of hypertension. Cardiovasc Drugs Ther 2009;23:317–26.

48. Reny JL, Millot O, Vanderecamer T, et al. Admission NT-proBNP levels, renal insufficiency and age as predictors of mortality in elderly patients hospitalized for acute dyspnea. Eur J Intern Med 2009;20:14–9.

49. Svensson M, Gorst-Rasmussen A, Schmidt EB, et al. NT-pro-BNP is an independent predictor of mortality in patients with end-stage renal disease. Clin Nephrol 2009;71:380–6.

50. Park S, Cho GY, Kim SG, et al. Brain natriuretic peptide levels have diagnostic and prognostic capability for cardio-renal syndrome type 4 in intensive care unit patients. Crit Care 2009;13:R70.

51. Hickman PE, McGill DA, Talaulikar G, et al. Prognostic efficacy of cardiac biomarkers for mortality in dialysis patients. Intern Med J 2008. DOI:10.1111/j.1445-5994.2008.01846.x.

52. Wu AH. Serial testing of B-type natriuretic peptide and NT pro-BNP for monitoring therapy of heart failure: the role of biologic variation in the interpretation of results. Am Heart J 2006;152:828–34.

53. Kellihan HB, Oyama MA, Reynolds CA, et al. Weekly variability of plasma and serum NT-proBNP measurements in normal dogs. J Vet Cardiol 2009;11(Suppl 1): S93–7.

54. Thomas CJ, Woods RL. Haemodynamic action of B-type natriuretic peptide substantially outlasts its plasma half-life in conscious dogs. Clin Exp Pharmacol Physiol 2003;30:369–75.

55. Boswood A, Dukes-McEwan J, Loureiro J, et al. The diagnostic accuracy of different natriuretic peptides in the investigation of canine cardiac disease. J Small Anim Pract 2008;49:26–32.

56. Sisson DD. Neuroendocrine evaluation of cardiac disease. Vet Clin North Am Small Anim Pract 2004;34:1105–26.

Natriuretic Peptides: The Feline Experience

David J. Connolly, BVetMed, PhD, CertSAM, CertVC

KEYWORDS

• Feline cardiomyopathy • Congestive heart failure
• Respiratory distress • Natriuretic peptides • Clinical utility

HISTORICAL BACKGROUND

Natriuretic peptides (NP) are a group of hormones synthesized by cardiomyocytes, and include atrial natriuretic peptide (ANP) and brain natriuretic peptide (BNP). They are released into the circulation as a result of numerous stimuli, including myocardial stretch, ischemia, hypoxia, and neurohormonal upregulation. NPs are responsible for the regulation of body fluid homeostasis and blood pressure.[1,2] In human patients, they are increasingly being used as markers for the diagnosis and prognosis of cardiac disease and failure.[3–5] Nesiritide, a product of recombinant DNA technology that has the same amino acid sequence as human BNP, may have a role in the treatment of people with heart failure.[6]

The translation of the BNP gene results in the production of a large pre-pro hormone that is rapidly processed to form the pro hormone proBNP by removal of its signal peptide. Subsequently proBNP is cleaved in two by the proteolytic enzymes corin, which is expressed in the myocardium, or furin, which is ubiquitously expressed, to form the larger biologically inert amino-terminal part NT-proBNP and the biologically active peptide BNP.[7–10] Post-translation modification of pre-proANP occurs in a similar fashion. The ELISA assays in current use measure circulating concentrations of the N-terminal portion of the protein rather than the biologically active peptide because the former is less rapidly eliminated or degraded and reaches a higher concentration than the C-terminal portion.[11]

The initial studies on NP in cats were hampered by the lack of homology between feline and human BNP and the cumbersome processes of extraction, validation, and quality control required for radioimmunoassay assessment of peptide concentration.[12] The possibility of using feline-specific BNP antibodies for assay analysis was realized following the cloning and sequencing of the feline BNP gene in 2002.[13] Because there is a high level of homology between human, canine, and feline ANP, accurate measurement of circulating feline ANP has been performed using antibodies directed against the human peptide even though the feline sequence has been determined.[14]

Department of Veterinary Clinical Sciences, Royal Veterinary College, Hawkshead Lane, Hatfield, Hertfordshire AL9 7TA, UK
E-mail address: dconnolly@rvc.ac.uk

Vet Clin Small Anim 40 (2010) 559–570
doi:10.1016/j.cvsm.2010.03.003
0195-5616/10/$ – see front matter © 2010 Elsevier Inc. All rights reserved.

vetsmall.theclinics.com

Early investigations evaluated the immunohistochemical distribution of ANP and BNP in the hearts of healthy control cats and those with hypertrophic cardiomyopathy (HCM) using antibodies directed against the C-terminal of human ANP and the N-terminal of feline BNP.[11] In control cats, ANP and BNP immunoreactivity was restricted to the atria and concentrated on the endocardial surface. In the cats with HCM, atrial immunoreactivity for ANP and BNP was more diffusely distributed and ventricular immunoreactivity was negative for ANP, but ventricular myocytes stained lightly and diffusely for BNP.[11] The first study to document circulating concentrations of NP in cats with cardiomyopathy used radioimmunoassay (RIA) to measure BNP concentrations and RIA and ELISA to measure ANP fragments. Relative to healthy cats, increased levels of NP were identified in cats with congestive heart failure (CHF) or systemic thromboembolism caused by cardiomyopathy (HCM, restrictive cardiomyopathy, or unclassified cardiomyopathy). Furthermore, BNP was found to be significantly increased in asymptomatic cats with cardiomyopathy compared with controls.[15]

INTRODUCTION OF THE ELISA

The availability of colorimetric sandwich ELISA technology has facilitated the measurement of circulating NP concentrations in feline samples.[16] The BNP assay uses immunoaffinity-purified sheep antibody for feline NT-proBNP. The sandwich comprises anti-NT–proBNP (1–20) bound to the wells of the plate and anti-NT–proBNP (60–80) conjugated to horseradish peroxidase. The ANP assay uses polyclonal sheep antihuman NT-proANP antibody. The sandwich comprises anti-NT–proANP (10–19) pre-coated to the wells of the plate and anti-NT–proANP (85–90) conjugated to horseradish peroxidase.[a,17]

ASSESSMENT OF CIRCULATING NATRIURETIC PEPTIDE CONCENTRATIONS IN CATS WITH MYOCARDIAL DISEASE

Following the introduction of these assays several preliminary studies have been performed to investigate their utility in the identification of feline cardiac disease. Plasma NT-proANP concentration was measured in 17 cats with HCM (two of which had CHF) and 19 healthy controls. No significant difference in concentrations was seen between the asymptomatic affected cats and the control population.[17] A second study investigated serum NT-proANP and NT-proBNP concentrations in 78 cats of which 28 were healthy controls, 17 had myocardial disease without signs of CHF and 33 had myocardial disease with CHF. In cats with heart disease, HCM was the most common myocardial disease followed by restrictive cardiomyopathy. Serum concentrations of NT-proANP and NT-proBNP were found to be significantly different between all three groups and the NT-proBNP assay appeared to have the greater discriminating power. The results from this study suggest that NP can distinguish cats with asymptomatic heart disease from healthy cats and those with CHF.[18] Several other studies have also convincingly shown that circulating NP concentrations in cats with CHF are significantly higher compared with healthy control animals.[19–21]

However the ability of these peptides to distinguish between healthy control animals and cats with myocardial disease but without signs of CHF remains controversial because of conflicting results from different studies. Two publications have suggested that the NT-proANP ELISA can distinguish asymptomatic cats with myocardial disease from controls[18,21] and one study showed no significant difference between controls and

[a] proANP(1–98), Feline cardioscreen NT-proBNP, IDEXX Laboratories, Westbrook (ME), USA

affected cats.[17] The literature regarding the NT-proBNP assay is also inconsistent. The results of three studies[18,22,23] suggest that the assay has the ability to identify cats with myocardial disease diagnosed by echocardiography but without signs of CHF. In contrast, an investigation of a colony of Maine Coon and Maine Coon cross cats genotyped as heterozygous or negative for the A31P myosin binding protein C mutation provided evidence that NT-proBNP measurement can identify asymptomatic cats with severe HCM with a high sensitivity and specificity, but is not useful for identifying cats with less severe disease because no differences in NT-proBNP concentrations were seen between normal cats and cats with equivocal or moderate HCM.[20]

Numerous factors may be responsible for these conflicting results: variation in sample handling, storage conditions, shipping conditions, and potential variation in NP concentration between plasma or serum samples.[24] Other comorbidities in the sample populations may also have influence on NT-proBNP concentration, such as renal dysfunction and systolic hypertension (these factors are described in more detail later in the article).[25] In two of the studies an attempt was made to rank the severity of hypertrophy ([normal, mild, moderate, and severe][23] or [normal, equivocal, moderate, and severe]).[20] These two studies showed considerable divergence of NT-proBNP concentration for all stages of hypertrophy as shown in **Table 1**. One possible explanation for this divergence is the way the data have been analyzed and presented. In the published study from Hsu and colleagues the data are presented as median and range, whereas in the study of Wess and colleagues the data is presented as mean and standard deviation. This difference in data analysis can markedly affect the results, so care must be taken when evaluating data from different studies to ensure that the influence of different statistical analysis is fully appreciated. Despite this, the author feels that inclusion of all relevant data is useful for comparison in view of the limited number of studies available. Other possible explanations for the discrepancy between the studies include the potential influence of the more restricted gene pool in the Maine Coon crossbred colony cats used in one study[20] that may have exerted an as yet undefined influence on circulating NT-proBNP concentrations at each stage of hypertrophy. A second issue maybe one of nomenclature given the somewhat arbitrary nature of categorization schemes used to define the severity of HCM. For instance all the cats with severe HCM in the study by Wess and colleagues[23] (43 out of 43) had enlarged left atria compared with only 3 out of 10 severely affected colony cats.[20] The diagnosis of mild or equivocal HCM using echocardiography is without doubt challenging even for experienced veterinary cardiologists who may place different emphasizes on subtle echocardiographic changes. This point is illustrated by the differences between these two studies with regard to criteria used to classify patients. In the investigation of Maine coon cats reported by Hsu and colleagues,[20] the presence of subjectively enlarged papillary muscles was considered equivocal evidence of disease whereas in the other study,[23] patients were included in the mildly affected category when ventricular wall thickness was in a range that Hsu and colleagues considered normal in the absence of enlarged papillary muscles.

A third explanation for the conflicting results in these studies could be that NT-proBNP does indeed lack the sensitivity to identify those cats with subtle echocardiographic changes suggestive of early disease in cats with a certain genotype.[20]

ASSESSMENT OF CIRCULATING NATRIURETIC PEPTIDE CONCENTRATIONS IN CATS WITH RESPIRATORY DISTRESS

Several studies in human patients have shown elevated circulating B-type NP concentration to be an accurate diagnostic marker of CHF, enabling patients with CHF to be

Table 1
Summary of results of studies investigating the utility of NT-proBNP to identify cats with asymptomatic myocardial disease

Echocardiographic Classification of Severity of HCM	Wess G et al[23] Plasma Mean (±SD) NT-proBNP (pmol/l)	Hsu A et al[20] Plasma (Range) NT-proBNP (pmol/l)	Clinical Classification	Connolly et al[18] Median (IQR 25th and 75th Percentiles) Serum NT-proBNP (pmol/ml)	Fox et al[22] Median (IQ Range) Serum NT-proBNP (pmol/ml)
Control	58 ± 65	21(10–79)	Control	33.6 (18.5, 11.5–30)	24 (24–45)
Mild/equivocal	333 ± 244	19 (5–53)	Cats with myocardial disease but not CHF	184.1 (217, 56–273)	283 (154–603)
Moderate	433 ± 299	22 (5–77)	Notes	NT-proBNP concentration was significantly greater in myocardial group compared with control group	NT-proBNP concentration was significantly greater in myocardial group compared with control group
Severe	835 ± 314	134 (12–252)	—		
Notes	NT-proBNP concentration was significantly greater in all HCM groups compared with control group. There was no significant difference between mild and moderate groups but both had significantly lower NT-proBNP concentration than the severe group.	NT-proBNP value was not significantly different between control, mild, or moderate groups. The NT-proBNP concentration in severe group was significantly greater than in all other groups.	—		

differentiated from those with non-cardiac causes of dyspnea.[26–32] Three feline studies have also investigated the utility of NP to aid diagnosis in cases of respiratory distress.[19,33,34] The ability to distinguish cardiac from non-cardiac causes of respiratory distress is a vital initial step in achieving an accurate diagnosis and appropriate treatment. It is often not possible to do this reliably on the basis of history and physical examination. Furthermore, the compromised state of any cat with severe respiratory distress often limits diagnostic evaluation.

Two of the three feline studies recruited cats with respiratory distress from their respective university hospitals in Europe[23,34] and the other was a multicenter study in which animals from 11 universities or private referral practices across the United States were recruited.[19] The studies included cats with a wide range of etiologies for their heart and primary respiratory disease. The results from the Investigations were reassuringly consistent (**Table 2**) and suggested that circulating NT-proBNP concentrations provide a reliable means of discriminating cats with CHF (caused by different types of cardiomyopathy) from those with primary respiratory causes of dyspnea.

It was also noted that cats with primary respiratory disease and no evidence of left ventricular hypertrophy also had increased concentrations of NT-proBNP over controls,[33,34] which was assumed to be a consequence of acquired pulmonary hypertension.[34]

OTHER FACTORS INFLUENCING CIRCULATING NATRIURETIC PEPTIDE CONCENTRATIONS

In cats, circulating NP concentrations are affected by several factors other than raised ventricular filling pressures, including renal function,[25,34] systolic blood pressure,[25] and sample handling.[24]

SAMPLE HANDLING

In a recent study, a poor correlation was seen between the concentration of feline NT-proBNP measured in serum and plasma, and furthermore, significant degradation of the peptide occurred if the sample was stored at 4°C for 24 hours or 25°C for 5 hours[24] Both NPs do appear stable if stored at −80°C for several years.[25] The stability of NT-proBNP in the presence of a protease inhibitor has also been recently investigated and preliminary results appear promising,[24] enabling the investigators to conclude that samples should either be transported to an external laboratory frozen or in tubes

Table 2
Summary of results of studies investigating the utility of NT-proBNP to distinguish cats with cardiac and non-cardiac causes of dyspnea

	Wess et al[33] Mean (±SD) Plasma NT-proBNP (pmol/l)	Fox et al[19] Median (IQR) Plasma NT-proBNP (pmol/l)	Connolly et al[34] Median (IQR 25th and 75th Percentiles) Serum NT-proBNP (pmol/l)
Respiratory dyspnea	170 ± 143	76.5 (24–180)	45 (75, 26–101)
CHF	686 ± 368	754 (437–1035)	532 (336, 347–683)
Sensitivity (sn), specificity (sp), and cutoff	277 sn, 95% sp, 84.6%	265 sn, 90.2% sp, 87.9%	220 sn, 93.9% sp, 87.8%

containing a protease inhibitor.[24] The potential influence of a protease inhibitor (not related to degradation rate) on circulating NP concentration will also require further investigation.

RENAL FUNCTION

Studies in humans have shown that circulating NT-proBNP concentrations increase as the glomerular filtration rate or creatinine clearance declines.[35–43] Two canine studies have also identified a positive correlation between NP and creatinine concentrations.[44,45] Mean serum NT-proBNP concentration was found to be significantly higher in dogs with renal disease but normal cardiac function compared with healthy control dogs suggesting that renal function should be considered when interpreting NT-proBNP results.[45] In a recent study evaluating plasma concentrations of NP in normotensive and hypertensive cats with chronic kidney disease (CKD), plasma NT-proANP and NT-proBNP concentration were significantly increased in cats with severe, normotensive CKD (International Renal Interest Society stage IV; creatinine >4.98 mg/dl)[46] compared with healthy controls. A significant difference in concentration was not seen for either NT-proANP or NT-proBNP between cats with mild-to-moderate, normotensive CKD (creatinine >2.00 mg/dl either repeatedly or in association with a urine specific gravity of less than 1.035 and compatible historical and physical examination finding) and healthy controls. The study also identified a significant positive correlation between NT-proANP and plasma creatinine concentrations but this correlation was not present with NT-proBNP.[25]

BLOOD PRESSURE

The same study also determined that plasma NT-proBNP concentrations were significantly higher in cats with hypertensive CKD compared with normal cats and those with normotensive CKD. Furthermore, in cats where treatment with the vasodilator amlodipine resulted in normalization of blood pressure, a significant reduction in plasma NT-proBNP concentration was noted suggesting that measurement of NT-proBNP shows potential as a diagnostic marker for systemic hypertension.[25] However, a major limitation of this study was that echocardiography was not performed in any of the cats.

OTHER FACTORS

In humans, circulating NP concentrations are influenced by obesity, pulmonary hypertension, pulmonary embolism, sepsis, hyperthyroidism, and age.[47–53] The influences of these factors on feline NP concentrations have not yet been established, however, a large, single-center study evaluating circulating NP in 500 cats with cardiac and noncardiac diseases is likely to investigate some of these comorbidities.[54]

NATRIURETIC PEPTIDES IN THE MANAGEMENT OF FELINE HEART DISEASE

A useful biomarker is one which may be used to assist in the diagnosis of a disease, the staging of a disease, the identification of a subpopulation requiring a specific intervention, the response to a particular intervention, or to assist with prognostication.[55] Over the last decade, NPs have emerged as established cardiac biomarkers in humans with wide potential application for diagnosis, disease staging, prognosis, and guide to therapeutic intervention.[29,56–62] To date there are insufficient feline studies published to determine whether NP will realize the full potential recognized in human clinical practice. There is substantial evidence supporting the utility of these peptides in aiding the diagnosis of myocardial disease in the cat and in association with other appropriate diagnostics increasing the probability of correctly distinguishing cats with CHF from those with non-cardiac dyspnea.[18,19,33,34] Furthermore, the clinical utility of measuring NP concentrations in the management of cats with respiratory distress will be significantly enhanced if the ELISA technology evolves toward a rapid cage side test.[31] Nevertheless, as with all other diagnostic tests, it is vital that NP concentrations are not interpreted blindly but rather in the context of good clinical judgment and experience based on an appropriate history, physical examination findings, and suitable differential diagnosis list.[56] The importance of this is illustrated by examining the results of one of the studies[34] shown in **Table 2** where measurement of NT-proBNP enabled CHF to be distinguished from non-cardiac cause of dyspnea in 74 cats with a sensitivity of 94% and a specificity of 88%. If this test was used as the sole means of diagnosis, then 6% of cats with CHF would have been misdiagnosed with respiratory disease as a cause of their dyspnea and 12% of cats with respiratory disease would have been incorrectly diagnosed with CHF. Therefore, in this scenario 13 out of 74 cats would have been given an erroneous diagnosis and potentially inappropriate treatment.

Common problems encountered in feline cardiology include how to interpret the presence of a systolic heart murmur in an otherwise healthy cat or how to definitively rule out cardiomyopathy on physical examination. In a recent study, heart murmurs were detected in 16 out of 103 (15.5%) apparently healthy cats and further assessment identified cardiomyopathy in 5 of the 16. Furthermore, in the same study 11 out of 16 cats with cardiomyopathy did not have a heart murmur.[63] Similarly, based on our present knowledge it is not possible to recommend measurement of NT-proBNP as the sole method of screening cats for silent myocardial disease. The results from the feline studies outlined in **Table 1** show some divergence with regard to the ability of NT-proBNP to identify asymptomatic cats with cardiomyopathy. Therefore, if a cat has an elevated NT-proBNP concentration and no other comorbidities, such as severe (but not mild or moderate) CKD or systemic hypertension,[25] further cardiac evaluation, such as echocardiography, should be performed whether a murmur has been detected or not. If a murmur is detected in a cat with normal circulating NT-proBNP concentration it is still not possible to completely rule out cardiomyopathy and so an echocardiogram would be recommended.

Measurement of NT-proBNP shows promise as a diagnostic maker for systemic hypertension, because it was able to distinguish hypertensive from normotensive cats with a sensitivity of 80% and a specificity of 93% using a cut-off value of greater than or equal to 203 pmol/l.[25] This test may have added benefit in those cats that develop transient high blood pressure caused by the"white coat effect" that results from the examination process. Such an effect may be marked in the cat and may not be predictable from the animal's behavior.[64] However, as previously emphasized, other comorbidities, such as severe chronic kidney disease and myocardial disease, must be ruled out before interpretation of the result is attempted.

The current recommendations from the manufacturer[a] of a feline NT-proBNP assay (Cardiopet proBNP Inc, ME, USA) are shown in **Table 3**. The recommendations are tempered with the warning that "there are cases where patients in heart failure may have NT-proBNP levels that are not significantly elevated. As with any test, these results should always be assessed within the context of the presenting clinical signs.[a]"

---

[a] IDEXX Laboratories, Inc, Westbrook (ME), USA

Table 3
Current recommendations from the manufacturer (Cardiopet proBNP) for the interpretation of the feline NT-proBNP assay

NT-proBNP Concentration (pmol/l)	Interpretation
<50	NT-proBNP concentration is not elevated. Heart disease is unlikely.
50–100	NT-proBNP concentration is elevated. Heart disease may be present. Consider an echocardiogram or repeating test in 3 months if clinical suspicion persists.
100–270	NT-proBNP concentration is elevated and consistent with heart disease or heart failure. An echocardiogram is recommended. If signs of heart failure are present, a chest radiograph is also recommended.
>270	NT-proBNP concentration is significantly elevated. Congestive heart failure is highly likely. Where clinically stable, a complete cardiac workup should be performed. Where clinically unstable, assess whether therapeutic stabilization is required if additional diagnostics prove stressful to the patient.

Given the emphasis the manufacturer places on not interpreting the test in isolation, these recommended cut-off values appear suitably cautious and broadly in agreement with the current literature.[18,19,22,23,25,33,34] However, in one study[20] evaluating NT-proBNP concentrations in a colony of Maine Coon and Maine Coon cross cats with equivocal and moderate HCM had median concentrations of 19 and 22 pmol/L respectively (see **Table 1**) and therefore within the range (<50 pmol/L) that the manufacturer suggests makes heart disease unlikely. Hopefully further refinement of the interpretation of NT-proBNP concentrations will be possible following the publication of more and larger studies, such as the single-center study evaluating circulating NP concentrations in 500 cats with cardiac and non-cardiac diseases.[54]

SUMMARY

The use of the ELISA to measure circulating NP concentrations in cats will provide many opportunities to evaluate the use of these peptides for diagnostic, prognostic, and therapeutic purposes in the management of feline cardiovascular, respiratory, and renal disease. Early studies have shown great potential and some conflict with regard to their use as diagnostic aids. The goal now is to refine the interpretation of NP concentrations through further scientific studies and clinical practice to determine their full potential as an important biomarker in the assessment and management of common feline diseases.

ACKNOWLEDGMENTS

The author acknowledges Simon Dennis BVetMed, MVM, CertVC, DipECVIM and Ricardo Soares Magalhaes DVM, MSc for help with the manuscript.

REFERENCES

1. Martinez-Rumayor A, Richards AM, Burnett JC, et al. Biology of the natriuretic peptides. Am J Cardiol 2009;101:3–8.

2. Wilkins MR, Redondo J, Brown LA. The natriuretic-peptide family. Lancet 1997; 349:1307–10.
3. Arteaga E, Araujo AQ, Buck P, et al. Plasma amino-terminal pro-B-type natriuretic peptide quantification in hypertrophic cardiomyopathy. Am Heart J 2005;150: 1228–32.
4. Tsutamoto T, Wada A, Maeda K, et al. Attenuation of compensation of endogenous cardiac natriuretic peptide system in chronic heart failure: prognostic role of plasma brain natriuretic peptide concentration in patients with chronic symptomatic left ventricular dysfunction. Circulation 1997;96:509–16.
5. Maisel A, Hollander JE, Guss D, et al. Primary results of the Rapid Emergency Department Heart Failure Outpatient Trial (REDHOT). A multicenter study of B-type natriuretic peptide levels, emergency department decision making, and outcomes in patients presenting with shortness of breath. J Am Coll Cardiol 2004;44:1328–33.
6. Jefferies JL, Denfield SW, Price JF, et al. A prospective evaluation of nesiritide in the treatment of pediatric heart failure. Pediatr Cardiol 2006;27:402–7.
7. Sudoh T, Kangawa K, Minamino N, et al. A new natriuretic peptide in porcine brain. Nature 2004;332:78–81.
8. Yan W, Wu F, Morser J, et al. Corin, a transmembrane cardiac serine protease, acts as a pro-atrial natriuretic peptide-converting enzyme. Proc Natl Acad Sci U S A 2000;97:8525–9.
9. Sawada Y, Suda M, Yokoyama H, et al. Stretch-induced hypertrophic growth of cardiocytes and processing of brain-type natriuretic peptide are controlled by proprotein-processing endoprotease furin. J Biol Chem 1997;272:20545–54.
10. Hunt PJ, Espiner EA, Nicholls MG, et al. The role of the circulation in processing pro-brain natriuretic peptide (proBNP) to amino-terminal BNP and BNP-32. Peptides 1997;18:1475–81.
11. Biondo AW, Ehrhart EJ, Sisson DD, et al. Immunohistochemistry of atrial and brain natriuretic peptides in control cats and cats with hypertrophic cardiomyopathy. Vet Pathol 2003;40:501–6.
12. Sisson DD. Neuroendocrine evaluation of cardiac disease. Vet Clin North Am Small Anim Pract 2004;34:1105–26.
13. Liu ZL, Wiedmeyer CE, Sisson DD, et al. Cloning and characterisation of feline brain natriuretic peptide. Gene 2002;292:183–90.
14. Biondo AW, Liu ZL, Wiedmeyer CE, et al. Genomic sequence and cardiac expression of atrial natriuretic peptide in cats. Am J Vet Res 2002;63:236–40.
15. Sisson DD, Oyama MA, Solter PF. Plasma levels of ANP, BNP, epinephrine, norepinephrine, serum aldosterone, and plasma renin activity in healthy cats and cats with myocardial disease [abstract]. J Vet Intern Med 2003;17:438.
16. Sisson DD. B-type natriuretic peptides. J Vet Cardiol 2009;11(S1):S5–7.
17. MacLean HN, Abbott JA, Ward DL, et al. N-terminal natriuretic peptide immunoreactivity in plasma of cats with hypertrophic cardiomyopathy. J Vet Intern Med 2006;20:284–9.
18. Connolly DJ, Magalhaes RJ, Syme HM, et al. Circulating natriuretic peptides in cats with heart disease. J Vet Intern Med 2008;22:96–105.
19. Fox FP, Oyama MA, Reynolds C, et al. Utility of plasma N-terminal pro-brain natriuretic peptide (NT-proBNP) to distinguish between congestive heart failure and non-cardiac causes of acute dyspnea in cats. J Vet Cardiol 2009;11(S1):S51–62.
20. Hsu A, Kittleson MD, Paling A. Investigation into the use of plasma NT-proBNP concentration to screen for feline hypertrophic cardiomyopathy. J Vet Cardiol 2009;11(S1):S63–70.

21. Zimmering TM, Meneses F, Nolte IJ, et al. Measurement of N-terminal proatrial natriuretic peptide in plasma of cats with and without cardiomyopathy. Am J Vet Res 2009;70:216–22.
22. Fox PR, Oyama MA, MacDonald K, et al. Assessment of NT-proBNP concentration in asymptomatic cats with cardiomyopathy [abstract]. J Vet Intern Med 2008;22:719.
23. Wess G, Daisenberger P, Hirschberger J, et al. The utility of NT-proBNP to detect early stages of hypertrophic cardiomyopathy in cats and to differentiate disease stages [abstract]. J Vet Intern Med 2009;23:687.
24. Carrier A, Beardow A, Farace G, et al. Analytical validation of a commercially available feline N-terminal prohormone brain natriuretic peptide ELISA [abstract]. J Vet Intern Med 2009;23:747.
25. Lalor SM, Connolly DJ, Elliott J, et al. Plasma concentrations of natriuretic peptides in normal cats and hypertensive cats with chronic kidney disease. J Vet Cardiol 2009;11(S1):S71–9.
26. Dao Q, Krishnaswamy P, Kazanegra R, et al. Utility of B-type natriuretic peptide in the diagnosis of congestive heart failure in an urgent-care setting. Am J Cardiol 2001;37:379–85.
27. Maisel AS, Krishnaswamy P, Nowak RM, et al. Breathing not properly multinational study investigators. Rapid measurement of B-type natriuretic peptide in the emergency diagnosis of heart failure. N Engl J Med 2002;347:161–7.
28. Mehra MR, Maisel A. B-type natriuretic peptide in heart failure: diagnostic, prognostic and therapeutic use. Crit Pathw Cardiol 2005;4:10–20.
29. Januzzi JL Jr, Camargo CA, Anwaruddin S, et al. The N-terminal Pro-BNP investigation of Dyspnea in the Emergency Department (PRIDE) study. Am J Cardiol 2005;95:948–54.
30. McCullough PA, Nowak RM, McCord J, et al. B-type natriuretic peptide and clinical judgment in emergency diagnosis of heart failure: analysis from Breathing Not Properly (BNP) multinational study. Circulation 2002;106:416–22.
31. Morrison LK, Harrison A, Krishnaswamy P, et al. Utility of rapid B-natriuretic peptide assay in differentiating congestive heart failure from lung disease in patients presenting with dyspnea. J Am Coll Cardiol 2002;39:202–9.
32. Mueller C, Scholer A, Laule-Kilian K, et al. Use of B-type natriuretic peptide in the evaluation and management of acute dyspnea. N Engl J Med 2004;350:647–54.
33. Wess G, Daisenberger P, Hirschberger J. The utility of NT-proBNP to differentiate cardiac and respiratory causes of dyspnea in cats [abstract]. J Vet Intern Med 2008;22:707–8.
34. Connolly DJ, Magalhaes RJ, Fuentes VL, et al. Assessment of the diagnostic accuracy of circulating natriuretic peptide concentrations to distinguish between cats with cardiac and non-cardiac causes of respiratory distress. J Vet Cardiol 2009;11(S1):S41–50.
35. Richards M, Nicholls MG, Espiner EA, et al. Comparison of B-type natriuretic peptides for assessment of cardiac function and prognosis in stable ischemic heart disease chronic coronary artery disease. J Am Coll Cardiol 2006;47:52–60.
36. Luchner A, Hengstenberg C, Lowel H, et al. Effect of compensated renal dysfunction on approved heart failure markers: direct comparison of brain natriuretic peptide (BNP) and N-terminal pro-BNP. Hypertension 2005;46:118–23.
37. Anwaruddin S, Lloyd-Jones DM, Baggish A, et al. Renal function, congestive heart failure, and amino-terminal pro-brain natriuretic peptide measurement. Results from the ProBNP Investigation of Dyspnea in the Emergency Department (PRIDE) study. J Am Coll Cardiol 2006;47:91–7.

38. McCullough PA, Kuncheria J, Mathur VS. Diagnostic and therapeutic utility of B-type natriuretic peptide in patients with renal insufficiency and decompensated heart failure. Rev Cardiovasc Med 2003;4:S3–12.
39. McCullough PA, Duc P, Omland T, et al. B-type natriuretic peptide and renal function in the diagnosis of heart failure: an analysis from the Breathing Not Properly Multinational Study. Am J Kidney Dis 2003;41:571–9.
40. deFillippi CR, Seliger SL, Maynard S, et al. Impact of renal disease on natriuretic peptide testing for diagnosing decompensated heart failure and predicting mortality. Clin Chem 2007;53:1511–9.
41. McCullough PA, Sandberg KR. B-type natriuretic peptide and renal disease. Heart Fail Rev 2003;8:355–8.
42. van Kimmenade RR, Januzzi JL, Baggish A, et al. Amino-terminal pro-brain natriuretic peptide, renal function, and outcomes in acute heart failure. J Am Coll Cardiol 2006;48:1621–7.
43. Bruch A, Reinecke H, Stypmann J, et al. N-terminal pro-brain natriuretic peptide, kidney disease and outcome in patients with chronic heart failure. J Heart Lung Transplant 2006;25:1135–41.
44. Boswood A, Dukes-McEwan J, Loureiro J, et al. The diagnostic accuracy of different natriuretic peptides in the investigation of canine cardiac disease. J Small Anim Pract 2008;49:26–32.
45. Schmidt MK, Reynolds CA, Estrada AH, et al. Effect of azotemia on serum N-terminal proBNP concentration in dogs with normal cardiac function: a pilot study. J Vet Cardiol 2009;11(S1):S81–86.
46. Syme HM, Markwell PJ, Pfeiffer D, et al. Survival of cats with naturally occurring chronic renal failure is related to severity of proteinuria. J Vet Intern Med 2006;20: 528–35.
47. Taylor JA, Christenson RH, Rao K, et al. B-type natriuretic peptide and N-terminal pro B-type natriuretic peptide are depressed in obesity despite higher left ventricular diastolic pressure. Am Heart J 2006;152:1071–6.
48. Horwich TB, Fonarow GC, Hamilton MA, et al. The relationship between obesity and mortality in patients with heart failure. J Am Coll Cardiol 2001;38:789–95.
49. Van Kimmenade R, van Dielen F, Bakker J. Is brain natriuretic peptide production decreased in obese subjects? J Am Coll Cardiol 2006;47:886–7.
50. Redfield MM, Rodeheffer RJ, Jacobsen SJ, et al. Plasma brain natriuretic peptide concentration: impact of age and gender. J Am Coll Cardiol 2002;40:976–82.
51. Dentali F, Donadini M, Gianni M. Brain natriuretic peptide as a preclinical marker of chronic pulmonary hypertension in patients with pulmonary embolism. Intern Emerg Med 2009;4:123–8.
52. Shah KB, Nolan MM, Rao K, et al. The characteristics and prognostic importance of NT-ProBNP concentrations in critically ill patients. Am J Med 2007; 120:1071–7.
53. Ozmen B, Ozmen D, Parildar Z, et al. Serum N-terminal-pro-B-type natriuretic peptide (NT-pro-BNP) levels in hyperthyroidism and hypothyroidism. Endocr Res 2007;32:1–8.
54. Ettinger S, Beardow A. Cardiac biomarkers measured in 500 cats with heart disease, heart failure and other diseases. In: Programs and abstracts of the 27th American College of Veterinary Internal Medicine Conference. Montreal, June 3–6, 2009.
55. Boswood A. The rise and fall of the cardiac biomarker [editorial]. J Vet Intern Med 2004;18:797–9.
56. Braunwald E. Biomarkers in heart failure. N Engl J Med 2008;358:2148–59.

57. Maisel AP, Krishnaswamy P, Nowak RM, et al. Rapid measurement of B-type natriuretic peptide in the emergency diagnosis of heart failure. N Engl J Med 2002; 347:161–7.

58. Januzzi JL Jr, Sakhuja R, O'Donoghue M, et al. Utility of amino-terminal pro-brain natriuretic peptide testing for prediction of 1-year mortality in patients with dyspnea treated in the emergency department. Arch Intern Med 2006;166:315–20.

59. Omland T, Persson A, Ng L, et al. N-terminal pro-B-type natriuretic peptide and long-term mortality in acute coronary syndromes. Circulation 2002;106:2913–8.

60. Omland T, Richards AM, Wergeland R, et al. B-type natriuretic peptide and long-term survival in patients with stable coronary artery disease. Am J Cardiol 2005; 95:24–8.

61. Troughton RW, Frampton CM, Yandle TG, et al. Treatment of heart failure guided by plasma aminoterminal brain natriuretic peptide (N-BNP) concentrations. Lancet 2000;355:1126–30.

62. Jourdain P, Jondeau G, Funck F, et al. Plasma brain natriuretic peptide-guided therapy to improve outcome in heart failure: the STARS–BNP Multicenter Study. J Am Coll Cardiol 2007;49:1733–9.

63. Paige CF, Abbott JA, Elvinger F, et al. Prevalence of cardiomyopathy in apparently healthy cats. J Am Vet Med Assoc 2009;234:1398–403.

64. Belew AM, Barlett T, Brown SA. Evaluation of then white coat-effect in cats. J Vet Intern Med 1999;13:134–42.

Current Use of Pimobendan in Canine Patients with Heart Disease

Adrian Boswood, MA, VetMB, DVC, MRCVS

KEYWORDS

- Pimobendan • DMVD • DCM • Heart failure

Pimobendan is a drug with both inotropic and vasodilatory properties and is widely used for the treatment of heart failure in dogs. It is a benzimidazole-pyridazinone derivative that exerts its inotropic and vasodilatory effects through a combination of calcium sensitization and phosphodiesterase inhibition. It is licensed for use in dogs in Japan, Canada, the United States, Australia, and several countries in Europe. It has been the subject of a previous review article in the *Veterinary Clinics of North America*.[1] This article is therefore largely restricted to developments in the knowledge of the benefits and risks associated with its use in the last 5 years.

The best evidence regarding its efficacy is derived from several clinical studies in dogs with the two most common conditions that result in heart failure: dilated cardiomyopathy (DCM) and degenerative mitral valve disease (DMVD). Given the differences that exist in the management of these two conditions, they are considered separately.

DILATED CARDIOMYOPATHY

DCM is characterized by systolic failure of the myocardium. It therefore seems intuitive that an inotropic agent might be effective in the treatment of this condition. Such intuitive support for the use of inotropes in the management of heart failure in human patients has frequently been contradicted by evidence from clinical trials, demonstrating detrimental effects of such therapy on outcomes including survival.[2,3] However, not all clinical trials involving the use of inotropes in human patients have been associated with increased mortality.[4] In contrast to the findings in human clinical trials, studies in dogs have demonstrated beneficial effects with pimobendan in the treatment of DCM.

There have been at least 3 clinical studies in which the effects of administering pimobendan to dogs with DCM have been compared with either placebo or a positive

Department of Veterinary Clinical Sciences, The Royal Veterinary College, Hawkshead Lane, North Mymms, Hatfield, Herts AL9 7TA, UK
E-mail address: aboswood@rvc.ac.uk

Vet Clin Small Anim 40 (2010) 571–580
doi:10.1016/j.cvsm.2010.04.003
0195-5616/10/$ – see front matter © 2010 Elsevier Inc. All rights reserved.

vetsmall.theclinics.com

control (benazepril). The first of these studies was the Pimobendan Trial in Congestive Heart Failure (PITCH) study. Dogs with both DMVD and DCM were recruited to the PITCH study; however, more than 75% of the dogs that were eventually enrolled had DCM.[1] The PITCH study compared 3 groups of dogs. All groups were able to receive background heart failure therapy (eg, diuretics). The first group received pimobendan, the second group received pimobendan and benazepril, and the third group received benazepril. Although the full data from the PITCH study have not been published, the results have been presented at several meetings[5] and previously described in summary.[1] The study concluded that there was a significant benefit associated with receiving pimobendan, but the design of the study, and its inherent weaknesses, left some unconvinced of the benefit; further studies have subsequently been conducted.

Two placebo-controlled, double-blind, randomized studies evaluating the benefit of pimobendan in DCM have been conducted.[6,7] The Kaplan-Meier survival curves for the time to primary endpoint for both the studies are illustrated in **Fig. 1**.

One of these studies enrolled cocker spaniels and Doberman pinschers,[6] whereas the other included only Doberman pinschers.[7] In the study by Luis Fuentes and colleagues,[6] a relatively small number of dogs (20) were recruited, of which half were Doberman pinschers. There were, therefore, only 5 Doberman pinschers receiving pimobendan and 5 Doberman pinschers receiving placebo. Despite these small numbers, the study demonstrated a significant difference in survival between the 2 groups, with a median survival time of 329 days in the pimobendan-treated group compared with 50 days in the placebo-treated group. Unfortunately, with low numbers of dogs in the study, randomisation failed to balance the groups with respect to some important characteristics of the dogs at enrolment. One consequence of this was that more dogs with atrial fibrillation, a factor considered to indicate poor prognosis, were randomized to the placebo group; therefore, there were some doubts whether the difference in outcome between the two groups was entirely attributable to the effects of pimobendan.

A similar study by O'Grady and colleagues[7] has analyzed the efficacy of pimobendan compared with placebo in the treatment of Doberman pinschers with DCM. There are not only important differences but also striking similarities between the studies. The O'Grady study was also a prospective, randomized, double-blind, placebo-controlled

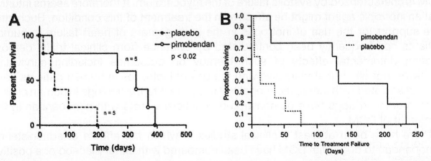

Fig. 1. Kaplan-Meier survival curves from the studies by Luis Fuentes and colleagues (*A*) and O'Grady and colleagues (*B*) illustrating the increased survival time associated with the administration of pimobendan to Doberman pinschers with heart failure secondary to DCM. (*From* Fuentes VL, Corcoran B, French A, et al. A double-blind, randomized, placebo-controlled study of pimobendan in dogs with dilated cardiomyopathy. J Vet Intern Med 2002;16:258; with permission; and O'Grady MR, Minors SL, O'Sullivan ML, et al. Effect of pimobendan on case fatality rate in Doberman Pinschers with congestive heart failure caused by dilated cardiomyopathy. J Vet Intern Med 2008;22:900; with permission.)

study. Importantly, in this study, the presence of atrial fibrillation was an exclusion criterion. The study compared groups with respect to time to a composite endpoint, which
was either death or the development of refractory pulmonary edema. It was originally
intended to recruit 20 dogs to the study, resulting in 10 dogs in each treatment group;
however, an interim analysis of the study demonstrated such strong evidence to
suggest a beneficial effect of pimobendan that the study was prematurely terminated
with only 16 dogs having been enrolled, with 8 dogs in each group. The median time
for the dogs receiving pimobendan was 130.5 days and for the dogs receiving placebo
was 14 days (see **Fig. 1**).

The combined evidence from these 3 studies suggests that there is strong
evidence to support the use of pimobendan in the treatment of almost all dogs
with congestive heart failure secondary to DCM. Although the study by Luis Fuentes
and colleagues[6] failed to demonstrate a benefit in cocker spaniels, the study was
not adequately powered to draw a negative conclusion; there was no evidence of
a detrimental effect, and therefore, the value of therapy in this breed should remain
subject to doubt.

So What if Any Questions Remain Regarding the Efficacy of Pimobendan in the Treatment of Dogs with this Disease?

Is pimobendan indicated before the onset of congestive heart failure?
In all the 3 studies referred to earlier, in which dogs with DCM were studied,
current or prior evidence of congestive heart failure was an inclusion criterion.
Thus it can only be concluded that pimobendan is efficacious in the treatment
of dogs with DCM that are suffering from congestive heart failure. At present,
there is no good-quality evidence regarding the effect of pimobendan in the occult
or preclinical stage of this disease. There is currently a study ongoing in Europe
and North America (the Pimobendan Randomized Occult DCM Trial to Evaluate
Clinical symptoms & Time to heart failure [PROTECT] study) examining the effect
of pimobendan compared with placebo in Dobermans with DCM before the onset
of heart failure.[8] The current lack of evidence means that no recommendations
can be made at this stage and a beneficial effect of therapy cannot be assumed
simply because the drug is efficacious after patients have gone into heart failure
(cf, angiotensin-converting enzyme [ACE] inhibitors in DMVD). The results of the
PROTECT study are awaited with interest.

Are results of studies conducted in Doberman pinschers applicable only to them?
The 2 most convincing studies of the benefit of pimobendan in DCM have been conducted exclusively in Doberman pinschers.[1,7] Adopting the most skeptical evidence-
based-medicine position might lead one to conclude that the evidence for benefit is
restricted to this breed. This hard-line position would only be sustainable, if there
was evidence to suggest that there was something so fundamentally different about
DCM in Doberman pinschers that it precluded extrapolation from this breed to others.
Although differences in the clinical and histopathologic features of DCM have been
described between breeds,[9] differences in response to cardiovascular therapies
have not been shown other than in the study referred to earlier.[6] The ability of genetic
differences between individuals to predict differences in response to medication is an
area of considerable interest and active research in human patients,[10] but until such
differences are demonstrated, it is probably more pragmatic to assume that dogs of
other breeds with DCM will also respond to pimobendan, until proved otherwise,
than to adopt the position of hard-line skepticism. It should also be borne in mind
that the original PITCH study included dogs with DCM from various breeds.

DMVD

The use of an inotropic agent for the treatment of dogs with heart failure secondary to DMVD seems rather less intuitive, and consequently, this initially proved to be a more controversial indication for the administration of pimobendan. The rationale for the use of pimobendan for DMVD includes the fact that dogs with this condition develop systolic dysfunction in the later stages of the disease[11] and that afterload reduction associated with arteriodilation may result in improved forward flow of blood and reduce the regurgitant fraction. There have been several studies in the last few years, examining the benefit of pimobendan in dogs with this condition, and our knowledge has been improved substantially in recent years.

The main studies addressing the effectiveness of pimobendan in dogs with clinical signs secondary to DMVD include the study by Smith and colleagues,[12] the Veterinary Study for the Confirmation of Pimobendan in Canine Endocardiosis (VetSCOPE) study,[13] and the QUality of life and Extension of Survival Time (QUEST) study.[14] The study by Smith and colleagues[12] compared pimobendan to the ACE inhibitor ramipril and addressed the tolerability of pimobendan therapy and the likelihood of development of an adverse heart failure outcome. A dog was considered to have had an adverse heart failure outcome if it died, was euthanized, or was discontinued from the study due to heart failure. Dogs in the ramipril group were 4 times more likely to reach this endpoint, suggesting a significant benefit of pimobendan in this group. Despite randomization, the dogs in the ramipril group were significantly different to the ones in pimobendan group in ways that might have been expected to lead to a worse outcome (eg, having a higher mobility score at enrollment). There were insufficient number of dogs experiencing events in the study to allow for a multivariate analysis to adjust for these factors, and therefore, some of the apparently beneficial effects of pimobendan could be attributable to other factors.

The VetSCOPE study[13] enrolled dogs with International Small Animal Cardiac Health Council class II and III heart failure secondary to DMVD. Dogs in this study initially received either pimobendan (plus standard therapy) or benazepril (plus standard therapy). The study consisted of 2 periods: a 56-day prospective double-blind, placebo-controlled period and an open-label long-term follow-up period. During the initial 56 days, the methodologically more rigorous part of the study, 2 dogs in the pimobendan group and 7 in the benazepril group died or were euthanized due to cardiac disease (**Fig. 2**). This was a significant difference in outcome favoring the pimobendan group. The long-term follow-up period of the study also demonstrated a more favorable outcome in the pimobendan group, but this part of the study was open-label and allowed for potentially unequal treatment of the groups thus its conclusions were rendered rather less robust.

The QUEST study[14] was a prospective, single-blind, positive-controlled study that compared the use of pimobendan (plus standard therapy) and benazepril (plus standard therapy) in dogs that were in, or had been in, modified New York Heart Association (NYHA) class III or IV. The principal outcome of interest in this study was survival. The primary endpoint was a composite of spontaneous cardiac death, euthanasia for cardiac reasons, or treatment failure. The study enrolled 260 dogs, of which 252 contributed to the final analysis. The number of dogs that reached the primary endpoint was 190, resulting in an event rate of 75%. This outcome makes the QUEST study the largest prospective treatment study to date in veterinary cardiology. The high event rate means that the outcome of interest occurs in most of the population and that conclusions are drawn from a large proportion of the population adding to their validity.

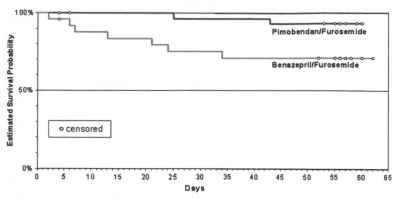

Fig. 2. Estimated survival probabilities for the 2 groups of dogs in the VetSCOPE study. (*From* Lombard CW, Jons O, Bussadori CM. Clinical efficacy of pimobendan versus benazepril for the treatment of acquired atrioventricular valvular disease in dogs. J Am Anim Hosp Assoc 2006;42:255; with permission.)

The QUEST study demonstrated that survival time in the group receiving pimobendan was significantly longer than that in the group receiving benazepril. The median time to the primary endpoint was 267 days for the pimobendan group and 140 days for the benazepril group (ie, pimobendan group survived on an average of 91% longer) (**Fig. 3**). The beneficial effect of pimobendan persisted even after adjustment for the effect of all of the variables recorded at baseline in the multivariate analysis.

A sufficient number of dogs reached each component part of the primary endpoint to allow comparisons to be drawn, regarding time to spontaneous death, euthanasia, and treatment failure for each of the dogs reaching that endpoint. Although none of these individual analyses had sufficient power to demonstrate a significant difference between the groups, there was no evidence of a detrimental effect of pimobendan on any of the outcomes that might be obscured by a combination of 3 different outcomes in the primary endpoint. The median time to all 3 subendpoints was longer in the dogs receiving pimobendan (**Fig. 4**). This finding was reassuring given the previous concerns about possible proarrhythmic effects of inotropic agents and possible detrimental effects of pimobendan on survival in human patients with heart failure.[15]

There have been several other studies examining the effect of pimobendan in dogs with DMVD on outcomes other than survival. One recent study examined the effect of pimobendan on N-terminal pro-B-type natriuretic peptide (NTproBNP) concentrations, velocity of the tricuspid regurgitation jet (TR velocity), and quality of life in dogs with pulmonary hypertension secondary to DMVD.[16] This study demonstrated an acute reduction in both TR velocity and NTproBNP concentrations and an acute improvement in quality of life. Only the reduction of TR velocity was sustained for the duration of follow-up. This study suggests that pimobendan may have specific benefits in dogs with pulmonary hypertension. These benefits may be mediated through pulmonary vasodilatory effects or may simply reflect decreases in left ventricular filling pressures, and hence pulmonary venous pressures, as a result of improved medical management of the left-sided heart failure.

Evidence now seems to overwhelmingly support the use of pimobendan in dogs that have developed clinical signs of heart failure secondary to DMVD. This is reflected in the fact that the American College of Veterinary Internal Medicine's (ACVIM's) publication "Guidelines for the diagnosis and treatment of canine chronic valvular heart

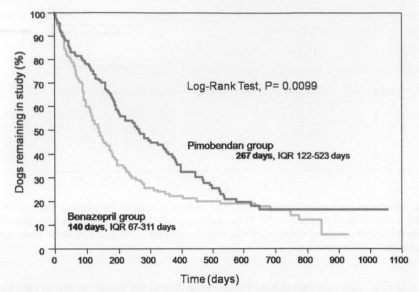

Fig. 3. Kaplan-Meier plot of percentage of dogs in the QUEST study as a function of time in 124 dogs treated with pimobendan and 128 dogs treated with benazepril. The pimobendan-treated dogs had a significantly longer median time period when compared with the benazepril-treated dogs (pimobendan for 267 days [interquartile range, 122–523 days] vs benazepril for 140 days [interquartile range, 67–311 days]; *P* = .0099). (*Adapted from* Haggstrom J, Boswood A, O'Grady M, et al. Effect of pimobendan or benazepril hydrochloride on survival times in dogs with congestive heart failure caused by naturally occurring myxomatous mitral valve disease: the QUEST study. J Vet Intern Med 2008;22:1129; with permission.)

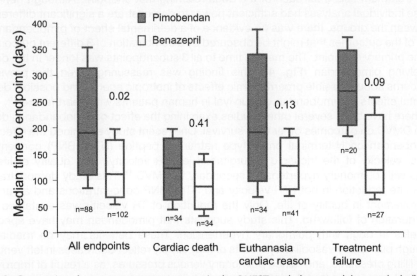

Fig. 4. Comparison between treatment groups in the QUEST study (censored dogs excluded) for the median time (interquartile range) to reach the endpoint for each of the individual endpoints, which were combined to create the composite primary endpoint of the study. (*Data from* Haggstrom J, Boswood A, O'Grady M, et al. Effect of pimobendan or benazepril hydrochloride on survival times in dogs with congestive heart failure caused by naturally occurring myxomatous mitral valve disease: the QUEST study. J Vet Intern Med 2008;22:1124–35.)

disease" recommends pimobendan for the management of heart failure secondary to DMVD both acutely and chronically.[17]

As was the Case for DCM there are Several Other Questions that Persist

Is there a benefit to the administration of pimobendan before the onset of heart failure in dogs with DMVD?

Inevitably, the demonstration of beneficial effects associated with pimobendan once dogs have developed heart failure has raised the question of whether it will be efficacious before heart failure. There is currently no large, prospective, well-controlled study available to determine whether therapy before the onset of heart failure would be of benefit. Given that many dogs with DMVD never develop such signs,[18] it is unlikely that all dogs with early DMVD would benefit from such therapy. Some studies have suggested a potential detrimental effect of pimobendan therapy when administered chronically to dogs with mild disease.[19,20] These studies evaluated either histopathologic or echocardiographic endpoints rather than demonstrating a detrimental effect on an outcome such as survival. Although the study by Chetboul and colleagues has proved controversial,[21,22] evidence from toxicologic studies has demonstrated that when administered intravenously at high doses, pimobendan can result in histopathologically demonstrable changes in the endocardium, valve, and myocardium.[23] It is right therefore to be cautious before administering pimobendan to animals that may not require treatment or to patients at a stage of disease where evidence of a beneficial effect of therapy is lacking.

Ultimately, the question of whether and which patients with DMVD, before the onset of signs of heart failure, will benefit from the administration of pimobendan should be settled by conducting a well-powered, prospective, controlled clinical trial measuring meaningful outcomes.

Should ACE inhibitors be administered concurrently with pimobendan in the treatment of dogs with heart failure secondary to DMVD?

The QUEST study compared the administration of pimobendan **or** benazepril in conjunction with other standard therapy. In this direct comparison, pimobendan had superior outcomes. Thus it can be concluded that when choosing between pimobendan and benazepril, outcomes will be superior if pimobendan is chosen. What the QUEST study cannot inform veterinarians is whether the outcome would be better still if the combination of pimobendan and ACE inhibitors was used. There is currently no well-designed study to help answer this question, and therefore controversy, conjecture, and mechanism-based arguments prevail. The study by Sayer and colleagues[24] has demonstrated that in normal dogs, although pimobendan alone does not lead to an increase in urinary aldosterone to creatinine ratio, the combination of furosemide and pimobendan does. The investigators, therefore, argue that an ACE inhibitor should also be administered when furosemide and pimobendan are being coadministered to protect against the detrimental effects of increased renin-angiotensin-aldosterone system activation. Again the solution to the persisting controversy would be a well-designed and adequately powered prospective study, and until such a study exists, no definitive answer can be given on this point.

In reality, for DMVD as for many other cardiac diseases treatment is usually administered chronically and requires adjustment during the course of a patient's disease. Evidence from the QUEST study should alter the priority with which drugs are administered. Dogs with signs caused by congestive heart failure should always receive a diuretic. In light of the QUEST study, if for any reason only a solitary additional agent is to be chronically administered in addition to diuretics, then pimobendan should be the agent of first choice. In practice, most cardiologists believe that ACE inhibitors are also indicated at this point in time, and this view is reflected in the ACVIM guidelines.[17] Furthermore, there is evidence to suggest there may also be a benefit of administering spironolactone in this circumstance.[25]

WHAT EVIDENCE SUPPORTS THE USE OF PIMOBENDAN IN OTHER FORMS OF HEART DISEASE AND FAILURE?

As mentioned previously, the best evidence to support the use of pimobendan exists for the most common acquired cardiovascular diseases of dogs for which good-quality evidence has been obtained. Clearly, not all cases of heart failure in dogs are caused by these two conditions. Pimobendan is only licensed for use in the treatment of DMVD and DCM; however, many cardiologists have the experience of using the drug in treating heart failure secondary to other conditions. The conditions in which pimobendan would be most likely to help are those with evidence of systolic dysfunction, either as a primary problem or secondary to chronic volume loading, contributing to the development of clinical signs. The conditions for which it is least likely to help and for which there may be some contraindications for its administration include heart failure secondary to pericardial effusions, arrhythmias, and conditions with obstructive lesions, such as aortic stenosis, leading to clinical signs.

SUMMARY

Since the introduction of ACE inhibitors, the advent of pimobendan for the medical management of dogs with congestive heart failure represents the single most significant advance in treating heart failure. Veterinarians understanding of when and how to use this agent is improving as more evidence is obtained. At present, pimobendan can be recommended for the treatment of any dog with signs of congestive heart failure secondary to DMVD or DCM. Evidence of benefit before the onset of heart failure is lacking. Further studies need to be conducted or concluded to address some of the current deficiencies in our knowledge.

REFERENCES

1. Luis Fuentes V. Use of pimobendan in the management of heart failure. Vet Clin North Am Small Anim Pract 2004;34:1145–55.
2. Feldman AM, Bristow MR, Parmley WW, et al. Effects of vesnarinone on morbidity and mortality in patients with heart failure. Vesnarinone Study Group. N Engl J Med 1993;329:149–55.
3. Packer M, Carver JR, Rodeheffer RJ, et al. Effect of oral milrinone on mortality in severe chronic heart failure. The PROMISE Study Research Group. N Engl J Med 1991;325:1468–75.
4. Metra M, Eichhorn E, Abraham WT, et al. Effects of low-dose oral enoximone administration on mortality, morbidity, and exercise capacity in patients with advanced heart failure: the randomized, double-blind, placebo-controlled, parallel group ESSENTIAL trials. Eur Heart J 2009;30:3015–26.
5. Lombard CW, Svoboda M. Therapy of congestive heart failure in dogs with inodilators. In: Svoboda M, editor. World Small Animal Association Congress, Prague, Czech Republic, 2006. World Small Animal Veterinary Association. p. 23–5.

6. Luis Fuentes V, Corcoran B, French A, et al. A double-blind, randomized, placebo-controlled study of pimobendan in dogs with dilated cardiomyopathy. J Vet Intern Med 2002;16:255–61.
7. O'Grady MR, Minors SL, O'Sullivan ML, et al. Effect of pimobendan on case fatality rate in doberman pinschers with congestive heart failure caused by dilated cardiomyopathy. J Vet Intern Med 2008;22:897–904.
8. Summerfield N, Dukes-McEwan J, Swift S, et al. Preclinical dilated cardiomyopathy in the dobermann. Vet Rec 2006;158:742–3.
9. Dukes-McEwan J, Borgarelli M, Tidholm A, et al. Proposed guidelines for the diagnosis of canine idiopathic dilated cardiomyopathy. J Vet Cardiol 2003;5: 7–19.
10. Ginsburg GS, Donahue MP, Newby LK. Prospects for personalized cardiovascular medicine: the impact of genomics. J Am Coll Cardiol 2005;46:1615–27.
11. Borgarelli M, Tarducci A, Zanatta R, et al. Decreased systolic function and inadequate hypertrophy in large and small breed dogs with chronic mitral valve insufficiency. J Vet Intern Med 2007;21:61–7.
12. Smith PJ, French AT, Van Israel N, et al. Efficacy and safety of pimobendan in canine heart failure caused by myxomatous mitral valve disease. J Small Anim Pract 2005;46:121–30.
13. Lombard CW, Jons O, Bussadori CM. Clinical efficacy of pimobendan versus benazepril for the treatment of acquired atrioventricular valvular disease in dogs. J Am Anim Hosp Assoc 2006;42:249–61.
14. Haggstrom J, Boswood A, O'Grady M, et al. Effect of pimobendan or benazepril hydrochloride on survival times in dogs with congestive heart failure caused by naturally occurring myxomatous mitral valve disease: the QUEST study. J Vet Intern Med 2008;22:1124–35.
15. Lubsen J, Just H, Hjalmarsson AC, et al. Effect of pimobendan on exercise capacity in patients with heart failure: main results from the Pimobendan in Congestive Heart Failure (PICO) trial. Heart 1996;76:223–31.
16. Atkinson KJ, Fine DM, Thombs LA, et al. Evaluation of pimobendan and N-terminal probrain natriuretic peptide in the treatment of pulmonary hypertension secondary to degenerative mitral valve disease in dogs. J Vet Intern Med 2009;23:1190–6.
17. Atkins C, Bonagura J, Ettinger S, et al. Guidelines for the diagnosis and treatment of canine chronic valvular heart disease. J Vet Intern Med 2009;23:1142–50.
18. Borgarelli M, Savarino P, Crosara S, et al. Survival characteristics and prognostic variables of dogs with mitral regurgitation attributable to myxomatous valve disease. J Vet Intern Med 2008;22:120–8.
19. Chetboul V, Lefebvre HP, Sampedrano CC, et al. Comparative adverse cardiac effects of pimobendan and benazepril monotherapy in dogs with mild degenerative mitral valve disease: a prospective, controlled, blinded, and randomized study. J Vet Intern Med 2007;21:742–53.
20. Tissier R, Chetboul V, Moraillon R, et al. Increased mitral valve regurgitation and myocardial hypertrophy in two dogs with long-term pimobendan therapy. Cardiovasc Toxicol 2005;5:43–51.
21. Le Bobinnec G. Concerns about "Comparative adverse cardiac effects of pimobendan and benazepril monotherapy in dogs with mild degenerative mitral valve disease: a prospective, controlled, blinded and randomized study". J Vet Intern Med 2008;22:243–4 [author reply: 245–6].
22. Corcoran B, Culshaw G, Dukes-McEwan J, et al. Concerns about "Comparative adverse cardiac effects of pimobendan and benazepril monotherapy in dogs

with mild degenerative mitral valve disease". J Vet Intern Med 2008;22:243 [author reply: 245].

23. Available at: http://www.fda.gov/downloads/AnimalVeterinary/Products/Approved AnimalDrugProducts/FOIADrugSummaries/ucm062328.pdf. Accessed October 25, 2009.

24. Sayer MB, Atkins CE, Fujii Y, et al. Acute effect of pimobendan and furosemide on the circulating renin-angiotensin-aldosterone system in healthy dogs. J Vet Intern Med 2009;23:1003–6.

25. Bernay F, Bland JM, Haggstrom J, et al. Efficacy of spironolactone on survival in dogs with naturally occurring mitral regurgitation caused by myxomatous mitral valve disease. J Vet Intern Med 2010;24:331–41.

Minimally Invasive Per-Catheter Occlusion and Dilation Procedures for Congenital Cardiovascular Abnormalities in Dogs

Anthony H. Tobias, BVSc, PhD*, Christopher D. Stauthammer, DVM

KEYWORDS

- Minimally invasive per-catheter occlusion
- Minimally invasive per-catheter dilation • Balloon dilation
- Congenital cardiovascular abnormalities

With ever-increasing sophistication of veterinary cardiology, minimally invasive per-catheter occlusion and dilation procedures for the treatment of various congenital cardiovascular abnormalities in dogs have become not only available, but mainstream. This evolution is as much driven by science as by public demand for minimally invasive options in the care of their companion animals. Minimally invasive per-catheter occlusion of left-to-right shunting patent ductus arteriosus, the most common congenital cardiovascular abnormality of dogs, is offered as a routine procedure by specialty and referral veterinary medical centers throughout North America, the European Union, and beyond. Per-catheter occlusion procedures are also available for less common abnormalities in dogs, such as atrial and ventricular septal defects. Minimally invasive balloon dilation is routinely performed to treat pulmonic stenosis. Balloon dilation is also performed for other obstructive cardiovascular abnormalities such as subvalvular aortic stenosis, cor triatriatum dexter, and atrioventricular valve stenosis.

Much new information about minimally invasive per-catheter patent ductus arteriosus occlusion has been published and presented during the past few years.

Veterinary Clinical Sciences Department, College of Veterinary Medicine, University of Minnesota, 1365 Gortner Avenue, St Paul, MN 55108, USA
* Corresponding author.
E-mail address: tobia004@umn.edu

Vet Clin Small Anim 40 (2010) 581–603
doi:10.1016/j.cvsm.2010.03.009
0195-5616/10/$ – see front matter © 2010 Elsevier Inc. All rights reserved.

Consequently, patent ductus arteriosus occlusion is the primary focus of this article. Occlusion of other less common congenital cardiac defects is also briefly reviewed. Balloon dilation of pulmonic stenosis, as well as other congenital obstructive cardiovascular abnormalities is discussed in the latter part of the article.

OCCLUSION PROCEDURES FOR PATENT DUCTUS ARTERIOSUS

Patent ductus arteriosus (PDA) occurs when the ductus arteriosus fails to close in the immediate postnatal period. The defect is inherited in a complex manner consistent with a polygenic threshold trait.[1] This mode of inheritance was established in a breeding colony of poodles, and extrapolation to other dog breeds should be made with appropriate circumspection. The defect is more common in females, and at least 13 dog breeds have been identified as predisposed. Relative to the general hospital population, the 3 breeds that have the greatest odds of ductal patency, that is, have the highest prevalence odds ratios, are the Maltese, toy poodle, and miniature poodle.[2]

The most characteristic physical examination finding in affected dogs is a continuous murmur, commonly associated with a thrill, with its point of maximal intensity high over the left heart base. Excessively strong or bounding pulses are frequently present. Radiographs typically demonstrate pulmonary overperfusion and left heart enlargement, and the diagnosis is readily confirmed by echocardiography.[3]

Puppies with PDA are usually clinically unaffected by their defect at the time of diagnosis. However, if left uncorrected, PDA typically leads to complications ascribable to chronic left-to-right shunting (ie, enlargement of the left-sided cardiac chambers, mitral valve regurgitation, arrhythmias, left-sided congestive heart failure, and death). To our knowledge, the natural history of untreated PDA in small animals is limited to a single study of 100 sequential cases in which the defect was not occluded in 14 affected dogs; 64% of these 14 dogs died within 1 year of examination.[4] In contrast, occlusion of uncomplicated PDA confers an outstanding long-term prognosis and it is considered to be curative.[5] Furthermore, PDA occlusion results in an immediate decrease in left-sided volume overload, followed by reversal of left ventricular eccentric hypertrophy over the longer term.[6]

Ductal morphology in dogs is classified according to its angiographic appearance as type I, IIA, IIB, and III (**Fig. 1**). The most common type is IIA (54.5% of affected dogs), where the PDA has a large ostium at its junction with the aorta, and a wide ampulla that abruptly narrows to a much smaller ostium at its junction with the main pulmonary artery. The ductus typically joins the main pulmonary artery at the level at which it bifurcates into the left and right pulmonary arteries. The minimal ductal diameter (MDD) of the ductus is most commonly at its junction with the pulmonary artery. The least common form of PDA in dogs is type III (8% of affected dogs), which has a tubular shape and an average MDD that is significantly greater than that of all other ductal types.[7]

PDA occlusion in affected dogs confers important clinical benefits, but the best method for PDA occlusion has yet to be identified. A variety of occlusion procedures have been described and these will be discussed in the following sections with the perspective that the ideal occlusion procedure should

- be feasible in dogs of various ages, weights, and somatotypes.
- be associated with no mortality, and no or few and inconsequential complications.
- completely and permanently occlude a wide range of ductal shapes and sizes.

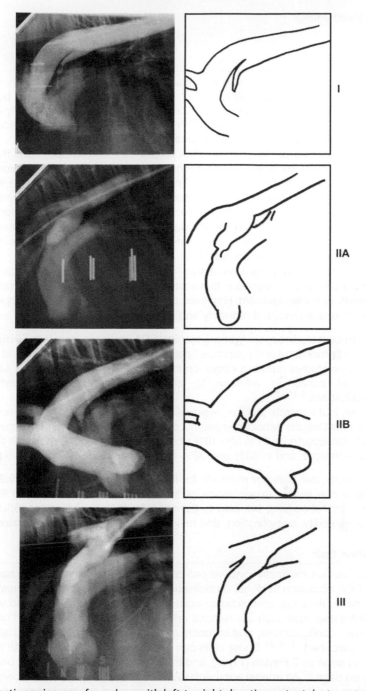

Fig. 1. Aortic angiograms from dogs with left-to-right shunting patent ductus arteriosus. To the right of each angiogram is a corresponding line drawing illustrating morphologic features. *Type I:* The diameter of the ductus gradually decreases in size from the aorta to the pulmonary artery. *Type IIA:* The walls of the ductus essentially parallel one another, and the ductal diameter abruptly decreases at the pulmonic ostium. *Type IIB:* The diameter of the ductus decreases markedly from the aortic to pulmonic side. *Type III:* The ductus is tubular with little or no change in diameter throughout its length. (*From* Miller MW, Gordon SG, Saunders AG, et al. Angiographic classification of patent ductus arteriosus morphology in the dog. J Vet Cardiol 2006;8:109–14; with permission.)

Surgical Occlusion

Surgical occlusion of PDA in a dog was first reported in 1952.[8] Since then, surgical occlusion has been, and probably remains the most common method by which PDA is treated in small animals. Although the focus of this article is minimally invasive per-catheter procedures, any review of PDA occlusion methods would be incomplete without at least a brief discussion of surgical occlusion.

The use of hemoclips for PDA occlusion has been described,[9] but the most common method for surgical PDA occlusion involves circumferential ligation of the ductus after a left-sided thoracotomy. The standard ligation technique involves dissection cranial and caudal to the ductus. This is followed by carefully creating a tunnel on the medical aspect of the ductus by blind dissection with right-angle forceps, through which ligature material is passed. The Jackson (or Jackson and Henderson) technique is considered to be a safer procedure because it avoids high-risk blind dissection medial to the ductus.[10]

Surgical ligation is regarded as a very successful method for PDA occlusion. Although the procedure involves a thoracotomy, recovery is usually very rapid with contemporary pain management. However, published data disclose that surgical ligation is by no means devoid of mortality and important complications:

- Three recent studies each involving surgical PDA ligation in more than 50 dogs have reported procedural and periprocedural mortality rates of 0%, 3.0%, and 5.6%.
- The same studies reported intraoperative ductal hemorrhage in 11%, 12%, and 15% of cases, in addition to an array of other major and minor complications.[5,11,12]
- Further, in 2 separate studies, residual or recurrent ductal flow (documented by color flow Doppler echocardiography, the presence of a continuous murmur, or both) was reported in 21% and 49% of dogs following PDA ligation with the standard technique, and in 53% and 36% of dogs with the Jackson technique.[11,13]

Consequently, per-catheter methods for PDA occlusion in dogs have evolved not only in response to the expectations of increasingly sophisticated and informed companion animal owners, but also to the need for PDA occlusion procedures that have lower mortality, complication, and residual or recurrent ductal flow rates.

Embolization Coils

Among the various minimally invasive per-catheter–delivered devices that have been used for PDA occlusion in dogs, embolization coils have been studied most extensively. In North America, embolization coils are most commonly deployed using an arterial (left-sided) approach via femoral arterial catheterization (**Fig. 2**). The use of various sizes, configurations, and numbers of both free-release and detachable coils has been described.[11,14–21] Some coils can be delivered via catheters with an outer diameter as small as 3 French (1 mm), and the procedure can therefore be performed in very small dogs.[22] An arterial approach via the carotid artery has also recently been described as a potentially useful alternative for vascular access in smaller dogs in which the diameter of the femoral artery may preclude performing this procedure.[23]

Embolization coils may also be deployed by a venous (right-sided) approach via the femoral or brachial vein.[24,25] A venous approach for the deployment of coils and other PDA occlusion devices is preferred by some because it allows for the use of larger-diameter delivery catheters, and avoids potential complications associated with arterial catheterization. However, the arterial approach avoids passing device delivery systems through the right heart chambers, which can be associated with difficult

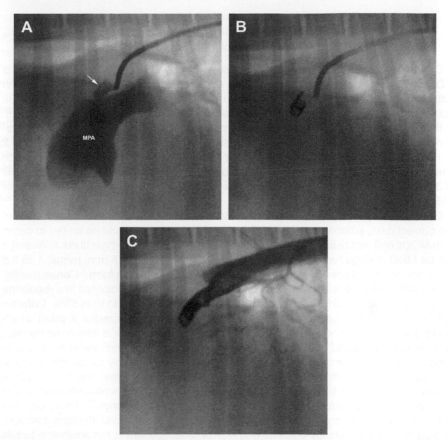

Fig. 2. Patent ductus arteriosus (PDA) occlusion with an embolization coil in a dog. (A) An angiogram shows a small PDA (*arrow*). The size of the PDA can be estimated by comparing it to the 4-French (outer diameter = 1.33 mm) catheter located within the aorta. (B) A free-release embolization coil has been delivered per-catheter into the ductal ampulla. (C) Following deployment of the embolization coil, an aortic angiogram shows complete ductal occlusion. MPA, main pulmonary artery.

retrograde PDA access, kinking of the delivery system within the right ventricle, and arrhythmias.[20,25–28]

Outcomes with coil occlusion of PDA in dogs have recently been reported in the largest and most comprehensive study to address this subject to date. The dogs in that study (n = 125) ranged in age from 2 to 108 months (median, 6 months) and weighed 1.2 to 40.0 kg (median, 5 kg)[29]:

- Procedural and periprocedural mortality was 2.4%.
- Complications included procedure abandonment in 11% because of coil instability in the ductus, aberrant coil migration in 22%, and other less common complications (transient hemolysis and aberrant coil placement).
- Residual or recurrent flow demonstrated by color flow Doppler echocardiography within 24 hours after the procedure was present in 66% of cases, and continuous murmurs were ausculted in 44%. However, delayed closure following coil embolization led to a reduction in the proportion of cases with residual flow

over time. Actuarial analysis of the outcomes data estimated a 54% ± 6% prevalence of any grade of residual ductal flow at 6 months, 41% ± 7% at 12 months, and 30% ± 9% at 24 months after coil occlusion.

Outcomes with embolization coils are generally better in dogs with smaller ductal MDDs.[25,29] This is consistent with a large study of coil occlusion of PDA in human patients (n = 1258) where increasing MDD and tubular shape (analogous to type III ductal morphology in the dog) were positively associated with unfavorable outcomes. In this study, ducti with MMDs larger than 2 mm all carried an increased risk of an unfavorable outcome and the effect was progressive. Compared to ducti with MDDs of 2 mm or smaller, those with MDDs of 4 mm or larger had an odds ratio of 24 (confidence interval, 12 to 48) of producing an unfavorable outcome. With a tubular PDA and MDD of 3 mm or larger, the risk of a poor outcome was particularly high with an odds ratio of 155 (confidence interval, 15 to 1521).[30]

Our experience with coil occlusion is limited. However, based on our assessment of the current data, embolization coil occlusion of PDA in dogs should be limited to cases with MDDs of 2 mm or smaller, and should not be considered for type III ducti. Average ductal MDD in dogs has been reported as 2.9 mm (median, 2.5 mm; range, 1 to 9.5 mm), and, as noted previously, type III PDA is the least common form.[7] Consequently, a favorable outcome with coil occlusion can be reasonably anticipated in a moderate proportion of dogs with PDA, but that proportion is probably less than 50%. Unfortunately, without angiography, it is not possible to accurately predict a priori which cases will be good candidates for coil occlusion, because there is little or no correlation between MDD and patient weight and age.[7,28] Further, transthoracic echocardiographic measurement of MDD cannot substitute for angiography for device selection for PDA occlusion. The mean difference or average bias between the 2 methods is small, but agreement between MDD measurements made by echocardiography and angiography in individual dogs is frequently unacceptably large.[31] Thus, any coil occlusion procedure should always be initiated with a backup plan in place, because angiography will frequently disclose ductal size or shape that is not amenable to this method of ductal closure.

Amplatzer Duct Occluder

The Amplatzer Duct Occluder (AGA Medical Corporation, Plymouth, MN, USA) is designed for minimally invasive per-catheter closure of PDA in human patients regardless of ductal shape or size (Fig. 3). It is a self-expanding device made from a nitinol (nickel titanium alloy) wire mesh. Nitinol has super-elastic properties, together with excellent memory and strength, making it particularly attractive for medical devices where compact configurations are required for device insertion and placement. The Amplatzer Duct Occluder is available in a range of sizes, and depending on the size, a 2- to 3-mm-wide retention flange ensures secure positioning of the device in the ductus. Polyester patches, which are sewn into the device, facilitate ductal occlusion by inducing thrombosis. The device and deployment procedure requires the use of a fairly large-diameter delivery system and in the "Instructions for Use" provided with the device, this method of PDA occlusion is listed as contraindicated for human patients who weigh less than 6 kg and are younger than 6 months old.

Use of the Amplatzer Duct Occluder for PDA occlusion in dogs has been described.[27,28,32] The procedure in dogs is similar to that for humans. It involves both left- and right-sided catheterization (via the femoral artery and vein, Fig. 4), and is well-described on the device manufacturer's Web site (http://www.amplatzer.com).

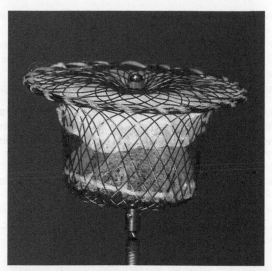

Fig. 3. An Amplatzer Duct Occluder, a self-expanding device made from nitinol wire mesh. The retention flange ensures secure positioning of the device in the ductus. Polyester patches, which are sewn into the device, facilitate ductal occlusion by inducing thrombosis.

A study of the use of the Amplatzer Duct Occluder in dogs with PDA reported very encouraging results. The client-owned dogs in that study (n = 23) ranged in age from 9 weeks to 7 years (median, 6 months), and weighed 3.4 to 32.0 kg (median, 6.3 kg)[28]:

- There was no procedural mortality. There were 2 postprocedural deaths in dogs with heart failure; both deaths were thought to be unrelated to the use of the duct occluder.

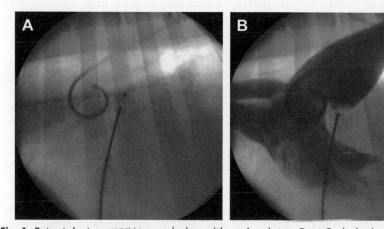

Fig. 4. Patent ductus arteriosus occlusion with an Amplatzer Duct Occluder in a dog. (*A*) The occluder attached to the delivery cable is deployed and positioned with the retention flange within the ductal ampulla. The barrel assumes an hourglass shape as it protrudes through the narrow pulmonic ostium of the ductus into the main pulmonary artery. A pigtail angiographic catheter is located within the aorta. (*B*) An aortic angiogram shows complete ductal occlusion.

- Complications were limited to 2 deployment failures, both of which were attributed to operator errors.
- Angiography performed after device deployment demonstrated complete PDA closure in 13 (65%) of 20 dogs. Complete PDA occlusion was confirmed in 17 of 19 dogs within 3 months and in 1 additional dog within 1 year, resulting in ductal closure in 18 of the 19 dogs that completed the study protocol.

Our experience with the Amplatzer Duct Occluder at the University of Minnesota Veterinary Medical Center, albeit more limited, has been less sanguine. We have evaluated the device and deployment procedure in 11 dogs that ranged in age from 3 to 64 months (median, 7 months), and weighed 3.4 to 35.0 kg (median, 7 kg).

- Procedural success and complete ductal occlusion was achieved in only 6 cases (55%).
- We experienced complications in the remaining 5 cases, of which some, but not all, could be attributed to operator error. Complications in each of these cases were the following:
1. sepsis
2. femoral vessels too small for the required delivery system
3. deployment failure because of persistent kinking of the delivery system in the right heart
4. residual ductal flow around occluder and right bundle branch block
5. smallest Amplatzer Duct Occluder too large resulting in excessive protrusion of the retention flange into the aorta.

We ultimately concluded that, in our hands, the device and procedure is effective for PDA occlusion in larger and generally older dogs with large ducti. Further, the device has less potential for residual flow and migration than embolization coils. However, the deployment procedure is substantially more difficult than coil occlusion and requires larger-diameter delivery systems. Consequently, we do not consider deployment of the Amplatzer Duct Occluder intended for use in humans to be a feasible routine method for PDA occlusion in dogs. This is especially true for dogs weighing less than 5 kg, which is consistent with the lower-weight cut-off for this procedure in human patients.

Amplatzer Vascular Plug

The Amplatzer Vascular Plug (AGA Medical Corporation) is intended for arterial and venous embolizations in the peripheral vasculature (**Fig. 5**). It is a self-expandable, cylindrical device made from a single layer of nitinol wire mesh. A more recent version, the Amplatzer Vascular Plug II, is a multilayered nitinol device with a multisegmented design. Both versions of these vascular plugs are available in a variety of sizes. Two additional multilayer, multisegment versions of the Amplatzer Vascular Plug (III and 4) are available in European Union countries, but neither are currently approved for use in the United States.

The "Instructions for Use" for the Amplatzer Vascular Plug has the following warning: "The safety and effectiveness of this device for cardiac uses (for example, patent ductus arteriosus or paravalvular leak closure) and neurological uses have not been established." Further, inadvertent stenting open of PDAs and unacceptable residual flow have been documented in some human patients when PDA occlusion with this device has been attempted.[33,34] Nevertheless, off-label use of the Amplatzer Vascular Plug for PDA occlusion in dogs has been reported in 2 studies each involving several dogs,[35,36] and in a single case report.[37] The deployment procedure involves

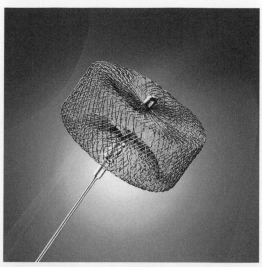

Fig. 5. An Amplatzer Vascular Plug, a self-expandable, cylindrical device constructed from a single layer of nitinol wire mesh.

either left-sided catheterization (via the femoral artery, **Fig. 6**), or left- and right-sided catheterization (via the femoral artery and vein), and is well described in these reports.

The first study involved 6 client-owned dogs that ranged in age from 16 weeks to 7.5 years, and weighed 2.9 to 27.6 kg (median, 6 kg)[35]:

- There was no procedural or periprocedural mortality.
- Successful device implantation was achieved in all dogs.
- Minor complications included mild lameness and bruising and pruritis around the vascular access site.
- Complete PDA occlusion was achieved in only 4 of the dogs. In 2 dogs, residual ductal flow was demonstrated by postdeployment angiography. Residual flow persisted in both dogs as demonstrated by color flow Doppler echocardiography and by the presence of continuous murmurs 24 hours after the procedure, as well as at follow-up examinations performed 8 to 18 weeks after the procedure.

The second study involved 31 client-owned dogs that ranged in age from 2.5 to 91.0 months (median, 6 months), and weighed 2.4 to 22.0 kg (median, 6.4 kg). All of these dogs had type II PDA (type IIA in 27 and type IIB in 4)[36]:

- There was no procedural or periprocedural mortality.
- Successful device deployment was achieved in 29 cases.
- Complications in the other 2 dogs were procedure abandonment because the femoral artery was too small for the required delivery system, and device migration to the pulmonary circulation.
- Postdeployment angiography, which was performed and recorded 5 to 15 minutes after device deployment in 21 dogs, documented some degree of residual flow in 11 (52%). However, transthoracic color flow Doppler echocardiography performed on all dogs the following day disclosed complete ductal occlusion in 22 (76%). Some degree of residual flow persisted in the remaining 7 dogs (24%), which is similar to the proportion of dogs with residual flow reported in the previous study.

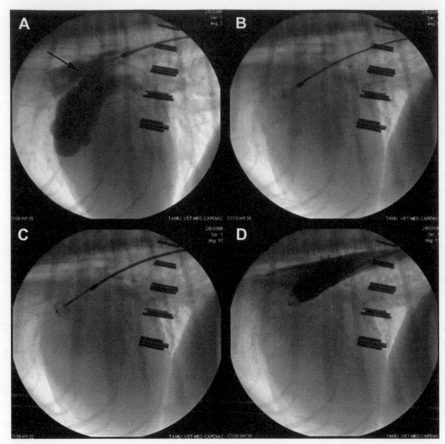

Fig. 6. Patent ductus arteriosus (PDA) occlusion with an Amplatzer Vascular Plug in a dog. (*A*) A long delivery sheath is advanced into the descending aorta and an angiogram demonstrates the PDA *(arrow)*. (*B*) An Amplatzer Vascular Plug is advanced to the tip of the sheath and partially extruded. (*C*) The Amplatzer Vascular Plug is then fully extruded and advanced to the distal PDA. (*D*) A final angiogram, which is performed after detaching and removing the device delivery cable, demonstrates complete ductal occlusion. (*From* Achen SE, Miller MW, Gordon SG, et al. Transarterial ductal occlusion with the Amplatzer Vascular Plug in 31 dogs. J Vet Intern Med 2008; 22:1348–52; with permission.)

- Two of the dogs with residual flow had complete occlusion several months post-procedure, although residual flow persisted in 1. Unfortunately, the remaining dogs with residual flow (4 of 7) were subsequently lost to follow-up making it difficult to ascertain whether delayed closure with this device should be regarded as a reasonable expectation. Further, lack of systematic long-term follow-up to assess for ductal recannalization was acknowledged as a limitation of this study.

In the case report of PDA occlusion with an Amplatzer Vascular Plug, complete occlusion was achieved.[37] In contrast, in the single case in which the authors used an Amplatzer Vascular Plug for PDA occlusion in a dog, color flow Doppler echocardiography disclosed mild but persistent (>12 months) residual ductal flow through the center of the device.

The procedure for deployment of Amplatzer Vascular Plugs for PDA occlusion is technically similar to that for embolization coils, although delivery of the device requires a fairly large-diameter delivery system, and vascular access limits its use in particularly small dogs. Further, the available data suggest that the procedure is associated with fewer complications than with embolization coils, and results in complete ductal occlusion in a higher proportion of cases.

Despite these encouraging results, we have adopted a wait-and-see approach before considering this method for routine PDA occlusion in dogs for several reasons. First, the reported incidence of residual ductal flow with this device, albeit apparently lower than with embolization coils, remains an important and persistent concern, as it is in human patients. Amplatzer Vascular Plugs II, III, and 4 are multilayered devices and this construction would probably result in a lower frequency of residual flow. However, their multisegmented design is unlikely to conform satisfactorily to the more common ductal shapes and sizes in dogs. Second, the Amplatzer Vascular Plug is deployed in the ductal ampulla and narrowing of the ductus at the pulmonic ostium is a prerequisite for device stability. Consequently, as is the case with embolization coils, this device should not be used for PDAs with type III morphology. Finally, no results of systematic long-term studies that investigate the potential for PDA recannalization following deployment of Amplatzer Vascular Plugs have been published, and recannalization has been reported experimentally with this device in the peripheral veins of dogs.[38]

Amplatz Canine Duct Occluder

The most recent addition to the armamentarium for minimally invasive per-catheter PDA occlusion in dogs is the Amplatz Canine Duct Occluder (AGA Medical Corporation) which became commercially available for worldwide distribution in January 2007 (**Fig. 7**). The Amplatz Canine Duct Occluder is a self-expanding multilayered nitinol mesh device, composed of a short waist that separates a flat distal disc from a cupped proximal disc. Devices are sized according to their waist diameters (from 3 to 10 mm in

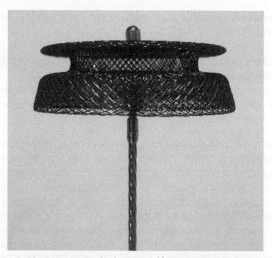

Fig. 7. An Amplatz Canine Duct Occluder, a self-expanding multi-layered nitinol mesh device, is composed of a short waist that separates a flat distal disc from a cupped proximal disc. The device is designed specifically to conform to the shape of the canine ductus.

1-mm increments, as well as 12 and 14 mm). A delivery cable attaches to a micro screw in the center of the cupped proximal disc. The Amplatz Canine Duct Occluder is designed specifically to conform to the shape of the canine PDA, and it is deployed via a left-sided (via the femoral artery) approach (**Fig. 8**).[39]

A recent study evaluated prototype Amplatz Canine Duct Occluders and the deployment procedure. The study involved 18 client-owned dogs of various breeds that ranged in age from 5 to 104 months (median, 13 months) and weighed 3.8 to 32.3 kg (median, 17.8 kg). Ductal morphologies included types IIA (n = 14), IIB (n = 3), and III (n = 1), and angiographic MDDs ranged from 1.1 to 6.9 mm (median, 3.7 mm). After device deployment, the presence of any residual or recurrent ductal flow was assessed by angiography, followed by color flow Doppler echocardiography at 1 day, 3 months, and 12 months or longer postprocedure[31]:

- There was no procedural or periprocedural mortality.
- Successful device placement was achieved in all 18 dogs; however, 1 dog required a second procedure with a larger prototype Amplatz Canine Duct Occluder after the first device migrated to the pulmonary vasculature without any apparent adverse consequences.
- Complete ductal occlusion was confirmed in 17 (94%) of 18 dogs by angiography, as well as by color flow Doppler echocardiography 1 day and 3 months after the procedure. In 1 dog, ductal flow through the prototype Amplatz Canine Duct Occluder was present at the 1-day, 3-month, and 12-month or later evaluations. However, complete occlusion persisted in all the other dogs that had undergone 12-month or later evaluations (n = 12) by the time the study was submitted for publication.

The Amplatz Canine Duct Occluder and its deployment procedure were first reported relatively recently,[40] and large studies reporting outcomes with the device are consequently not yet available. However, to date at the our veterinary medical center, we have successfully performed more than 40 PDA occlusion procedures with this device:

- There has been no procedural or periprocedural mortality, or any instance of procedure abandonment.
- We have had no major or minor complications subsequent to the single case of device migration that occurred during the early investigational stage of device and procedure development.
- Except for the 1 case of persistent or recurrent ductal flow that occurred with a prototype device, PDA occlusion has been immediate, complete, and permanent.

The Amplatz Canine Duct Occluder has proven to be effective over a wide range of ductal shapes and sizes, although our experience with type III ductal morphology is limited and we urge caution with this ductal shape. The deployment procedure, which is straightforward and technically similar to left-sided deployment of embolization coils and Amplatzer Vascular Plugs, is feasible in dogs of widely varying weights and somatotypes. There is no change in occlusion status after 3 months, obviating the need to evaluate patients for recurrent ductal flow beyond this time frame. Similar favorable results and conclusions with this device and procedure were recently reported in a study involving 23 client-owned dogs with PDA from Texas A&M University.[41] These outcomes are better than any achieved with surgical or other minimally invasive per-catheter methods for PDA occlusion in dogs to date. Consequently, at our veterinary medical center, deployment of an Amplatz Canine Duct Occluder is the current treatment of choice for canine PDA.

An important limitation of the use of the Amplatz Canine Duct Occluder is the relatively large diameter delivery systems that are required for device delivery and deployment. We preserve the femoral artery and repair the arteriotomy site at the end of each procedure, and in our hands, adequately gentle vascular handling for the required delivery systems can be challenging in dogs weighing less than 4 kg. We do not attempt this procedure in dogs weighing less than about 3 kg with the currently available Amplatz Canine Duct Occluders because the diameters of the required delivery systems are too large. However, research is ongoing to design and manufacture low-profile devices and smaller diameter delivery systems, as well as to develop a novel deployment procedure specifically for PDA occlusion in small dogs.

OCCLUSION PROCEDURES FOR OTHER CONGENITAL CARDIOVASCULAR DEFECTS

Atrial septal defect (ASD) is an uncommon congenital cardiac abnormality in dogs (0.7% to 3.7% of canine congenital heart defects). Predisposed breeds include the boxer, standard poodle, Doberman, and Samoyed. Atrial septal defects are classified according to their location in the septum, with a midseptal defect or ostium secundum ASD being the most common in dogs. The presence of an ASD results in the shunting of blood from the left atrium to the right, leading to volume overload of the right-sided chambers. Sequelae depend on the size of the defect and the amount of left-to-right shunting, and may include right-sided heart failure, pulmonary hypertension, and death. Dogs with ASD may demonstrate exercise intolerance, failure to thrive, respiratory distress, and ascites. However, clinical signs may not manifest until dogs are older than 3 to 5 years. The most common abnormality noted on cardiac auscultation is a left basilar systolic murmur attributable to increased pulmonary arterial blood flow (relative pulmonic stenosis). Surgical ASD repair is rarely performed in dogs because of limited cardiac bypass availability, expense, and high perioperative morbidity and mortality.[3]

Minimally invasive per-catheter ASD occlusion with an Amplatzer Atrial Septal Occluder (AGA Medical Corporation) has recently been reported in dogs.[42,43] The Amplatzer Atrial Septal Occluder is a self-expanding, double-disk, nitinol wire mesh device filled with thrombogenic polyester material. It is deployed across the defect via a sheath-based delivery system. The device is specifically designed for ostium secundum ASD closure in human patients, and secure device placement requires a rim of tissue around 75% or more of the defect.

The results of a study of 13 dogs with ASD in which closure with Amplatzer Atrial Septal Occluders was attempted were encouraging[43]:

- There was no procedural or periprocedural mortality.
- Successful device deployment was achieved in 10 (77%) of the 13 dogs.
- Complications included device migration in 2 dogs, accidental device release in the right atrium in 1 dog, and development of a small thrombus on the device in 1 dog.
- Short-term results in the 10 dogs in which successful device deployment was achieved were complete ASD occlusion in 5, trivial to mild residual shunting in 4, and moderate persistent shunting in 1.
- Longer-term follow-up (11.2 ± 8.0 months) disclosed complete occlusion in 7 dogs and residual shunting that was assessed to be hemodynamically inconsequential in the remaining 3.

Thus, although the data are limited and further research is required, ASD in dogs appears to be amenable to minimally invasive per-catheter occlusion with currently available devices.

Ventricular septal defect (VSD) in the dog is relatively common (7% to 12% of congenital heart defects). Predisposed breeds include the English bulldog, springer

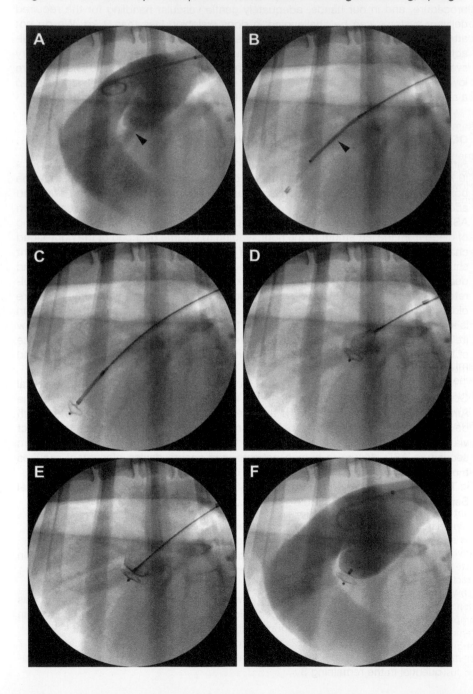

spaniel, and West Highland white terrier. Most VSDs are located in the membranous portion of the interventricular septum immediately below the aortic valve but some occur in the muscular portion of the septum. The defect results in a direct communication between the ventricles, allowing for blood to shunt from one ventricle to the other. Shunt severity depends on the size of the defect, the pressure gradient between the left and right ventricles, and the presence of other concurrent cardiovascular abnormalities. Typically, blood shunts from left-to-right with subsequent pulmonary overcirculation, left-sided volume overload, and congestive heart failure. Dogs with VSD may demonstrate failure to thrive, exercise intolerance, coughing, respiratory distress, and other signs attributed to congestive heart failure. However, VSDs in dogs are frequently small and well-tolerated. Cardiac auscultation of affected individuals commonly discloses a right-sided systolic murmur. A left basilar systolic murmur may also be heard owing to relative pulmonic stenosis. Surgical VSD repair has the same limitations as those for ASD.[3]

Per-catheter delivered devices for minimally invasive occlusion of VSDs in experimental canine models has been reported. The studies concluded that successful per-catheter VSD occlusion is feasible in dogs with surgically created VSD.[44,45] However, very limited data are available for per-catheter occlusion of naturally occurring VSDs in dogs:

- Embolization coils were successfully deployed across membranous VSDs in 4 dogs, for which long-term follow-up (1 year after the procedure) was reported for 3. At these follow-up evaluations, murmurs consistent with VSD were present and color flow Doppler identified recurrent or residual VSD flow in all cases.[46,47]
- A recent case report documented complete muscular VSD closure with a per-catheter–deployed Amplatzer Muscular Ventricular Septal Defect Occluder (AGA Medical Corporation). Complete occlusion was confirmed at follow-up approximately 2 years postprocedure.[48]

Per-catheter VSD closure in dogs is investigational at present. Outcomes with embolization coil occlusion of naturally occurring VSD have been disappointing, whereas occlusion of a hemodynamically significant muscular VSD with an Amplatzer Muscular Ventricular Septal Defect Occluder appears feasible. The available data, however, are very limited, and much more research is required before minimally invasive per-catheter VSD closure in dogs can be considered as a routine procedure.

Fig. 8. Patent ductus arteriosus occlusion with an Amplatz Canine Duct Occluder in a dog. (A) An aortic angiogram is performed via a pigtail angiographic catheter. A narrow jet of contrast emerges from the pulmonic ostium of the ductus (arrowhead) to enter the main pulmonary artery. (B) From the aorta, a delivery catheter is advanced across the patent ductus arteriosus and into the main pulmonary artery. The compressed device (arrowhead) is advanced via the catheter. (C) The flat distal disc is deployed within the main pulmonary artery. The Amplatz Canine Duct Occluder, delivery cable, and guiding catheter are then retracted as a single unit until the flat distal disc engages the pulmonic ostium of the ductus. (D) While maintaining tension on the delivery cable, the delivery catheter is withdrawn to deploy the device waist across the pulmonic ostium and proximal disc within the ductal ampulla. (E) The proximal disc assumes its native cupped shape. (F) After detaching and removing the device delivery cable and catheter, a final angiogram performed via a pigtail angiographic catheter demonstrates complete ductal occlusion. (Modified from Nguyenba TP, Tobias AH. The Amplatz canine duct occluder: a novel device for patent ductus arteriosus occlusion. J Vet Cardiol 2007;9:109–17; with permission.)

BALLOON DILATION OF PULMONIC STENOSIS

Pulmonic stenosis (PS) is the third most common congenital cardiovascular abnormality of dogs after PDA and subvalvular aortic stenosis. As with PDA, the mode of inheritance of PS is complex and most consistent with a polygenic threshold trait.[1] This mode of inheritance was established in a breeding colony of beagles, and extrapolation to other dog breeds should be made with appropriate circumspection. The defect most frequently occurs as a primary malformation (dysplasia) of the pulmonic valve, although concurrent or isolated right ventricular outflow tract obstructions may be subinfundibular (double-chambered right ventricle), infundibular, subvalvular, and supravalvular. It commonly occurs as an isolated heart defect, but PS may be accompanied by other cardiac abnormalities such as tricuspid valve dysplasia, and may form part of more complex congenital cardiac disorders such as Tetralogy of Fallot. Eight dog breeds have been identified as predisposed to PS. The 3 breeds with the highest odds ratios for being affected are the English bulldog, Scottish terrier, and wirehaired fox terrier.[2]

Most dogs with PS are asymptomatic in the first year of life, during which the condition is discovered through detection of a systolic heart murmur that is frequently, but not invariably loud. The point of maximal intensity of the murmur is typically over the left heart base. Thoracic radiographs often demonstrate right heart enlargement, and poststenotic dilation of the main pulmonary artery may be a prominent and diagnostically supportive finding in ventrodorsal or dorsoventral views. Electrocardiogram findings consistent with right ventricular enlargement (deep S waves in leads I, II, III, and aVF, and right orientation of the mean electrical axis of ventricular depolarization) are common.[3]

A thorough echocardiographic examination that includes color flow and spectral Doppler is crucial in the evaluation of any dog with suspected PS. Echocardiography is required to confirm the diagnosis, assess for concurrent cardiac abnormalities, and determine the location and severity of the stenosis. Even in apparently uncomplicated cases of valvular PS, a detailed echocardiographic examination that includes imaging following venous injection of agitated saline (ie, a "bubblegram" or contrast echocardiogram) may disclose patency of the foramen ovale. Right-to-left shunting of sufficient quantity via a patent foramen ovale causes arterial oxygen desaturation and even cyanosis in some dogs with PS, especially if there is concurrent tricuspid regurgitation and likely increases the risk of complications during per-catheter intervention. Echocardiography is also necessary to check that the left coronary artery originates from its correct location behind the left coronary cusp of the aortic sinus of Valsalva. Single right coronary artery, associated with an abnormal origin and course of the left coronary artery, has been reported mainly (but not exclusively) in English bulldogs with PS,[49,50] and the anomalous course of the artery complicates surgical and balloon dilation procedures to relieve PS.[49,51] Finally, if a balloon dilation procedure is anticipated, a thorough echocardiogram is necessary to measure the diameter of the pulmonic valve annulus (for cases with valvular PS), or the diameter of the stenosis and outflow tract at the locations of infundibular, subvalvular, and supravalvular stenoses, to guide selection of an appropriately sized valvuloplasty catheter.

The natural history of untreated PS has not been definitively established, and some dogs with mild or even moderate PS lead normal or near-normal lives. However, this generalization does not extend to dogs with severe PS, and dogs with associated complicating conditions such as tricuspid valve dysplasia. Those cases frequently develop right-sided heart failure, exertional syncope, and serious arrhythmia (eg, atrial fibrillation), and sudden death occurs in some cases.[3]

Firm guidelines for recommending balloon dilation in dogs with PS have not been established. We recommend the procedure when 1 or more of the following are present:

- Clinical signs (especially exertional syncope) ascribable to the defect.
- Significant right-to-left shunt via a patent foramen ovale, especially if this causes cyanosis.
- Substantial tricuspid regurgitation attributable to either concurrent tricuspid valve dysplasia or as a secondary consequence of PS.
- Substantial right ventricular concentric hypertrophy and evidence of myocardial fibrosis, necrosis, and ischemia (subendocardial and papillary muscle hyperechogenicity and/or ST segment abnormalities on electrocardiogram).
- A Doppler-derived pressure difference across the stenosis of 50 mm Hg or greater.

Balloon dilation of valvular PS in the dog was first described in 1988.[52] The procedure involves inflating the balloon of a valvuloplasty catheter that is positioned across the stenosis (**Fig. 9**). The procedure is performed either via the jugular or femoral vein. A valvuloplasty catheter is selected with an inflated balloon diameter 1.2 to 1.5 times the diameter of the pulmonic valve annulus.[53] A double ballooning technique has been described as an alternative in small dogs with a pulmonic annulus size that would otherwise require a large dilation catheter and large-diameter introducer.[54] Maneuvering guidewires and catheters through the right heart and positioning the balloon of the valvuloplasty catheter across the stenosis can be challenging in dogs weighing less than 4 kg. This is especially true in cases with substantial concentric right ventricular hypertrophy. However, with currently available equipment and low-profile valvuloplasty catheters, the procedure is feasible in dogs of virtually any size.

A unique and interesting challenge arises in dogs with PS where correct origin of the left coronary artery is not identified during echocardiography. In such cases, aortic root angiography or selective coronary arteriography is performed before PS balloon dilation to delineate coronary artery anatomy. The left coronary artery in some dogs arises aberrantly from the right coronary artery and courses circumpulmonic to the left heart. This coronary artery anomaly has been described in the English bulldog and boxer, where it appears to contribute to subvalvular pulmonic stenosis.[49,50] We have also identified this coronary artery anomaly in an American Staffordshire terrier with valvular PS. The best approach to treating PS in these cases is not known. Our current strategy is to proceed with the balloon dilation procedure, but to use a valvuloplasty catheter with a balloon diameter that is equal to (rather than 1.2 to 1.5 times) the diameter of the pulmonic valve annulus, and a similar approach has recently been described by others.[55]

Balloon dilation is a relatively benign minimally invasive per-catheter procedure that successfully alleviates clinical signs and prolongs survival in dogs with severe PS (pressure difference across the stenosis greater than 80 mm Hg).[56] Ideally, we strive to decrease the pressure difference across the stenosis to less than 50 mm Hg on follow-up Doppler echocardiography at 1 day and 3 months postprocedure, although many cases show substantial improvement in clinical signs even when this end point is not achieved. The most favorable results with this procedure are achieved with the most common form of PS, ie, isolated valvular PS. However, salutary outcomes are also achieved with balloon dilation of stenotic lesions in other right ventricular outflow tract locations. Supravalvular PS is particularly challenging, but successful balloon dilation with stenting of supravalvular PS in a dog has recently been reported.[57]

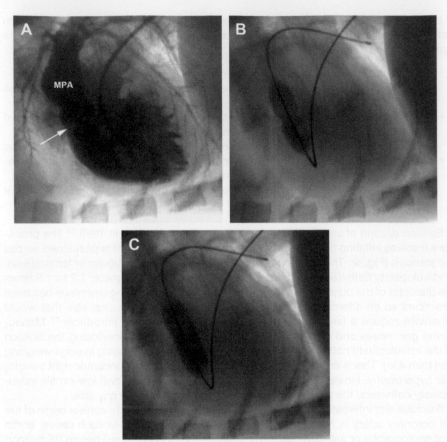

Fig. 9. Balloon dilation of valvular pulmonic stenosis in a dog. (*A*) Right ventricular angiogram showing the location of the stenotic pulmonic valve (*arrow*) and poststenotic dilation of the main pulmonary artery (MPA). (*B*) The balloon of the valvuloplasty catheter is positioned across the stenosis and inflated. During inflation the balloon initially assumes an hourglass shape because of constriction at its mid-length by the stenotic valve. (*C*) With further inflation, the hourglass shape disappears as the stenosis is relieved.

BALLOON DILATION OF OTHER OBSTRUCTIVE CONGENITAL CARDIOVASCULAR ABNORMALITIES

Subvalvular aortic stenosis (SAS) is the second most common congenital heart defect in dogs. Newfoundlands, boxers, rottweilers, golden retrievers, and German shepherds are most commonly affected. The stenosis typically results from a ring of fibrous tissue within the left ventricular outflow tract immediately below the aortic valve. Obstruction to ejection results in elevated left ventricular systolic pressure, with concentric hypertrophy and myocardial ischemia as a consequence. Affected dogs are commonly asymptomatic when the diagnosis is first made, but may exhibit exercise intolerance, syncope, and left-sided congestive heart failure. Sudden death is common in dogs with severe SAS, often occurring during the first 3 years of life.[3] Surgical resection of the stenotic lesion results in significant reductions in the pressure gradient across the stenosis but fails to improve survival times.[58]

Balloon dilation has been investigated for the treatment of severe SAS. In a recent study, 28 dogs with severe SAS were randomly assigned to a balloon dilation (n = 15) or atenolol therapy (n = 13) group[59]:

- In the balloon dilation group, the peak systolic pressure gradient reduced significantly (P<.001) from 147.0 ± 43.9 mm Hg at baseline to 86.7 ± 36.3 mm Hg 6 weeks postprocedure.
- In the atenolol group, there was no significant change in the peak systolic pressure gradient at baseline and at a 6-week recheck (122.2 ± 41.0 vs 113.0 ± 46.2 mm Hg, respectively, P = .765).
- Survival for dogs in the balloon dilation group (median, 55 months; range, 12 to 108 months) was not significantly different (P = .952) from the atenolol group (median, 56 months; range, 10 to 99 months).

Although a significant decrease in the peak systolic pressure gradient in dogs with severe SAS is achieved with balloon dilation, at least in the short term, this procedure does not confer a survival benefit compared with therapy with atenolol. This lack of survival benefit is consistent with the results of surgical resection of the lesion, and indicates that reduction in pressure gradient has no significant effect on the clinically relevant end point of cardiac mortality. Consequently, based on the currently available data, we do not advocate balloon dilation for dogs with SAS.

Cor triatriatum dexter is a rare congenital heart defect in dogs in which the right atrium is divided into a cranial and caudal chamber by a fibromuscular septum (persistent sinus venosus valve). Affected dogs show congestion of the caudal half of the body (ascites) without jugular distention. The diagnosis is confirmed by echocardiography and cardiac catheterization (angiography and pressure measurements).[60] The defect may be addressed by surgical resection of the anomalous septum,[60,61] but balloon dilation of the defect is a very effective minimally invasive option.[62–65]

Atrioventricular valve stenosis affecting the mitral or tricuspid valve is a rare congenital heart defect in the dog. It is characterized by fibrosis of the affected valve leaflets and fusion of the leaflet commissures, resulting in reduced leaflet mobility and effective valve orifice size. Atrioventricular valve stenosis limits ventricular filling and increases atrial pressure with subsequent supraventricular arrhythmias, congestive heart failure, and death. Clinical signs include exercise intolerance, syncope, and left- or right-sided congestive heart failure.[3] Balloon dilation has been successfully performed in dogs with mitral and tricuspid valve stenosis with a reduction in both the pressure gradient across the stenotic valve, and the associated clinical signs.[66,67]

SUMMARY

Over the past approximately 2 decades, minimally invasive per-catheter occlusion and dilation procedures for the treatment of congenital cardiovascular disease in dogs have become an integral and routine part of veterinary cardiology. These procedures initially evolved to reduce the morbidity and mortality associated with cardiovascular surgery, and in response to public demand for less invasive treatment options for their companion animals. However, as outcomes data emerge, some of these procedures are proving to be more effective than cardiovascular surgery for certain abnormalities, and this is especially true for PDA occlusion. Minimally invasive occlusion procedures also show promise for dogs with ostium secundum ASD and muscular VSD, defects for which routine surgical options are realistically not available. Similarly, balloon dilation is now considered by most, if not all veterinary cardiologists to be the standard of care for pulmonic stenosis, as well as for several other obstructive cardiovascular abnormalities. The development of minimally invasive per-catheter procedures in veterinary cardiology is an extremely active and exciting area of research. An ever-increasing array of practical and effective options is available for the minimally invasive treatment of cardiovascular disorders in companion animals, and our profession, our patients, and their owners all benefit greatly from this evolution.

REFERENCES

1. Patterson DF. Hereditary congenital heart defects in dogs. J Small Anim Pract 1989;30:153–65.
2. Buchanan JW. Prevalence of cardiovascular disorders. In: Fox PR, Sisson D, Moïse NS, editors. Textbook of canine and feline cardiology. 2nd edition. Philadelphia: WB Saunders Company; 1999. p. 457–70.
3. Oyama MA, Sisson DD, Thomas WP, et al. Congenital heart disease. In: Ettinger SJ, Feldman EC, editors. Textbook of veterinary internal medicine. 6th edition. St. Louis (MO): Elsevier Saunders; 2005. p. 972–1021.
4. Eyster GE, Eyster JT, Cords GB, et al. Patent ductus arteriosus in the dog: characteristics of occurrence and results of surgery in one hundred consecutive cases. J Am Vet Med Assoc 1976;168:435–8.
5. Bureau S, Monnet E, Orton EC. Evaluation of survival rate and prognostic indicators for surgical treatment of left-to-right patent ductus arteriosus in dogs: 52 cases (1995–2003). J Am Vet Med Assoc 2005;227:1794–9.
6. Stauthammer CD, Nguyenba TP, Tobias AH. Short and long term cardiac changes following complete occlusion of uncomplicated patent ductus arteriosus in dogs [abstract]. J Vet Intern Med 2007;21:609.
7. Miller MW, Gordon SG, Saunders AG, et al. Angiographic classification of patent ductus arteriosus morphology in the dog. J Vet Cardiol 2006;8:109–14.
8. Walters B, Bramer CN. Patent ductus arteriosus. North Am Vet 1952;33:252–5.
9. Corti LB, Merkley D, Nelson OL, et al. Retrospective evaluation of occlusion of patent ductus arteriosus with hemoclips in 20 dogs. J Am Anim Hosp Assoc 2000;36:548–55.
10. Fossum TW. Surgery of the cardiovascular system. In: Fossum TW, editor. small animal surgery. 3rd edition. St. Louis (MO): Mosby Elsevier; 2007. p. 775–816.
11. Van Israël N, French AT, Dukes-McEwan J, et al. Review of left-to-right shunting patent ductus arteriosus and short term outcomes in 98 dogs. J Small Anim Pract 2002;43:395–400.
12. Goodrich KR, Kyles AE, Kass PH, et al. Retrospective comparison of surgical ligation and transarterial catheter occlusion for treatment of patent ductus arteriosus in two hundred and four dogs (1993–2003). Vet Surg 2007;36:43–9.
13. Stanley BJ, Luis-Fuentes V, Darke PG. Comparison of the incidence of residual shunting between two surgical techniques used for ligation of patent ductus arteriosus in the dog. Vet Surg 2003;32:231–7.
14. Snaps FR, McEntree K, Saunders JH, et al. Treatment of patent ductus arteriosus by placement of intravascular coils in a pup. J Am Vet Med Assoc 1995;207:724–5.
15. Fox PR, Bond BR, Sommer RJ. Nonsurgical transcatheter coil occlusion of patent ductus arteriosus in two dogs using a preformed nitinol snare delivery technique. J Vet Intern Med 1998;12:182–5.
16. Saunders JH, Snaps FR, Peeters D, et al. Use of a balloon occlusion catheter to facilitate transarterial coil embolization of a patent ductus arteriosus in two dogs. Vet Rec 1999;145:544–6.

17. Stokhof AA, Sreeram N, Wolvekamp WT. Transcatheter closure of patent ductus arteriosus using occluding spring coils. J Vet Intern Med 2000;14:452–5.
18. Tanaka R, Hoshi K, Nagashima Y, et al. Detachable coils for occlusion of patent ductus arteriosus in 2 dogs. Vet Surg 2001;30:580–4.
19. Tanaka R, Nagashima Y, Hoshi K, et al. Supplemental embolization coil implantation for closure of patent ductus arteriosus in a beagle dog. J Vet Med Sci 2001; 63:557–9.
20. Glaus TM, Martin M, Boller M, et al. Catheter closure of patent ductus arteriosus in dogs: variation in ductal size requires different techniques. J Vet Cardiol 2003;5:7–12.
21. Gordon SG, Miller MW. Transarterial coil embolization for canine patent ductus arteriosus occlusion. Clin Tech Small Anim Pract 2005;20:196–202.
22. Hogan DF, Green HW III, Miller GS. Transarterial coil embolization of patent ductus arteriosus in small dogs with 0.025-inch vascular occlusion coils: 10 cases. J Vet Intern Med 2004;18:325–9.
23. Miller SJ, Thomas WP. Coil embolization of patent ductus arteriosus via the carotid artery in seven dogs. J Vet Cardiol 2009;11:129–36.
24. Fellows CG, Lerche P, King G, et al. Treatment of patent ductus arteriosus by placement of two intravascular coils in a puppy. J Small Anim Pract 1998;39: 196–9.
25. Schneider M, Hildebrandt N, Schweigl T, et al. Transvenous embolization of small patent ductus arteriosus with single detachable coils in dogs. J Vet Intern Med 2001;15:222–8.
26. Bilkis AA, Alwi M, Hasri S, et al. The Amplatzer duct occluder: experience in 209 patients. J Am Coll Cardiol 2001;37:258–61.
27. Tobias AH, Jacob KA, Fine DM, et al. Patent ductus arteriosus occlusion with Amplatzer duct occluders. In: Proceedings of the 20th Annual American College of Veterinary Internal Medicine Forum. Dallas, TX, May 29–June 1, 2002. p. 100–1.
28. Sisson D. Use of a self-expanding occluding stent for nonsurgical closure of patent ductus arteriosus in dogs. J Am Vet Med Assoc 2003;223:999–1005.
29. Campbell FE, Thomas WP, Miller SJ, et al. Immediate and late outcomes of transarterial coil occlusion of patent ductus arteriosus in dogs. J Vet Intern Med 2006; 20:83–96.
30. Magee AG, Huggon IC, Seed PT, et al. Transcatheter coil occlusion of the arterial duct. Eur Heart J 2001;22:1817–21.
31. Nguyenba TP, Tobias AH. Minimally invasive per-catheter patent ductus arteriosus occlusion in dogs using a prototype duct occluder. J Vet Intern Med 2008; 22:129–34.
32. Glaus TM, Berger F, Amman FW, et al. Closure of large patent ductus arteriosus with a self-expanding duct occluder in two dogs. J Small Anim Pract 2002;43:547–50.
33. Cheatham JP. Not so fast with that novel use: does AVP = PDA? [editorial]. Catheter Cardiovasc Interv 2005;65:581–3.
34. Javois AJ, Husayni TS, Thoele D, et al. Inadvertent stenting of patent ductus arteriosus with Amplatzer vascular plug. Catheter Cardiovasc Interv 2006;67: 485–9.
35. Smith PJ, Martin MW. Transcatheter embolization of patent ductus arteriosus using an Amplatzer vascular plug in six dogs. J Small Anim Pract 2007;48:80–6.
36. Achen SE, Miller MW. Transarterial ductal occlusion with the Amplatzer vascular plug in 32 dogs. J Vet Intern Med 2008;22:1348–52.
37. Hogan DF, Green HW, Sanders RA. Transcatheter closure of patent ductus arteriosus in a dog with a peripheral vascular occlusion device. J Vet Cardiol 2006;8: 139–43.

38. Sharafuddin MJ, Gu X, Urness M, et al. The nitinol vascular occlusion plug: preliminary experimental evaluation in peripheral veins. J Vasc Interv Radiol 1999;10:23–7.

39. Nguyenba TP, Tobias AH. The Amplatz canine duct occluder: a novel device for patent ductus arteriosus occlusion. J Vet Cardiol 2007;9:109–17.

40. Nguyenba TP, Tobias AH. Patent ductus arteriosus occlusion with an investigational Amplatzer canine ductal occluder [abstract]. J Vet Intern Med 2006;20:730.

41. Achen SE, Gordon SG, Saunders AB, et al. Transarterial ductal occlusion using the Amplatz canine duct occluder in 23 cases [abstract]. J Vet Intern Med 2008;22:762.

42. Sanders RA, Hogan DF, Green HW III, et al. Transcatheter closure of an atrial septal defect in a dog. J Am Vet Med Assoc 2005;227:430–4.

43. Gordon SG, Miller MW, Roland RM. Transcatheter atrial septal defect closure with the Amplatzer atrial septal occluder in 13 dogs: short- and mid-term outcome. J Vet Intern Med 2009;23:995–1002.

44. Amin Z, Gu X, Berry JM, et al. New device for closure of muscular ventricular septal defects in a canine model. Circulation 1999;100:320–8.

45. Ding ZR, Qin YW, Hu JQ, et al. A new pan-nitinol occluder for transcatheter closure of ventricular septal defects in a canine model. J Interv Cardiol 2009; 22:191–8.

46. Fujii Y, Fukuda T, Machida, et al. Transcatheter closure of congenital ventricular septal defects in 3 dogs with a detachable coil. J Vet Intern Med 2004;18:911–4.

47. Shimizu M, Tanaka R, Hirao H, et al. Percutaneous transcatheter coil embolization of a ventricular septal defect in a dog. J Am Vet Med Assoc 2005;226:69–72.

48. Margiocco ML, Bulmer BJ, Sisson DD. Percutaneous occlusion of a muscular ventricular septal defect with an Amplatz muscular VSD occluder. J Vet Cardiol 2008;10:61–6.

49. Buchanan JW. Pulmonic stenosis caused by single coronary artery in dogs: four cases (1965–1984). J Am Vet Med Assoc 1990;196:115–20.

50. Buchanan JW. Pathogenesis of single coronary artery and pulmonic stenosis in English bulldogs. J Vet Intern Med 2001;15:101–4.

51. Kittleson M, Thomas W, Loyer C, et al. Single coronary artery (type R2A) [letter to the editor]. J Vet Intern Med 1992;6:250–1.

52. Sisson DD, MacCoy DM. Treatment of congenital pulmonic stenosis in two dogs by balloon valvuloplasty. J Vet Intern Med 1988;2:92–9.

53. Estrada A, Moïse NS, Erb HN, et al. Prospective evaluation of the balloon-to-annulus ratio for valvuloplasty in the treatment of pulmonic stenosis in the dog. J Vet Intern Med 2006;20:862–72.

54. Estrada A, Moïse NS, Renaud-Farrell S. When, how and why to perform a double ballooning technique for dogs with valvular pulmonic stenosis. J Vet Cardiol 2005; 7:41–51.

55. Fonfara S, Martinez Pareira Y, Swift S, et al. Balloon valvuloplasty for treatment of pulmonic stenosis in English bulldogs with aberrant coronary artery. J Vet Intern Med 2010;24:354–9.

56. Stafford Johnson M, Martin M, Edwards D, et al. Pulmonic stenosis in dogs: balloon dilation improves clinical outcome. J Vet Intern Med 2004;18:656–62.

57. Griffiths LG, Bright JM, Chan KC. Transcatheter intravascular stent placement to relieve supravalvular pulmonic stenosis. J Vet Cardiol 2006;8:145–55.

58. Orton EC, Herndon GD, Boon JA, et al. Influence of open surgical correction on intermediate-term outcome in dogs with subvalvular aortic stenosis: 44 cases (1991–1998). J Am Vet Med Assoc 2000;216:364–7.

59. Meurs KM, Lehmkuhl LB, Bonagura JD. Survival times in dogs with severe sub-valvular aortic stenosis treated with balloon valvuloplasty or atenolol. J Am Vet Med Assoc 2005;227:420–4.

60. Tobias AH, Thomas WP, Kittleson MD, et al. Cor triatriatum dexter in two dogs. J Am Vet Med Assoc 1993;202:285–90.

61. Tanaka R, Hoshi K, Shimizu M, et al. Surgical correction of cor triatriatum dexter in a dog using extracorporeal circulation. J Small Anim Pract 2003;44:370–3.

62. Adin DB, Thomas WP. Balloon dilation of cor triatriatum dexter in a dog. J Vet Intern Med 1999;13:617–9.

63. Atkins C, DeFrancesco T. Balloon dilation of cor triatriatum dexter in a dog. J Vet Intern Med 2000;14:471–2.

64. Mitten RW, Edwards GA, Rishniw M. Diagnosis and management of cor triatriatum dexter in a Pyrenean mountain dog and an Akita Inu. Aust Vet J 2001;79: 177–80.

65. Johnson MS, Martin M, De Giovanni JV, et al. Management of cor triatriatum dexter by balloon dilatation in three dogs. J Small Anim Pract 2004;45:16–20.

66. Kunze P, Abbott JA, Hamilton SM, et al. Balloon valvuloplasty for palliative treatment of tricuspid stenosis with right-to-left atrial-level shunting in a dog. J Am Vet Med Assoc 2002;220:491–6.

67. Oyama MA, Weideman JA, Cole SG. Calculation of pressure half-time. J Vet Cardiol 2008;10:57–60.

Surgery for Cardiac Disease in Small Animals: Current Techniques

Leigh G. Griffiths, VetMB, MRCVS, PhD

KEYWORDS

- Cardiac surgery • Cardiopulmonary bypass
- Open heart surgery • Inflow occlusion

The complexity and inherent risks associated with cardiovascular surgical procedures necessitate a team-based approach to consistently achieve successful outcomes. As a minimum, the cardiac surgical team consists of the primary surgeon, surgical assistant, scrub nurse, circulating nurse, anesthesiologist, and perfusionist (cardiopulmonary bypass). Members of the intensive care unit (ICU) should also be included in the team because transfer and recovery in ICU are critical steps in effective case management. The importance of effective teamwork has been studied in medical cardiovascular surgical units.[1–3] Cardiac surgery teams that work together consistently are less likely to make surgical technical errors. Correlation has been demonstrated between breakdown in teamwork and occurrence of surgical technical errors.[2] Correlation between number of teamwork errors and surgical mortality rate has also been identified.[1] The most common cause for teamwork error is inaccurate communication between the surgeon, technical support staff, anesthesiologist, and perfusionist.[2] Consequently the cardiac surgical team should strive to develop excellent communication, with pre- and postoperative case briefings, to improve teamwork and minimize intraoperative errors.

In 1999 Dr Lawrence Cohn[4] detailed the qualities necessary for excellence in cardiac surgery in his American Society of Thoracic Surgery Presidential Address. These same qualities are essential for excellence in veterinary cardiac surgery. Importantly, leadership of the cardiac surgery team is critical to success. Knowledge of inherent risks associated with cardiac surgical procedures has a tendency to generate stress in all members of the cardiac surgical team. The successful cardiac surgeon must maintain a calm, relaxed working environment regardless of case progress. Even the most talented surgeon will falter if they allow teamwork and communication to breakdown in the face of surgical complications.

Department of Veterinary Medicine and Epidemiology, University of California, One Shields Avenue, 2108 Tupper Hall, Davis, CA 95618, USA
E-mail address: lggriffiths@ucdavis.edu

Vet Clin Small Anim 40 (2010) 605–622
doi:10.1016/j.cvsm.2010.04.001
0195-5616/10/$ – see front matter. Published by Elsevier Inc.

PREOPERATIVE ASSESSMENT

Presence of cardiovascular disease usually necessitates use of additional diagnostic evaluations prior to commencement of the surgical procedure. Preoperative determination and understanding of the pathophysiologic effects of the cardiovascular condition is essential to a successful outcome. Patients may range from those with early subclinical cardiac disease and minimal functional impairment, to those with end-stage cardiovascular disease that has resulted in severe structural and functional derangement. The intraoperative acute hemodynamic effects of the proposed surgery must also be considered in the preoperative plan. For example, in patients undergoing inflow occlusion procedures, it is not uncommon for a small amount of blood loss to occur during the open-heart portion of the procedure. Such blood loss is generally well tolerated unless it becomes excessive. However, in toy and small breeds even minimal blood loss may be sufficient to induce hypovolemic shock and consequently the preoperative plan should include immediate volume replacement and blood transfusion following the period of inflow occlusion.

INFLOW OCCLUSION

Inflow occlusion temporarily interrupts venous return to the heart, allowing for open heart surgery and direct intracardiac visualization in a bloodless field. In human patients who are normothermic, periods of inflow occlusion of 4 minutes or less are well tolerated.[5] Addition of mild hypothermia (30°C) reduces basal metabolic rate, increasing safe occlusion time to 8 minutes. In normothermic canine experimental models, periods of inflow occlusion of 8 minutes are well tolerated, with no apparent neurologic dysfunction following recovery.[6–8] Cardiac massage following the period of inflow occlusion is critical in ensuring survival.[7] Additionally, the descending aorta can be digitally occluded during resuscitation to direct available cardiac output to the heart and brain. Initial studies demonstrated that moderate hypothermia (20–25°C) extended the tolerated duration of inflow occlusion.[9,10] However, the risk for development of spontaneous ventricular fibrillation increases dramatically with body temperatures below 30°C.[10] Under conditions of moderate hypothermia, ventricular fibrillation is commonly induced by minor mechanical stimuli.[10] Because of the risk for spontaneous ventricular fibrillation, the author prefers to perform inflow occlusion procedures at normothermic or mildly hypothermic conditions. The hypothermia durations cited previously represent the maximal time period tolerated by normal dogs. It is likely that the duration of inflow occlusion tolerated by patients with preexisting cardiovascular disease is significantly shorter. Additionally, a safety margin should be incorporated in the plan to allow time to address complications if they occur. Consequently, at normothermia inflow occlusion times of 2 minutes or less are ideal. Hyperventilation with 100% oxygen for 5 minutes prior to initiation of inflow occlusion improves outcomes.

Inflow occlusion can be performed through sternotomy, left or right intercostal thoracotomy. Left fourth intercostal approach provides optimal right ventricular outflow tract (RVOT) exposure for patch graft placement in pulmonic stenosis. Right fourth intercostal approach provides optimal RVOT exposure for resection of RVOT tumors.[11] However, caudal vena caval dissection is challenging via the fourth intercostal approach. A fifth intercostal space approach improves exposure of the caudal vena cava, but RVOT exposure is more limited. Consequently, for procedures involving the RVOT, patient factors (cardiac displacement, tumor location) and surgeon preference dictate the choice of approach.

Surgical procedures utilizing inflow occlusion have been documented in dogs and cats with spontaneous cardiac disease.[11–15] Individual umbilical tapes are passed around the cranial vena cava, caudal vena cava, and azygous vein (**Fig. 1**A). Because the azygous vein joins the cranial vena cava within the cranial mediastinum, outside of the pericardial space, an alternative technique is to approach the cranial vena cava intrapericardially (**Fig. 2**). However, an intrapericardial approach to the cranial vena cava is challenging from a left thoracotomy requiring retraction of the pulmonary artery, RVOT, and aorta.

CARDIOPULMONARY BYPASS

The primary function of cardiopulmonary bypass (CPB) is to divert systemic venous return away from the heart and return it to the systemic arterial system. Cardiopulmonary bypass therefore allows open heart surgical procedures to be performed in a bloodless field, without the severe time constraints imposed by inflow occlusion. Additionally, the surgeon may opt to use cardioplegia solution delivered via the coronary vasculature to induce diastolic cardiac arrest, eliminating myocardial motion and allowing for surgery on a stationary heart. The general principle and components of the CPB circuit are simple. Venous cannulation allows for gravity drainage of systemic venous return to the CPB machine. The venous reservoir then serves as a buffer for venous drainage, allowing the perfusionist time to balance venous return with cardiac output (machine flow rate). The machine pumps the blood through an oxygenator that acts as an artificial lung and heat exchanger, allowing for patient ventilation and manipulation of patient body temperature throughout the procedure. Finally, the blood is returned to the systemic vasculature via the arterial cannula. Placement of an aortic cross clamp on the ascending aorta completes the isolation of the heart and lungs from the systemic vasculature (with the exception of bronchial pulmonary blood flow, see requirement for venting).

Initial attempts to perform CPB in humans met with almost universal failure, despite acceptable results in experimental animals. The majority of failures were related to the high flow rates used during the procedure (165 mL/kg/min), which resulted in excessive blood in the surgical field and high risk for air embolus. The critical advance in achieving the promise of CPB is attributed to a 1954 paper, which demonstrated 100% survival for 30 minutes in anesthetized dogs subjected to cranial and caudal

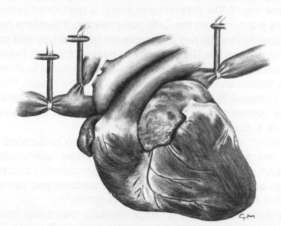

Fig. 1. Heart and vasculature as viewed from left, showing extrapericardial tape positions for inflow occlusion. Umbilical tapes are placed to encircle the azygous vein, cranial, and caudal vena cavae. Tapes are passed through rubber tubing to create Rummel tourniquets. The Rummel tourniquets are tightened to temporarily interrupt venous return.

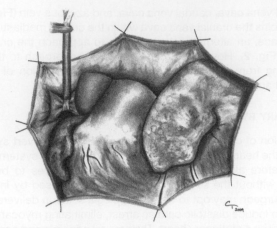

Fig. 2. Heart and vasculature from a left-thoracotomy approach with the pericardium opened and sutured to the incision. Cranial vena caval umbilical tape is placed intrapericardially, allowing a single tape to occlude cranial vena caval and azygous flow.

vena cava ligation.[16] The explanation for this seemingly incredible finding is that normal venous oxygen saturation is 65% to 75% at basal cardiac output. Full oxygen extraction from arterial blood results in absolutely no physiologic harm. Consequently, when cardiac output is limited to azygos flow (8–14 mL/kg/min), oxygen extraction increases and tissue oxygenation is maintained. This landmark discovery introduced the concept of "physiologic flow", which is still critical to the success of CPB today. Physiologic flow rates (50–65 mL/kg/min for adults, 100–150 mL/kg/min for pediatric or canine patients) combined with reduction of basal metabolic rate using hypothermia, have become standard practice in CPB.

Cannulation: Because of concerns regarding canine aortic fragility, arterial cannulation is accomplished through the femoral or carotid artery.[17–23] Heparin (initial dose 400 IU/kg) is given prior to arterial cannulation, with the goal of maintaining activated clotting time greater than 400s. Arterial cannulation is performed prior to thoracotomy allowing for patient support from the CPB pump should it become necessary.

Arterial cannulation technique requires exposure of the artery and placement of two silk sutures around the vessel. The sutures are passed through Rummel tourniquets and tightened, isolating a segment of the vessel. The vessel is incised using a No. 11 blade, the hole dilated and the cannula inserted into the vessel. The proximal Rummel tourniquet is released to allow cannula passage, and re-tightened to secure the cannula within the vessel. Finally, the cannula is affixed to the Rummel tourniquets using encircling silk suture (**Fig. 3**).

Venous Cannulation: Venous cannulation configuration is dictated by the intracardiac procedure being performed. Although cavoatrial cannulation is generally preferred, right heart procedures require bi-caval cannulation. Cavoatrial cannulation has the advantage of being particularly simpler to perform and provides right-sided decompression that is lacking with bi-caval cannulation.[24]

Cavoatrial cannulation utilizes a two-stage cannula, with distal holes placed in the caudal vena cava and proximal holes in the right atrium. Two purse string sutures are placed around the auricular appendage and secured with Rummel tourniquets. The auricular appendage is amputated and trabeculae within the auricle are transected allowing unimpeded passage of cannula. The cannula is inserted into the atrium,

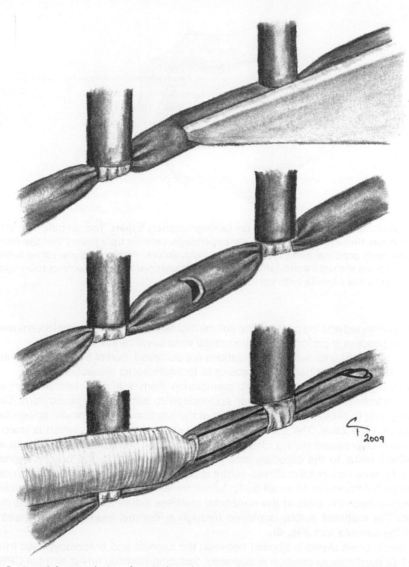

Fig. 3. Arterial cannulation for cardiopulmonary bypass. Two encircling Rummel tourniquets are placed around the artery, proximal and distal to the proposed arteriotomy incision (*top*). The vessel is incised using a No. 11 and the hole dilated (*middle*). The proximal Rummel tourniquet is released to allow cannula passage, and re-tightened to secure the cannula within the vessel (*bottom*). Finally, the cannula is affixed to the Rummel tourniquet's using encircling silk suture.

with the tip passed into the caudal vena cava. The Rummel tourniquets are tightened and secured to the cannula with encircling silk suture (**Fig. 4**).

Bi-caval cannulation requires umbilical tape placement around the cranial and caudal vena cavae. A double purse string suture is placed in the right atrial wall, a stab incision is made in the center of the purse string, and the hole is dilated. The caudal caval

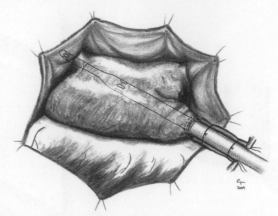

Fig. 4. Cavoatrial venous cannulation for cardiopulmonary bypass. The cannula is inserted into the atrium through the right auricular appendage. Cannula tip is passed into the caudal vena cava, with proximal holes located in the right atrium. Preplaced purse string sutures placed in around the right auricular appendage are tightened through Rummel tourniquets and secured to the cannula with encircling silk suture.

cannula is inserted and the purse string sutures tightened through Rummel tourniquets. The same process is performed for the cranial vena caval cannula (**Fig. 5**).

Once the arterial and venous cannulations are achieved, partial bypass can be initiated to stabilize patient hemodynamics or to facilitate aortic dissection.

Cardioplegia Cannula: Aortic root cannulation from the right lateral approach requires retroflection of the auricular appendage to expose the aortic root. Care must be taken to avoid traction and tearing at the junction of the auricular appendage and cranial vena cava. The aorta is encircled with umbilical tape, which is used to apply counter pressure during cross clamp application. An aortic root cannula site is selected, distal to the coronary artery ostia but proximal to the brachiocephalic trunk. A Prolene horizontal mattress suture is placed in the aortic wall, with each needle bite partial thickness to avoid aortic lumen penetration. The aortic root cannula is inserted between the bites of the horizontal mattress suture and flow in the cannula verified. The mattress suture is placed through a Rummel tourniquet and used to secure the cannula foot (**Fig. 6**).

The aortic cross clamp is applied between the cannula and brachiocephalic trunk. Cold (4°C) cardioplegia solution is delivered, inducing diastolic arrest and full CPB is initiated. Numerous cardioplegia strategies have been investigated, including crystalloid solutions versus blood cardioplegia, intermittent versus continuous administration, intracellular versus extracellular electrolyte composition, cold versus hot shot cardioplegia, and various additions to the range of basic electrolyte solutions utilized to induce diastolic arrest.[25–27] The author's preference is to employ an intermittent blood-based cardioplegia strategy, utilizing the Buckberg cardioplegia solutions. With this strategy the majority of patients require no defibrillation on removal of the aortic cross clamp, and postoperative ventricular arrhythmias are rarely evident.

Requirement for Venting: Venting is necessary to prevent dilation of cardiac chambers on the side of the heart that is unopened during the procedure. Delivery of cardioplegia solution results in coronary sinus venous return to the right atrium. This result is rarely problematic because with cavoatrial cannulation, this return drains via the venous cannula; whereas with bi-caval cannulation the right heart is open

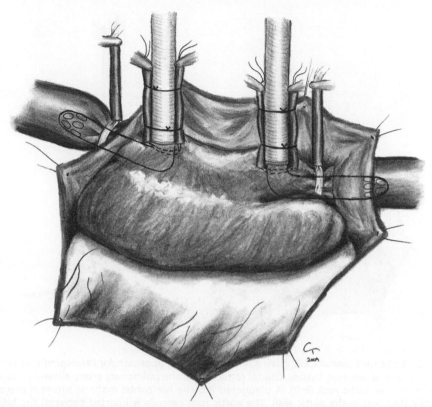

Fig. 5. Bi-caval venous cannulation for cardiopulmonary bypass. Cranial and caudal vena caval right angled venous cannulae placed through purse string sutures in the right atrial wall. Encircling cranial and caudal vena caval umbilical tapes are tightened through Rummel tourniquets preventing venous return around the cannulae.

allowing direct suction of coronary sinus flow. Venous return to the left atrium during bypass is more problematic. A large proportion of bronchial artery flow drains via the pulmonary veins.[28] This physiologic shunt results in progressive left-sided dilation unless adequate venting is ensured. Insertion of a flexible vent cannula through a pledgeted purse string suture in the left atrium is essential to procedural success in cases where the left heart is unopened.

CONGENITAL HEART DEFECTS
Patent Ductus Arteriosus

With the advent of catheter-based methods for closure of patent ductus arteriosus (PDA), the indications for surgical closure are becoming increasingly rare. Catheter-based procedures have success rates comparable to those reported for surgical closure, low mortality risk, low incidence of complication, and minimal morbidity.[29–33] The technique for surgical ligation of PDA has been extensively described.[30,34–39]

Pulmonic Stenosis

Although valvular lesions are the most common form of pulmonic stenosis (PS) in canine patients, subvalvular and supravalvular lesions have been described.[12,40–45] Although catheter-based balloon dilation is successful in addressing valvular PS in

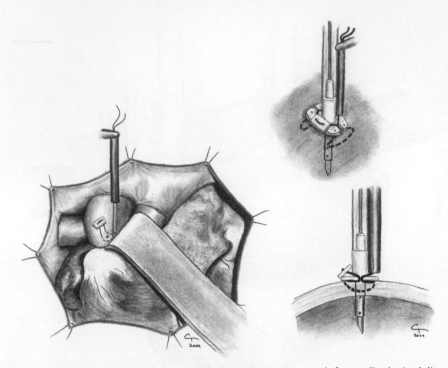

Fig. 6. Aortic root cannulation, from a left-thoracotomy approach, for cardioplegia delivery during cardiopulmonary bypass. Caudal retraction of the pulmonary artery allowing visualization of the aortic root (*left*). A pledgeted Prolene horizontal mattress suture is placed partial thickness in the aortic wall. The aortic root cannula is inserted between the bites of the horizontal mattress suture and flow in the cannula verified (*top right*). The pledgeted mattress suture is used to secure the foot of the aortic root cannula and the Rummel tourniquet tightened. Cross section of the aortic wall and aortic root cannula demonstrating ideal cannula placement (*bottom right*).

many patients, specific lesions exist that necessitate a surgical option. Severe annular hypoplasia or thickened immobile leaflets are associated with less favorable outcomes following catheter-based intervention.[40] Approximately 50% of such patients respond acceptably to balloon dilation. However, it is rarely possible to predict which patients will fail balloon dilation.[40] Because of the inherent risk associated with surgical correction of such lesions, surgery is generally reserved for patients in which balloon dilation has failed. Subvalvular PS represents an exception to this approach, because results of balloon dilation are poor for this lesion.[46]

Surgical correction of pulmonic stenosis can be accomplished using either inflow occlusion or CPB. CPB has the advantage of allowing abundant time for infundibular myectomy or valvulectomy if these are deemed necessary.

Coronary Artery Anatomy: It is essential to determine coronary artery anatomy preoperatively in cases of PS, particularly in breeds that are predisposed to coronary artery anomalies.[47,48] The patch-graft technique involves incision of the right ventricular outflow tract (RVOT), pulmonary valve annulus, pulmonary valve, and pulmonary artery. In cases of R2A-type anomalous left coronary artery, the left coronary artery arises from the right coronary and traverses the RVOT/pulmonary valve annulus before forming the left circumflex coronary artery.[48] The proposed incision for patch grafting therefore leads to transection of the anomalous left coronary artery, resulting in patient death.[49] In such cases, either pulmonary valvulectomy or placement of a right ventricular to pulmonary artery conduit is required.[50–52]

Patch Graft (inflow occlusion): The patch-graft technique has been reported using either PTFE (Bard Peripheral Vascular Inc, Tempe, AZ, USA); Gore-Tex patch (W.L. Gore and Associated, Flagstaff, AZ, USA); or autogenous pericardium.[12,14,52] Inflow occlusion is preferred over the closed technique because it allows direct valve visualization, valvulectomy if necessary, and allows more accurate incision of the RVOT, pulmonary annulus, and valve.[12]

Several modifications of the original patch-graft technique have been described. The author currently prefers the incised-patch technique, utilizing a Gore-Tex patch and suture. Although the original technique described partial thickness incision of the RVOT prior to patch placement, this step is generally not performed because it can result in significant arrhythmia and hemorrhage. The patch is sutured onto the surface of the RVOT, pulmonary valve annulus, and pulmonary artery leaving redundant patch between the suture lines (**Fig. 7**). The patch is incised along its long axis and stay sutures are placed at the borders of this incision. Inflow occlusion is initiated and the heart allowed to empty. The published technique described pulmonary artery incision that is extended into the RVOT; however, the author has found that this technique risks incomplete transection of the pulmonary valve leaflets or hypertrophied RVOT. Full thickness incision of the RVOT is critical to successful reduction of the pressure gradient. Consequently, the procedure is modified using an initial RVOT stab incision that is then extended through the pulmonary valve and pulmonary artery. Care must be taken to avoid incision of the interventricular septum with the initial stab incision. The patch incision is clamped with a preselected, side-biting vascular clamp and inflow occlusion is released. The procedure is completed by closure of the patch incision using Gore-Tex suture (see **Fig. 7**).

Patch Graft (CPB): Patch graft for PS is simple when performed under CPB.[53] The RVOT, pulmonary artery, and valve are incised prior to patch placement. Myectomy or valvulectomy are performed and the patch sutured to the incision. This method achieves a more reliable reduction in pressure gradient; however, access to CPB is limited and expensive.

Double Chambered Right Ventricle

The terminology and classification of double chambered right ventricle (DVRC) has been recently questioned.[54,55] However, regardless of the terminology used or suspected lesion etiology, the pathophysiology of mid-right ventricular obstruction is identical. The lesion is a mid-ventricular obstruction of the right ventricle (RV), with a concentrically hypertrophied inflow portion and normal outflow portion of the RV. Although lesions may appear muscular on echocardiography, they are almost invariably associated with a fibrous ring when visualized directly. This fibrous constriction is likely the reason for the poor respond documented for balloon dilation of DCRV.[46,54] In the author's experience, full resection of the fibrous band requires CPB. The resection is combined with myectomy and patch-graft placement over the region of stenosis. Brockman and colleagues[14] recently reported a method for patch-graft placement combined with elliptical resection of the RV wall over the DCRV lesion, utilizing inflow occlusion. Whether this procedure can be performed consistently without damaging the tricuspid valve apparatus is yet to be demonstrated.

Subaortic Stenosis

Unlike other congenital cardiac diseases, the lesion of subaortic stenosis (SAS) is not present at birth and instead develops during the first 3 to 8 weeks of life. In human

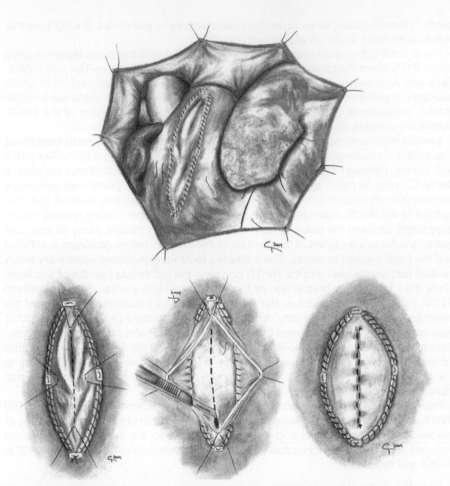

Fig. 7. Patch-graft placement for treatment of pulmonic stenosis under inflow occlusion. A Gore-Tex patch sutured onto the surface of the RVOT, pulmonary valve annulus, and pulmonary artery, leaving redundant patch between the suture lines (*top*). The patch is incised along its long axis and stay sutures placed at the borders of this incision (*bottom left*). A stab incision is made in the RVOT, extended through the pulmonary valve annulus and into the pulmonary artery (*bottom center*). Following re-institution of flow, the patch incision is closed using Gore-Tex suture (*bottom right*).

patients, several anatomic precursors have been suggested to be important causative factors in the development of SAS, although the definitive etiology remains unknown.[56] A spectrum of disease is recognized with discrete SAS lesions defined as a thin fibrous membrane, whereas tunnel SAS is associated with a thicker fibromuscular narrowing of the left ventricular outflow tract (LVOT).

Orton and colleagues[21] utilized a transaortic approach for membranectomy, with or without quadratic septal myectomy, for surgical correction of SAS in 22 dogs. Although this approach resulted in significant reduction in LVOT pressure gradient, surgical resection failed to improve survival time when compared to patients treated with beta-blocker therapy alone.

Results of surgical correction of SAS in humans vary according to anatomy of the lesion. Discrete SAS has been reported to have a 10-year mortality rate around 6%

and reoperation rates of 11% to 16.5%.[57,58] Results for tunnel SAS lesions are significantly less promising with 40-year mortality rates of 16% and reoperation rate of 70% reported.[57] Although these results exceed those published for canine patients, SAS in humans is still associated with a high risk for mortality or reoperation even after a successful surgical resection. Although it is possible that more aggressive surgical resection, including early intervention, routine use of myectomy, and intervention, in patients with mild-to-moderate gradients (30–50 mmHg pressure gradient) may improve survival rates in canine patients, the results from human studies suggest that surgical intervention is unlikely to ever be considered curative in all patients.

Atrial Septal Defect

Failure of the complex embryologic development of the atrial septum results in atrial septal defect (ASD). Knowledge of this embryology is critical in understanding the anatomical variations described for ASD.[59,60] Ostium primum ASD is located directly above the atrioventricular (AV) valve annulus. Ostium secundum ASD is located in the middle of the interatrial septum, in the location of the normal fossa ovalis. Patent foramen ovale is a failure of permanent closure of the fossa ovalis. Finally, sinus venosus ASD is located at the junction of the right atrium and cranial vena cava.[60,61]

Patients with small isolated ASDs have a good long-term prognosis and do not require treatment.[62] The decision to surgically intervene for ASD is based on presence of clinical signs or assessment of hemodynamic significance of the lesion. Development of significant pulmonary hypertension caused by elevated pulmonary vascular resistance represents a contraindication to surgical ASD closure. Consequently, pulmonary artery pressure and vascular resistance should be assessed prior to ASD closure.[63–65]

Surgical closure of ASD requires CPB. Atrial septal defect is often a concurrent lesion and should be closed at the same time as the primary lesion.[62] Careful inspection of pulmonary vein anatomy is required to identify and correct partial anomalous pulmonary drainage. Closure is achieved using horizontal mattress sutures for small defects or a patch of pericardium or Gore-Tex for larger defects.[61,66]

Ventricular Septal Defect

Embryologic development of the ventricular septum involves complex interplay between the developing trabecular, inlet, membranous, and conal/infundibular septal regions.[59,60] Failure of embryologic development of the ventricular septum results in muscular (trabecular septum); inlet (inlet septum, commonly associated with ostium primum ASD resulting in AV septal defect); perimembranous (membranous septum); or infundibular/supracristal/subaortic (conal/infundibular septum) VSD, respectively.[60,67] Hemodynamic significance and secondary consequences of ventricular septal defect must be assessed prior to formulating the therapeutic plan.[68]

Although hemodynamically significant VSD can be palliated with pulmonary artery banding, definitive repair requires CPB. Closure is best accomplished via right atriotomy, however, with complex lesions or supracristal VSDs right ventriculotomy may be required.[68] Closure of VSD is achieved by placement of a Gore-Tex or pericardial patch. The bundle of His is located on the left side of the septum at the caudal border of perimembranous VSD lesions. Knowledge of this anatomy is essential for avoiding conduction system damage during VSD repair.[68]

Tetralogy of Fallot

Tetralogy of Fallot is one of several complex congenital heart defects resulting from abnormal embryologic conotruncal development. Tetralogy of Fallot is comprised of PS, subaortic VSD, overriding aorta, and right ventricular hypertrophy. The degree of right ventricular outflow tract obstruction is critical in determining patient hemodynamics and clinical presentation. Indications for surgical intervention include development of progressive polycythemia or syncopal episodes (tet spells).

Palliative and definitive surgical procedures have been described for treatment of tetralogy of Fallot.[69–72] Palliative procedures aim to increase pulmonary blood flow through creation of an extracardiac systemic to pulmonary shunt. Although several techniques have been described, the modified Blalock-Taussig shunt is generally preferred.[69] Definitive correction under CPB comprises combined VSD and PS closure.[71]

Tricuspid Dysplasia

Congenital tricuspid valve malformation results in stenosis or regurgitation. The natural history of tricuspid valve dysplasia is difficult to predict, because a large proportion of patients remain subclinical despite severe valvular insufficiency.[73] Documentation of progressive right atrial and ventricular enlargement by sequential radiographic studies is thus essential before scheduling surgical correction.

Septal leaflet elongation; septal leaflet adherence to the interventricular septum; short/absent chordae; direct papillary muscle insertion onto the leaflets; papillary muscle fusion; and hypertrophy are all commonly reported in dogs with tricuspid dysplasia.[74] Results of valve repair have been disappointing because of the severity of the valve abnormalities (Leigh G. Griffiths, VetMB, MRCVS, PhD, unpublished data, 2010). Replacement with a glutaraldehyde-fixed bioprosthetic valve is currently the treatment of choice for tricuspid dysplasia.[75]

Mitral Dysplasia

Mitral valve dysplasia most commonly leads to valvular insufficiency, valve stenosis is less common. Surgical intervention is reserved until patients have shown progressive left atrial and ventricular dilation, or more commonly left-sided congestive heart failure.

The most common findings are restrictive septal or parietal leaflet motion, short thick primary chordae, chordal fusion, direct leaflet to papillary muscle attachment, hypertrophied or fused papillary muscles, and secondary annular dilation.[18,76] Mitral valve replacement and mitral repair have been successfully used for treatment of mitral dysplasia.[18,77,78] Mitral valve repair utilizes annuloplasty to correct secondary annular dilation.[18] Chordal and papillary muscle fenestration are used to correct restrictive leaflet motion.[18] In cases where leaflet prolapse or chordal absence are found, artificial chordae or edge-to-edge repair may be utilized.[18]

ACQUIRED HEART DEFECTS
Degenerative Mitral Valve Disease

The prevalence of myxomatous mitral valve degeneration is reported to be 58% in dogs greater than or equal to 9 years of age.[79] Prevalence of left apical holosystolic murmur in adult small breed dogs is 14.4%, with the majority of these patients having international small animal cardiac health council (ISACHC)[80] class I disease.[81] Because a large proportion of patients remain subclinical for throughout their lifetime, surgical correction is currently reserved for patients showing clinical signs (ISACHC class II or above).

The anatomic lesions of myxomatous mitral valve degeneration include nodular thickening of the valve apposition surfaces, chordal elongation or rupture, contraction of the remaining valve tissue, and secondary annular dilation.[79] Surgical intervention aims to correct the primary leaflet abnormality and secondary annular dilation.[18] These surgical goals can be achieved either by valve replacement[20,23,75,77,78] or mitral valve repair.[18]

Mitral valve replacement can be accomplished via sternotomy, right or left lateral thoracotomy.[20,23,75,77,78] The author prefers left lateral thoracotomy with cavoatrial venous cannulation because this affords simple aortic root dissection and excellent mitral valve visualization. The native mitral valve can either be completely resected[23,75,77,78] or the parietal leaflet can be preserved to maintain chordal and papillary muscle geometry.[20] Pledgeted horizontal mattress sutures are preplaced around the valve annulus and the valve parachuted into position.[20] Alternatively, valve placement can be achieved using a continuous suture pattern around the annulus. Short-term results of valve replacement are encouraging; however, bioprosthetic and mechanical replacement valves have significant limitations. Mechanical valves require lifelong anticoagulation that has proven challenging to consistently provide in veterinary patients.[20] The initial generation of glutaraldehyde-fixed bioprosthetic valves suffered from early calcification, thrombus formation, and pannus

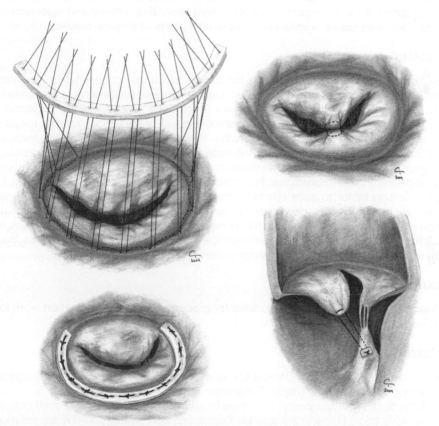

Fig. 8. Techniques reported for mitral valve repair in dogs. Mitral annuloplasty ring placement using a series of horizontal mattress sutures placed in the annulus of the mitral valve (*top left*). The ring is parachuted onto the valve annulus and the mattress sutures tied, resulting in placation of the mitral annulus (*bottom left*). Suture placement for edge-to-edge (Alfieri) repair of leaflet prolapse (*top right*). This repair utilizes the chordae of the unaffected leaflet to stabilize the affected leaflet, creating a double orifice valve in the process. Artificial chordae placement from the papillary muscle to the septal leaflet of the mitral valve (*bottom right*).

encroachment in dogs.[75] The current generation of glutaraldehyde-fixed bioprosthetic valves may have been largely alleviated these problems.[82] However, even with the current generation of glutaraldehyde-fixed bioprosthetic valves and improved postoperative care strategies, the author has observed postoperative valve failure caused by thrombus or pannus formation (Leigh G. Griffiths, VetMB, MRCVS, PhD, unpublished results, 2010).

Mitral valve repair is an attractive alternative to valve replacement because it maintains the native valve. However, valve repair is technically challenging and presence of even mild residual valvular insufficiency complicates postoperative recovery. In contrast to human patients, septal leaflet prolapse is the predominant leaflet abnormality identified at surgery.[18] Valve repair focuses on addressing the primary leaflet abnormality with a combination of artificial chordae or edge-to-edge repair (**Fig. 8**).[18] Secondary annular dilation is corrected by annuloplasty ring placement, which is parachuted onto the annulus in the same manner as described for valve replacement (see earlier discussion; see **Fig. 8**).[18] Results of mitral valve repair are encouraging with approximately 70% of patients surviving surgery and resolution of congestive heart failure reported in approximately 75% of surgical survivors.[18]

SUMMARY

The feasibility of surgical correction for almost all canine congenital or acquired cardiac diseases has been demonstrated. Current surgical success rates are remarkably high considering the infrequency with which such procedures are performed. Such results are a testament to the dedication and skill of the various cardiac surgical teams offering these procedures worldwide. However, experience from the medical field indicates that the only way to increase success rates above those presently achieved will be to dramatically increase the frequency with which cardiac surgical teams perform these procedures. Fortunately, lack of case load does not appear to be the limiting factor to such efforts. Rather, lack of infrastructure and lack of man power are the major obstacles for expansion of cardiac surgical programs. The challenge in bringing cardiac surgery into the mainstream is to achieve a critical mass of expertise and personnel within each surgical program, to allow greater case load with its consequential increase in surgical consistency and success rates.

ACKNOWLEDGMENTS

Many thanks to Chrisoula Toupadakis for producing all of the original art work for this manuscript.

REFERENCES

1. de Leval MR, Carthey J, Wright DJ, et al. Human factors and cardiac surgery: a multicenter study. J Thorac Cardiovasc Surg 2000;119:661.
2. ElBardissi AW, Wiegmann DA, Henrickson S, et al. Identifying methods to improve heart surgery: an operative approach and strategy for implementation on an organizational level. Eur J Cardiothorac Surg 2008;34:1027.
3. Wiegmann DA, ElBardissi AW, Dearani JA, et al. Disruptions in surgical flow and their relationship to surgical errors: an exploratory investigation. Surgery 2007;142:658.
4. Cohn LH. What the cardiothoracic surgeon of the twenty-first century ought to be. J Thorac Cardiovasc Surg 1999;118:581.
5. Lillehei CW, Todd DB Jr, Levy MJ, et al. Partial cardiopulmonary bypass, hypothermia, and total circulatory arrest. A lifesaving technique for ruptured mycotic

aortic aneurysms, ruptured left ventricle, and other complicated cardiac pathology. J Thorac Cardiovasc Surg 1969;58:530.

6. Cohen M, Hammerstrom RN, Spellman MW, et al. The tolerance of the canine heart to temporary complete vena caval occlusion. Surg Forum 1953;(38th Congress):172–7.

7. Read RC, Lillehei CW, Varco RL. Cardiac resuscitation and neurologic tolerance to anoxia. Circ Res 1956;4:45.

8. Hunt GB, Malik R, Bellenger CR, et al. Total venous inflow occlusion in the normo-thermic dog: a study of haemodynamic, metabolic and neurological conse-quences. Res Vet Sci 1992;52:371.

9. Niazi SA, Lewis FJ. Resumption of heartbeat in dogs after standstill at low temper-atures. Surg Forum 1955;5:113.

10. Swan H, Zeavin I, Holmes JH, et al. Cessation of circulation in general hypo-thermia. I. Physiologic changes and their control. Ann Surg 1953;138:360.

11. Bracha S, Caron I, Holmberg DL, et al. Ectopic thyroid carcinoma causing right ventricular outflow tract obstruction in a dog. J Am Anim Hosp Assoc 2009;45:138.

12. Orton EC, Bruecker KA, McCracken TO. An open patch-graft technique for correction of pulmonic stenosis in the dog. Vet Surg 1990;19:148.

13. Bright JM, Toal RL, Blackford LA. Right ventricular outflow obstruction caused by primary cardiac neoplasia. Clinical features in two dogs. J Vet Intern Med 1990;4:12.

14. Brockman DJ, Borer KE, Baines SJ, et al. Partial right ventriculectomy using the incised patch technique to treat double chambered right ventricle and chylothor-ax in a cat. Vet Surg 2009;38:631.

15. Iizuka T, Hoshi K, Ishida Y, et al. Right atriotomy using total venous inflow occlu-sion for removal of heartworms in a cat. J Vet Med Sci 2009;71:489.

16. Cohen M, Lillehei CW. A quantitative study of the azygos factor during vena caval occlusion in the dog. Surg Gynecol Obstet 1954;98:225.

17. Soda A, Tanaka R, Saida Y, et al. Successful surgical correction of supravalvular pulmonary stenosis under beating heart using a cardiopulmonary bypass system in a dog. J Vet Med Sci 2009;71:203.

18. Griffiths LG, Orton EC, Boon JA. Evaluation of techniques and outcomes of mitral valve repair in dogs. J Am Vet Med Assoc 2004;224:1941.

19. Monnet E, Orton EC, Gaynor JS, et al. Open resection for subvalvular aortic stenosis in dogs. J Am Vet Med Assoc 1996;209:1255.

20. Orton EC, Hackett TB, Mama K, et al. Technique and outcome of mitral valve replacement in dogs. J Am Vet Med Assoc 2005;226:1508.

21. Orton EC, Herndon GD, Boon JA, et al. Influence of open surgical correction on intermediate-term outcome in dogs with subvalvular aortic stenosis: 44 cases (1991–1998). J Am Vet Med Assoc 2000;216:364.

22. Klement P, del Nido PJ, Mickleborough L, et al. Technique and postoperative management for successful cardiopulmonary bypass and open-heart surgery in dogs. J Am Vet Med Assoc 1987;190:869.

23. Klement P, Feindel CM, Scully HE, et al. Mitral valve replacement in dogs. Surgical technique and postoperative management. Vet Surg 1987;16:231.

24. Bennett EV Jr, Fewel JG, Grover FL, et al. Myocardial preservation: effect of venous drainage. Ann Thorac Surg 1983;36:132.

25. Follette D, Fey K, Becker H, et al. Superiority of blood cardioplegia over asangui-nous cardioplegia–an experimental and clinical study. Chir Forum Exp Klin Forsch 1980;142:279.

26. Buckberg GD, Allen BS, Beyersdorf F. Blood cardioplegia strategies during adult cardiac operations. In: Piper HM, Preusse CJ, editors. Ischemia-reperfusion in cardiac surgery. Boston: Kluwer Academic Publishers; 1992. p. 181.

27. Kronon MT, Allen BS, Bolling KS, et al. The role of cardioplegia induction temperature and amino acid enrichment in neonatal myocardial protection. Ann Thorac Surg 2000;70:756.

28. Ellis H. Lungs: blood supply, lymphatic drainage and nerve supply. Anaesth Intensive Care Med 2005;6:362.

29. Hogan DF, Green HW, Gordon S, et al. Transarterial coil embolization of patent ductus arteriosus in small dogs with 0.025-inch vascular occlusion coils: 10 cases. J Vet Intern Med 2004;18:325.

30. Goodrich KR, Kyles AE, Kass PH, et al. Retrospective comparison of surgical ligation and transarterial catheter occlusion for treatment of patent ductus arteriosus in two hundred and four dogs (1993–2003). Vet Surg 2007;36:43.

31. Campbell FE, Thomas WP, Miller SJ, et al. Immediate and late outcomes of transarterial coil occlusion of patent ductus arteriosus in dogs. J Vet Intern Med 2006; 20:83.

32. Stokhof AA, Sreeram N, Wolvekamp WT. Transcatheter closure of patent ductus arteriosus using occluding spring coils. J Vet Intern Med 2000;14:452.

33. Nguyenba TP, Tobias AH. Minimally invasive per-catheter patent ductus arteriosus occlusion in dogs using a prototype duct occluder. J Vet Intern Med 2008; 22:129.

34. Van Israel N, French AT, Dukes-McEwan J, et al. Review of left-to-right shunting patent ductus arteriosus and short term outcome in 98 dogs. J Small Anim Pract 2002;43:395.

35. Hunt GB, Simpson DJ, Beck JA, et al. Intraoperative hemorrhage during patent ductus arteriosus ligation in dogs. Vet Surg 2001;30:58.

36. Bellenger CR, Hunt GB, Goldsmid SE, et al. Outcomes of thoracic surgery in dogs and cats. Aust Vet J 1996;74:25.

37. Eyster GE, Eyster JT, Cords GB, et al. Patent ductus arteriosus in the dog: characteristics of occurrence and results of surgery in one hundred consecutive cases. J Am Vet Med Assoc 1976;168:435.

38. Birchard SJ, Bonagura JD, Fingland RB. Results of ligation of patent ductus arteriosus in dogs: 201 cases (1969–1988). J Am Vet Med Assoc 1990;196:2011.

39. Bureau S, Monnet E, Orton EC. Evaluation of survival rate and prognostic indicators for surgical treatment of left-to-right patent ductus arteriosus in dogs: 52 cases (1995–2003). J Am Vet Med Assoc 2005;227:1794.

40. Bussadori C, DeMadron E, Santilli RA, et al. Balloon valvuloplasty in 30 dogs with pulmonic stenosis: effect of valve morphology and annular size on initial and 1-year outcome. J Vet Intern Med 2001;15:553.

41. Estrada A, Moise NS, Erb HN, et al. Prospective evaluation of the balloon-to-annulus ratio for valvuloplasty in the treatment of pulmonic stenosis in the dog. J Vet Intern Med 2006;20:862.

42. Estrada A, Moise NS, Renaud-Farrell S. When, how and why to perform a double ballooning technique for dogs with valvular pulmonic stenosis. J Vet Cardiol 2005;7:41.

43. Griffiths LG, Bright JM, Chan KC. Transcatheter intravascular stent placement to relieve supravalvular pulmonic stenosis. J Vet Cardiol 2006;8:145.

44. Johnson MS, Martin M. Results of balloon valvuloplasty in 40 dogs with pulmonic stenosis. J Small Anim Pract 2004;45:148.

45. Johnson MS, Martin M, Edwards D, et al. Pulmonic stenosis in dogs: balloon dilation improves clinical outcome. J Vet Intern Med 2004;18:656.

46. Schrope DP. Primary pulmonic infundibular stenosis in 12 cats: natural history and the effects of balloon valvuloplasty. J Vet Cardiol 2008;10:33.

47. Buchanan JW. Pathogenesis of single right coronary artery and pulmonic stenosis in English Bulldogs. J Vet Intern Med 2001;15:101.
48. Buchanan JW. Pulmonic stenosis caused by single coronary artery in dogs: four cases (1965–1984). J Am Vet Med Assoc 1990;196:115.
49. Minami T, Wakao Y, Buchanan J, et al. A case of pulmonic stenosis with single coronary artery in a dog. Nippon Juigaku Zasshi 1989;51:453.
50. Fiore AC, Peigh PS, Sears NJ, et al. The prevention of extra cardiac conduit obstruction: an experimental study. J Surg Res 1983;34:463.
51. Khanna SK, Anstadt MP, Bhimji S, et al. Apico-aortic conduits in children with severe left ventricular outflow tract obstruction. Ann Thorac Surg 2002;73:81.
52. Hunt GB, Pearson MR, Bellenger CR, et al. Use of a modified open patch-graft technique and valvulectomy for correction of severe pulmonic stenosis in dogs: eight consecutive cases. Aust Vet J 1993;70:244.
53. Tanaka R, Shimizu M, Hoshi K, et al. Efficacy of open patch-grafting under cardiopulmonary bypass for pulmonic stenosis in small dogs. Aust Vet J 2009;87:88.
54. Minors SL, O'Grady MR, Williams RM, et al. Clinical and echocardiographic features of primary infundibular stenosis with intact ventricular septum in dogs. J Vet Intern Med 2006;20:1344.
55. Martin JM, Orton EC, Boon JA, et al. Surgical correction of double-chambered right ventricle in dogs. J Am Vet Med Assoc 2002;220:770.
56. Barkhordarian R, Wen-Hong D, Li W, et al. Geometry of the left ventricular outflow tract in fixed subaortic stenosis and intact ventricular septum: an echocardiographic study in children and adults. J Thorac Cardiovasc Surg 2007;133:196.
57. Ruzmetov M, Vijay P, Rodefeld MD, et al. Long-term results of surgical repair in patients with congenital subaortic stenosis. Interact Cardiovasc Thorac Surg 2006;5:227.
58. Erentug V, Bozbuga N, Kirali K, et al. Surgical treatment of subaortic obstruction in adolescent and adults: long-term follow-up. J Card Surg 2005;20:16.
59. Bishop SP. Embryologic development: the heart and great vessels. In: Fox PR, editor. Textbook of canine and feline cardiology. 2nd edition. Philadelphia: WB Saunders; 1999. p. 3.
60. Reller MD, McDonald RW, Gerlis LM, et al. Cardiac embryology: basic review and clinical correlations. J Am Soc Echocardiogr 1991;4:519.
61. Stark JF, Tsang VT. Secundum atrial septal defect and partial anomalous pulmonary venous return. In: Stark JF, deLeval MR, Tsang VT, editors. Surgery for congenital heart defects. 3rd edition. Chichester, West Sussex (UK): Wiley; 2006. p. 343.
62. Guglielmini C, Diana A, Pietra M, et al. Atrial septal defect in five dogs. J Small Anim Pract 2002;43:317.
63. Moake L, Ramaciotti C. Atrial septal defect treatment options. AACN Clin Issues 2005;16:252.
64. Marie Valente A, Rhodes JF. Current indications and contraindications for transcatheter atrial septal defect and patent foramen ovale device closure. Am Heart J 2007;153:81.
65. Gordon SG, Miller MW, Roland RM, et al. Transcatheter atrial septal defect closure with the Amplatzer atrial septal occluder in 13 dogs: short- and mid-term outcome. J Vet Intern Med 2009;23:995.
66. Eyster GE, Anderson LK, Krehbeil JD, et al. Surgical repair of atrial septal defect in a dog. J Am Vet Med Assoc 1976;169:1081.
67. Goor DA, Lillehei CW, Rees R, et al. Isolated ventricular septal defect. Development basis for various types and presentation of classification. Chest 1970; 58:468.

68. VanDoorn C, DeLeval MR. Ventricular septal defects. In: Stark JF, deLeval MR, Tsang VT, editors. Surgery for congenital heart defects. 3rd edition. Chichester, West Sussex (UK): Wiley; 2006. p. 355.
69. Brockman DJ, Holt DE, Gaynor JW, et al. Long-term palliation of tetralogy of Fallot in dogs by use of a modified Blalock-Taussig shunt. J Am Vet Med Assoc 2007; 231:721.
70. Weber UT, Carrel T, Lang J, et al. [Palliative treatment of tetralogy of Fallot using a PTFE (polytetrafluoroethylene) vascular graft]. Schweiz Arch Tierheilkd 1995; 137:480 [in German].
71. Orton EC, Mama K, Hellyer P, et al. Open surgical repair of tetralogy of Fallot in dogs. J Am Vet Med Assoc 2001;219:1089.
72. Lew LJ, Fowler JD, McKay R, et al. Open-heart correction of tetralogy of Fallot in an acyanotic dog. J Am Vet Med Assoc 1998;213:652.
73. Hoffmann G, Amberger CN, Seiler G, et al. [Tricuspid valve dysplasia in fifteen dogs]. Schweiz Arch Tierheilkd 2000;142:268 [in German].
74. Liu SK, Tilley LP. Dysplasia of the tricuspid valve in the dog and cat. J Am Vet Med Assoc 1976;169:623.
75. Breznock EM. Tricuspid and mitral valvular disease: valve replacement. Semin Vet Med Surg (Small Anim) 1994;9:234.
76. Litu SK, Tilley LP. Malformation of the canine mitral valve complex. J Am Vet Med Assoc 1975;167:465.
77. White RN, Stepien RL, Hammond RA, et al. Mitral valve replacement for the treatment of congenital mitral dysplasia in a bull terrier. J Small Anim Pract 1995;36:407.
78. Behr L, Chetboul V, Sampedrano CC, et al. Beating heart mitral valve replacement with a bovine pericardial bioprosthesis for treatment of mitral valve dysplasia in a Bull Terrier. Vet Surg 2007;36:190.
79. Whitney JC. Observations on the effect of age on the severity of heart valve lesions in the dog. J Small Anim Pract 1974;15:511.
80. International Small Animal Cardiac Health Council. Appendix A. Recommendations for diagnosis of heart disease and treatment of heart failure in small animals. In: Fox PR, Sisson D, Moise NS, editors. Textbook of canine and feline cardiology. 2nd edition. Philadelphia: W.B Saunders Co; 1999. p. 883.
81. Serfass P, Chetboul V, Sampedrano CC, et al. Retrospective study of 942 small-sized dogs: prevalence of left apical systolic heart murmur and left-sided heart failure, critical effects of breed and sex. J Vet Cardiol 2006;8:11.
82. Takashima K, Soda A, Tanaka R, et al. Long-term clinical evaluation of mitral valve replacement with porcine bioprosthetic valves in dogs. J Vet Med Sci 2008;70:279.

Pulmonary Hypertension in Dogs: Diagnosis and Therapy

Heidi B. Kellihan, DVM*, Rebecca L. Stepien, DVM, MS

KEYWORDS

- Sildenafil • Pulmonary disease • Syncope • Heart disease
- Echocardiographic • Right heart catheterization

> *"You see only what you look for. You recognize only what you know."*
> —*Merril C. Sosman*

In the veterinary literature, pulmonary hypertension (PH) has been echocardiographically defined as pulmonary arterial systolic pressure greater than approximately 30 mm Hg.[1–6] PH is a complex syndrome that has historically resulted in a poor prognosis. Pulmonary arterial pressure (PAP) is influenced by pulmonary blood flow, pulmonary vascular resistance (PVR), and pulmonary venous pressure. The elevated PAP of the syndrome of PH may be caused by pulmonary vascular abnormalities associated with increased blood flow (ie, "hyperkinetic" PH secondary to a patent ductus arteriosus), changes affecting resistance to flow (precapillary pulmonary arterial hypertension, PAH) or caused by increased "downstream" resistance (postcapillary pulmonary venous hypertension, PVH). Pulmonary arterial hypertension has a multifactorial pathophysiology that results from the imbalance of endogenous and exogenous pulmonary artery (PA) vasodilators and vasoconstrictors, ultimately resulting in vasoconstriction, vascular smooth-muscle-cell proliferation, and thrombosis. Diagnosis of PH requires diagnostic testing that quantifies the degree of elevation of PAP, determines the underlying disease process if possible, and identifies the degree of hemodynamic impairment. Significant advances in therapy that target the derangements of the PH pathophysiology have been made in animals and people, providing an improved prognosis for survival and better quality of life.

Department of Medical Sciences, School of Veterinary Medicine, University of Wisconsin, 2015 Linden Drive, Madison, WI 53706, USA
* Corresponding author.
E-mail address: kellihanh@svm.vetmed.wisc.edu

Vet Clin Small Anim 40 (2010) 623–641
doi:10.1016/j.cvsm.2010.03.011
0195-5616/10/$ – see front matter © 2010 Elsevier Inc. All rights reserved.

vetsmall.theclinics.com

CLASSIFICATION OF PULMONARY HYPERTENSION

Pulmonary hypertension can be classified as pre- or postcapillary PH, or can be classified based on the disease process causing PH. The categories include pulmonary arterial hypertension, pulmonary venous hypertension, hypoxic PH, PH secondary to respiratory disease, PH secondary to thromboembolic disease, and PH secondary to miscellaneous etiologies (**Table 1**).[1–36] The etiology of PH may affect therapeutic choices, as some causes of PH can be rectified (eg, patent ductus arteriosus occlusion), thereby eliminating the PH.

There have been a limited number of published studies that evaluated naturally occurring PH in dogs. Previous investigators have described PH in specific canine hospital populations (**Table 2**).[1,3,4,6,13] Left-sided heart disease is a common cause of PH in dogs in these studies. Pulmonary hypertension secondary to left-sided heart disease occurs from elevated left atrial pressure (pulmonary venous hypertension) and may be compounded by reactive PA vasoconstriction occurring in response to hypoxia from pulmonary edema if severe left heart failure is present. In contrast to the systemic vasculature that responds to hypoxia with vasodilation to better perfuse

Table 1
Classification of pulmonary hypertension with mechanisms indicated

1. Pulmonary Arterial Hypertension
 • Heartworm disease (↑PVRI)
 • Congenital systemic-to-pulmonary shunts (↑PA blood flow)
  Atrial septal defect (ASD)
  Ventricular septal defect (VSD)
  Patent ductus arteriosus (PDA)
 • Idiopathic
 • Necrotising vasculitis/arteritis

2. Pulmonary Hypertension with Left Heart Disease (↑pulmonary venous pressure) • Mitral valve disease • Myocardial disease • Miscellaneous left-sided heart diseases
3. Pulmonary Hypertension with Pulmonary Disease or Hypoxia (↑PVRI) • Chronic obstructive pulmonary disease • Interstitial pulmonary fibrosis • Neoplasia • High-altitude disease • Reactive pulmonary artery vasoconstriction (eg, hypoxia owing to pulmonary edema)

4. Pulmonary Hypertension owing to Thrombotic and/or Embolic Disease (↑PVRI)
 • Thromboembolism
  Immune-mediated hemolytic anemia
  Neoplasia
  Cardiac disease
  Protein-losing disease (nephropathy or enteropathy)
  Hyperadrenocorticism
  Disseminated intravascular coagulation
  Sepsis
  Trauma
  Recent surgery
 • Heartworm disease

5. Miscellaneous • Compressive mass lesions (neoplasia, granuloma)

Abbreviations: PA, pulmonary artery; PVRI, pulmonary vascular resistance index.

Table 2 Diseases associated with canine pulmonary hypertension in clinical canine populations (references noted)	Johnson 1999[3] N = 53	Pyle 2004[6] N = 54	Bach 2006[4] N = 13	Kellum 2007[1] N = 22	Serres 2007[13] N = 60
Left-sided heart disease	23 (43%)	24 (44%)	1 (8%)	9 (41%)	51 (85%)
Pulmonary disease	12 (23%)	22 (41%)	5 (38%)	11 (50%)	7 (12%)
Pulmonary overcirculation (ie, left to right cardiovascular shunts)	2 (4%)	1 (2%)	1 (8%)	2 (9%)	0
Heartworm disease	5 (9%)	3 (6%)	0	0	0
Pulmonary thromboembolism	5 (9%)	2 (4%)	1 (8%)	0	1 (2%)
Miscellaneous	6 (11%)	2 (4%)	5 (38%)	0	1 (2%)

hypoxic tissue, the pulmonary vasculature responds to hypoxia by pulmonary artery vasoconstriction. Presumably, pulmonary arteries constrict to divert blood from diseased lung and preserve arterial oxygen content. In studies of dogs with mitral valve disease, prevalence of PH has been reported to be as low as 14% and as high as 31%.[14,37]

SIGNALMENT AND CLINICAL SIGNS

With the exception of dogs with PH related to congenital heart diseases, the populations of dogs that have been reported with PH are of smaller breeds and typically middle-aged to older; this distribution may reflect the predisposition of older small-breed dogs for mitral valve disease and chronic pulmonary conditions.[1,3,4,6,13] The clinical history of dogs with symptomatic PH typically includes combinations of cough, dyspnea, lethargy, syncope or collapse episodes, exercise intolerance, or reported heart murmurs or abdominal distension (ascites).[1,3–6,12–16,21–23,25,31–33,35,36,38,39] These clinical signs may be caused by the elevated pulmonary pressures or reflect the underlying disease that led to PH (eg, chronic obstructive pulmonary disease [COPD]).

PHYSICAL EXAMINATION

Physical examination findings associated with PH in dogs are variable and again may reflect elevated pulmonary arterial pressure, the underlying disease condition, or a combination of the two. Typical physical examination abnormalities include heart murmurs of mitral and/or tricuspid insufficiency, split or abnormally loud second heart sounds, pulmonary crackles, increased bronchovesicular pulmonary sounds, cyanosis, and ascites.[1,3,5,6,14,16,23,25,30,36] In most cases, detection of these physical examination findings in patients with typical historical presentations leads the clinician to suspect PH as a clinical diagnosis, but confirmation of PH requires further diagnostic testing.

DIAGNOSIS

The goals of diagnostic testing in the syndrome of PH are to identify the underlying etiology or etiologies resulting in PH (ie, classification), to quantify the degree of PH, to assess evidence of hemodynamic impairment, and to assist in patient prognostication. Right heart catheterization is the most accurate method of diagnosing PH but is often unavailable for routine clinical use. Ancillary testing, including thoracic radiography, electrocardiography, and measurement of biomarkers may provide supportive evidence for PH and information about concurrent or causative diseases in an individual patient. Two-dimensional and echocardiographic examinations provide the diagnosis in most clinical veterinary patients.

Right Heart Catheterization

Right heart catheterization is the gold standard for diagnosing PH. In clinical veterinary medicine the right heart catheterization procedure may be considered unacceptably invasive in a compromised patient, but when available, provides multiple hemodynamic parameters that assist in the diagnosis and etiologic classification of PH. Introduction of a hemodynamic catheter into the right atrium, right ventricle, and main pulmonary artery provides hemodynamic information regarding the presence and degree of PH as well as information regarding the function of the right heart (eg, elevated end diastolic right ventricular pressures may indicate right ventricular systolic or diastolic impairment). The systolic, diastolic, and mean PAPs can be measured directly, and the pulmonary arterial wedge pressure (PAWP) can be measured to detect elevated pulmonary venous pressures.

In veterinary patients, the systolic PAP is often used to quantify the degree of PH because this value can also be estimated by noninvasive methods (Doppler echocardiography, see Echocardiography, later). Invasively measured mean PAP and PAWP can be used to calculate the PVR index (PVRI, per m^2), a measure of the vascular resistance to pulmonary blood flow that can assist in distinguishing precapillary (attributable to pulmonary vascular disease) from postcapillary (attributable to pulmonary venous hypertension) PH (**Table 3**).[40] PVRI is calculated according to the following equation and expressed as dynes*sec*cm^{-5}/m^2:

$$PVRI = [PAPm - PAWP] \times 80/CI,$$

where PAPm indicates mean pulmonary artery pressure; PAWP, pulmonary arterial wedge pressure; and CI, cardiac index.

The definition of pulmonary arterial hypertension (precapillary, elevated PAP with normal left atrial pressure, usually seen in pulmonary vascular diseases) is increased PAPm, increased PVRI, and normal PAWP. The definition of pulmonary venous hypertension (postcapillary, elevated PAP with elevated left atrial pressure, usually seen with left heart disease) is increased PAPm, increased PAWP, and normal PVRI. When reactive precapillary PAH (eg, attributable to hypoxia from pulmonary edema) there is increased PAPm, increased PAWP, and increased PVRI (see **Table 3**).[41]

Table 3
Invasive hemodynamic definitions of pulmonary hypertension

Definition	Characteristics	Clinical Group(s)
Pulmonary hypertension	↑ PAP	All
Precapillary PH (pulmonary arterial hypertension)	↑ PAP ↑ PVRI Normal PAWP	Pulmonary arterial hypertension (class 1) PH secondary to pulmonary disease or hypoxia (class 3) PH secondary to thromboembolic disease (class 4)
Postcapillary PH (pulmonary venous hypertension)	↑ PAP Normal PVRI ↑ PAWP	PH secondary to left-sided heart disease (class 2)

When noted, classes are as indicated in **Table 1**.

Abbreviations: PAP, pulmonary artery pressure; PAWP, pulmonary arterial wedge pressure; PH, pulmonary hypertension; PVRI, pulmonary vascular resistance index.

Thoracic Radiography

Pulmonary hypertension cannot be diagnosed based on thoracic radiographic findings alone, but radiographic findings suggestive or supportive of PH include pulmonary artery enlargement, pulmonary infiltrates, right-heart enlargement, pulmonary arterial tortuosity, and the pulmonary arterial "pruning" associated with heartworm (HW) disease. Conversely, in some severe cases of PH, the radiographic abnormalities may be minimal (**Fig. 1**). Often, the thoracic radiographic findings are complicated by underlying cardiopulmonary disease; these findings may help in determining the underlying etiology of the PH (ie, left-heart disease, patent ductus arteriosus [PDA], pulmonary neoplasia).

Electrocardiogram

Electrocardiographic findings are often normal in patients with pulmonary hypertension, but findings supportive of a diagnosis of PH include right axis deviation or other evidence of right-heart enlargement (**Fig. 2**). The electrocardiographic findings may also represent changes that have occurred secondary to the underlying disease process (ie, supraventricular or ventricular arrhythmias associated with left-sided cardiac disease, bradyarrhythmias and atrioventricular blocks associated with increased parasympathetic tone seen in pulmonary disease).

Biomarkers

NT-proBNP (N-terminal-pro-B-type natriuretic peptide), a peptide released by ventricular myocardium under circumstances of stress or strain, appears to have some potential in aiding in the diagnosis of PH. Typically, NT-proBNP has been used to discriminate between cardiac and respiratory disease in dogs.[42] In people, NT-proBNP is elevated in the presence of precapillary PH, and it has been used to stratify disease severity, monitor response to treatment, and serve as a prognostic parameter.[43-45] NT-proBNP measurements were found to be higher in canine clinical patients with precapillary PH than in normal dogs, and moderate to severe and severe PH resulted in higher NT-proBNP concentrations versus dogs with no or mild PH (Heidi B. Kellihan, DVM, unpublished data, Madison, WI, June 2009). There was

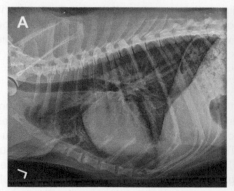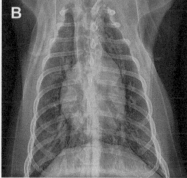

Fig. 1. Thoracic radiographs. Lateral (A) and ventral dorsal (B) thoracic radiographs from a dog with severe PH secondary to presumed pulmonary fibrosis. The cardiac silhouette and pulmonary vessels are normal in size and shape despite the presence of significant PH (systolic PAP estimated at 86 mm Hg). Interstitial to alveolar infiltrates cranial and caudal to the cardiac silhouette reflect the presence of chronic pulmonary disease.

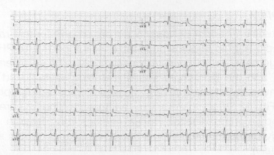

Fig. 2. Electrocardiogram. Electrocardiogram from a dog with severe PH secondary to a large thrombus in the main pulmonary artery. Right axis deviation consistent with right heart enlargement is present: 50 mm/s, 0.5 cm: 1 mV.

a strong positive correlation between the measured tricuspid regurgitation (TR) peak systolic gradient (estimated systolic pulmonary artery pressure) and NT-proBNP concentrations (r = 0.89, P = .0005) (Heidi B. Kellihan, DVM, unpublished data, Madison, WI, June 2009).

Echocardiography

Echocardiography is the standard, noninvasive method of diagnosing PH in clinical veterinary patients. Multiple echocardiographic modalities, including 2-dimensional imaging, Doppler flow examinations, and tissue Doppler examinations offer complementary information in the diagnosis of PH. Doppler flow interrogations of tricuspid insufficiency and pulmonary insufficiency jets provide estimates of systolic and diastolic PAP pressure respectively, allowing diagnosis and quantification of PH. Tissue Doppler imaging has been used to detect elevated PAP based on right ventricular myocardial movement.[13] Echocardiographic examination can be used to detect PH-related right-sided cardiac abnormalities, such as main pulmonary artery enlargement, functional changes, through the use of systolic time intervals, and concurrent left-sided heart disease. Two-dimensional echocardiography also allows identification of related disease findings such as thrombi or, occasionally, heartworms. Clinical signs such as respiratory distress may interfere with examination and limit the quality of individual echocardiographic recordings; the use of multiple echocardiographic imaging modalities for diagnosis is recommended to identify the maximum number of "supportive" findings in patients in whom direct estimation of PAP via Doppler flow interrogation is not possible.

Tricuspid regurgitation

In the absence of right ventricular outflow tract obstruction, right ventricular and pulmonary artery pressures are equivalent during systole and quantitative assessment of a TR jet provides an estimate of systolic PAP. The tricuspid transvalvular pressure gradient is estimated using the peak TR velocity (m/sec) in the modified Bernoulli equation (pressure gradient = 4 * [peak flow velocity]^2). This estimated pressure difference approximates the systolic PAP (**Fig. 3**). The TR systolic peak velocity and resulting estimated right ventricular systolic pressure is used to classify PH severity (**Table 4**).[1,3,5] In people, there is conflicting evidence as to the correlation of noninvasive TR gradient-derived estimations of PAP to invasively measured systolic PAP obtained by right heart catheterization.[46,47] The addition of estimated right atrial pressures to the measured TR peak gradient is performed by some investigators, and is

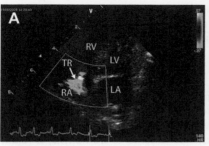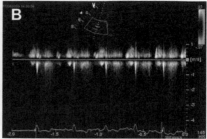

Fig. 3. Tricuspid regurgitation. Doppler echocardiographic images from a dog with moderate pulmonary hypertension secondary to presumed pulmonary fibrosis. (*A*) Color Doppler map of tricuspid regurgitation (TR). The TR flow is from the higher pressure right ventricle (RV) to the lower pressure right atrium (RA). The left ventricle (LV) and left atrium (LA) are also labeled. Image obtained from the left apical 4-chamber view. (*B*) Spectral Doppler trace of TR. Tricuspid systolic velocity of approximately 3.7 m/s, indicating a peak tricuspid gradient of approximately 54 mm Hg (moderate pulmonary hypertension). Velocities were recorded from the left apical 4-chamber view.

believed by some investigators to provide a more accurate assessment of PH.[5,46] More recent human data suggest that the addition of estimated right arterial (RA) pressure may lead to overestimation of PH severity, and confirmed that inaccurate TR jet velocity measurement (related to poor signal strength or poor jet alignment) leads to underestimation of PAP.[47] Difficulty obtaining an optimal peak systolic TR measurement is common in clinical patients and may be attributable to poor patient compliance with the echocardiographic procedure, poor image quality secondary to pulmonary disease/dyspnea, or poor jet alignment with the Doppler interrogation beam. Tricuspid insufficiency jet peak velocity is also affected by right ventricular function; in cases where right ventricular myocardial failure is present, PAPs assessed by echocardiography may inadequately reflect the severity of pulmonary vascular disease because of the inability of the right ventricular (RV) myocardium to generate high pressures.[8] Some patients with PH do not have identifiable TR and other findings (eg, pulmonary insufficiency peak velocity) must be used to identify elevated PAP. Peak TR systolic velocity gradients are the most frequently used echocardiographic surrogate for PAP in clinical patients, but the situational limitations of such estimates must be kept in mind during examination, and additional supportive information sought when a diagnosis of PH is contemplated.

Pulmonic insufficiency
The presence of pulmonic insufficiency (PI) allows for the quantitative assessment of estimated diastolic PAP. Pulmonic insufficiency occurs in diastole and allows estimation of the PA-to-RV pressure difference. Similar to TR measurements, the velocity of

Table 4
Pulmonary hypertension severity grading system based on peak tricuspid regurgitation velocity and associated TR gradient

	Mild	Moderate	Severe
TR peak systolic velocity (m/s)	≥ 2.8 to < 3.5	3.5–4.3	>4.3
TR systolic gradient (mm Hg)	≥ 31.4 to < 50	50–75	>75

Abbreviation: TR, tricuspid regurgitation.

the PI jet (m/s) is used to calculate the gradient (mm Hg) using the modified Bernoulli equation. This echocardiographic measurement is especially helpful in diagnosing PH if TR is not present. A PI velocity 2.2 m/s or more or a gradient of 19 mm Hg or higher is elevated and suggestive of PH (**Fig. 4**).[1]

Pulmonary artery systolic flow profiles

Scrutiny of PA systolic flow profiles has been used in people and dogs to estimate the severity of PH.[1,3,5,13,22,26,35,41,48,49] Pulmonary artery systolic flow profiles are obtained by measuring the PA blood flow with pulse wave Doppler immediately after the pulmonic valve in the PA. Type I PA flow (considered to be normal) is relatively symmetric in appearance, with the peak velocity occurring close to the middle of the envelope with relatively equal acceleration and deceleration times. Type II PA flow profile is typically associated with mild and moderate PH and is characterized by a peak velocity occurring earlier in systole with a longer deceleration phase. A Type III PA flow profile is associated with more severe PH. The pattern is similar to Type II but there is a "notch" in the deceleration phase, thought to be caused by flow reversal (**Fig. 5**). Although identifiable PA flow patterns may aid in the diagnosis of PH, it is often difficult to obtain "clean" signals in dyspneic clinical patients.

Tei index of myocardial performance of the right ventricle

The Tei index of myocardial performance is a computed value that combines Doppler-derived RV systolic and diastolic functional estimates to provide a quantitative assessment of RV function.[50,51] The Tei index has been used to aid in the diagnosis of PH in people and dogs.[13,51,52] The Tei index formula is as follows: (isovolumetric contraction + isovolumetric relaxation)/ejection time, and Tei index values are increased when PH is present.[50] Right ventricular Tei index can be calculated using the pulsed-wave Doppler of the tricuspid valve (TV) inflows measurements and the pulmonic valve ejection measurements. The index can be calculated from the formula (a − b)/b where "a" represents the interval from cessation to onset of the TV inflow (time from the end of the TV A wave to the beginning of the TV E wave, and "b" represents ejection time across the pulmonic valve (time from the beginning to the end of the PA flow profile). The inflow and outflow signals cannot be recorded

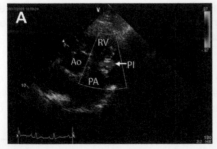 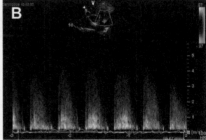

Fig. 4. Pulmonic insufficiency. Doppler echocardiographic images from a dog with severe pulmonary hypertension and a reversed patent ductus arteriosus. (*A*) Color Doppler map of a pulmonic insufficiency (PI) jet. The PI flow is from the higher pressure pulmonary artery (PA) to the lower pressure right ventricle (RV). The aorta (Ao) is also labeled. Image obtained from the right parasternal basilar short axis view. (*B*) Spectral Doppler trace of PI. Pulmonic insufficiency velocity of approximately 4.7 m/s, indicating a pulmonic gradient of approximately 86 mm Hg in early diastole. Velocities were recorded from the right parasternal basilar short-axis view.

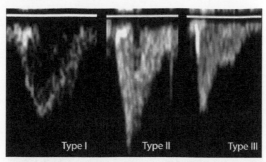

Type I   Type II   Type III

Fig. 5. Pulmonary artery systolic flow profiles. Pulmonary artery systolic velocity flow profiles: type I (normal, a domelike profile with the peak velocity flow occurring in the middle of systole with symmetric acceleration and deceleration phases), type II (the peak velocity flow occurring early in systole with a steep and rapid acceleration phase and slower deceleration phase), or type III (the same as type II but a notch occurs in the deceleration phase caused by PA flow reversal).

simultaneously, so both recordings are from unrelated cardiac cycles. Serres and colleagues[13] described a cutoff value of 0.25 as being predictive of PH in dogs with a sensitivity of 78% and a specificity of 80%. Drawbacks to the use of the Tei index to identify increased PAP in dogs include high intrapatient variability and the difficulty of obtaining good signals in a clinically dyspneic patient.[51]

Right ventricular tissue Doppler imaging
Tissue Doppler imaging (TDI) indices of RV function, such as Stdi (longitudinal peak velocity of the right myocardial wall measured during systole by the use of color TDI), E/Atdi (ratio of longitudinal peak velocities of the right myocardial wall measured in early [E] and late [A] diastole by using color TDI), and G-TDI (global TDI index defined as Stdi*E/Atdi) have been described in dogs with PH by Serres and colleagues.[13] A G-TDI value of less than 11.8 cm/s was predictive of PH with a sensitivity of 89% and a specificity of 93%.[13] An E/Atdi value of less than 1.12 was predictive of PH with a sensitivity of 89% and a specificity of 90%.[13] Detailed tissue Doppler interrogation of the RV can be difficult in patients with significant respiratory effort and TDI assessment of the RV can be considered supportive of PH rather than diagnostic.

2-Dimensional echocardiography
Right ventricular hypertrophy (concentric or eccentric) may occur in patients with PH owing to chronic increases in RV afterload. The presence of RV hypertrophy in a patient suspected of having PH is supportive evidence of the syndrome **(Fig. 6)**.[1,3,12,16,21,25,31]

Septal flattening can be noted in patients with moderate to severe PH if the RV pressure exceeds the left ventricular pressure. The presence of septal flattening in conjunction with RV eccentric or concentric hypertrophy is supportive of significantly increased RV pressure and is an indication for further investigations to identify PH (see **Fig. 6**).[1,39]

Main pulmonary artery enlargement may be noted in dogs with moderate to severe PH.[1,13,16,21] The diameter of the main pulmonary artery in relation to the diameter of the aorta in the right parasternal basilar short axis view (PA:Ao ratio) can be used to identify abnormal PA size. PA:Ao ratios exceeding 0.98 indicate PA enlargement (when the aorta is of normal diameter) and support a tentative diagnosis of PH **(Fig. 7)**.[13]

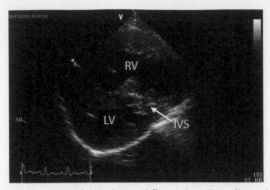

Fig. 6. Right ventricular hypertrophy and septal flattening. Two-dimensional imaging from a dog with severe pulmonary hypertension and a reversed patent ductus arteriosus. The right ventricle (RV) and the left ventricle (LV) are shown in short axis from the right parasternal view at the level of the papillary muscles in diastole. There is subjectively severe concentric (thickened RV walls and papillary muscles) and eccentric (dilated RV lumen) hypertrophy present. The RV walls appear "fluffy" and thickened owing to the extensive trabeculation of the RV walls associated with concentric hypertrophy. There is severe septal flattening of the interventricular septum (IVS) toward the LV lumen in diastole, which indicates high right ventricular pressure.

Right ventricular systolic time intervals

RV systolic time intervals (acceleration time [AT], ejection time [ET], AT:ET, and pre-ejection period [PEP]) have been used to support the diagnosis of PH in dogs and people.[1,5,13,26,35,48,49,53] These values, obtained from echocardiographic and electrocardiographic findings associated with the pulmonic outflow velocities (RV ejection), reflect changes in RV loading. Schober and Baade[5] demonstrated that AT:ET of 0.31 or less and AT value of 0.058 or less were predictive of PH. Abnormal RV systolic time intervals would be particularly supportive of the diagnosis of PH when other clinical findings suggest PH and a measurable TR Doppler gradient is absent.

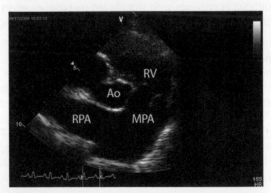

Fig. 7. Main pulmonary artery enlargement. Two-dimensional imaging from a dog with severe pulmonary hypertension and a reversed patent ductus arteriosus. The main pulmonary artery (MPA), right pulmonary artery (RPA), aorta (Ao), and right ventricle (RV) are shown in short axis from the right parasternal basilar view. The Ao:PA is 0.76 (indicating enlargement of the PA) and the RPA is subjectively enlarged suggestive of PH. The PA should be equal in size or smaller than the adjacent Ao in normal dogs.

TREATMENT

Pulmonary hypertension reflects abnormalities or imbalances in multiple signaling pathways, resulting in a final common pathway of medial hypertrophy, intimal proliferation, and a decrease in vascular compliance. The targets of PH therapy focus on these derangements.

The goals of treatment for PH patients are to ameliorate clinical signs, improve exercise tolerance, decrease the PAP, decrease the RV workload, prolong progression of disease (decrease hospitalization), improve survival, and improve quality of life. Because most cases of PH are secondary to an underlying disease process, treatment aimed at eliminating or improving the underlying disease status is the basis for therapy. If the PH is not controlled by primary disease therapy or if the etiology of the PH appears to be idiopathic, then direct PAP modulation through the use of pulmonary vasodilators should be implemented. Pulmonary vasodilating drugs currently in use target the pathophysiologic abnormalities associated with the pulmonary arterial endothelin pathway (endothelin receptor antagonists), prostanoid pathway (prostacyclin analogs), and nitric oxide pathway (specific or nonspecific phosphodiesterase inhibitors). More recently, calcium-sensitizing agents with phosphodiesterase-3 inhibiting actions have also been used for clinical PH, especially when left heart disease is a contributing cause.

Endothelin Pathway

Endothelin-1 (ET-1), released by the vascular endothelium, is a potent vasoconstrictor, stimulates PA smooth muscle cell proliferation, and can ultimately lead to vascular remodeling.[54] In patients with PH, clearance of ET-1 appears to be impaired in the pulmonary vasculature.[55] Plasma concentration of ET-1 is elevated in people with PH and ET-1 concentration correlates with the severity of PH and prognosis.[56]

Endothelin receptor antagonists (bosentan, sitaxsentan, ambrisentan) are oral medications and have had promising results in people with idiopathic PH,[57-61] but at present, are usually cost prohibitive for veterinary patients.

Prostanoid Pathway

Prostacyclin and thromboxane A2 are arachidonic acid metabolites. Prostacyclin is a potent vasodilator, inhibitors platelet activation, and has antiproliferative effects in the pulmonary artery. Thromboxane A2 is a potent vasoconstrictor and promotes platelet activation. In patients with idiopathic PH, there is an imbalance of these metabolites, favoring the production of thromboxane A2, leading to vasoconstriction, proliferation, and thrombosis.[45]

The administration of prostacyclin analogs (epoprostenol, treprostinil, iloprost) has been the mainstay of treatment for PAH in people.[62-64] Epoprostenol is administered to human patients as a continuous rate infusion with an ambulatory pump through a central venous indwelling catheter. Treprostinil is also administered intravenously or in frequent subcutaneous injections. Iloprost is in an inhaled formulation requiring dosing 6 to 12 times daily.[45] At present, these required methods of delivery prohibit the use of these medications in veterinary patients.

Nitric Oxide Pathway

Nitric oxide (NO) is a potent vasodilator, inhibitor of platelet activation, and inhibitor of vascular smooth muscle cell proliferation. NO is synthesized endogenously from L-arginine and oxygen by nitric oxide synthase (NOS) isoenzymes in the vascular endothelium. NO activates guanylate cyclase, which increases cyclic guanosine monophosphate (cGMP). cGMP enhances vascular relaxation and is rapidly inactivated by phospodiesterase (PDE), particularly PDE-5 isosenzymes.[54,55] PDE-5 inhibitors are used to block the inactivation of cGMP and use of PDE-5 inhibitors results in enhanced pulmonary artery vasodilation.

Selective phospodiesterase inhibitors

PDE-5 inhibitors (sildenafil, tadalafil, vardenafil) were originally investigated in coronary artery research with positive results, yet the short half-life and interaction with nitrates precluded sildenafil use in this clinical situation. PDE-5 is abundantly expressed in the lungs, hence the rationale for its use with PH.[65]

Sildenafil (Viagra, Revatio) is an orally active, highly selective PDE-5 inhibitor. Multiple studies have demonstrated the benefits of sildenafil in people with PH.[66-72] Sildenafil appears to produce beneficial effects in PH by multiple mechanisms,[73] but the primary mechanism operative in patients with PH appears to be direct pulmonary artery vasodilation. In mice, sildenafil blocks the intrinsic catabolism of cGMP within the myocardium by suppressing chamber and myocyte hypertrophy and improving in vivo cardiac function when exposed to chronic pressure overload.[74] Sildenafil also reversed preexisting hypertrophy in pressure-loaded mice hearts.[74] Sildenafil has been shown to decrease PVR, therefore preventing the increase in PAP by partially preventing an increase in medial thickness of pulmonary arteries in piglets with PAH.[75] Borlaug and colleagues[76] have demonstrated that sildenafil can modify or blunt the response to beta-adrenergic stimulation by suppressing cardiac contractility in people. In addition to improved PAP, Ghofrani and colleagues[77] showed that sildenafil also ameliorated ventilation-perfusion mismatch, which improved oxygen saturation in people. In people, chronic sildenafil usage has been shown to significantly improve the functional ability of exercise as represented by an improved 6-minute walk test, which is considered a surrogate measure of mortality.[66]

In dogs, sildenafil has been administered for PH with encouraging results.[1,4,39] Bach and colleagues[4] demonstrated that in the 8 of 13 dogs with PH for which follow-up data were available, sildenafil (1.9 mg/kg orally every 8–24 hours) significantly decreased the PAP (measured invasively or estimated by Doppler echocardiography). The median survival time for dogs that survived 1 day after initiation of therapy was 175 days (range: 28–693). Kellum and Stepien[1] did not find a significant reduction in PAP (based on TR estimations) after sildenafil (1 mg/kg orally every 8–12 hours), but there was a significant improvement in patients' (n = 22) clinical scores (clinical signs and quality of life). Dogs with PH in the latter study had a 95% probability of survival at 3 months, an 84% probability of survival at 6 months, and a 73% probability of survival at 1 year.[1] There were no limiting adverse side effects noted in either the Bach or Kellum studies. The only study evaluating survival times in dogs before sildenafil use was by Johnson and colleagues[3] in 1999, and the median survival times for dogs that died and were euthanized was 3.5 days and 3 days, respectively.

Tadalafil (Cialis) is a longer-acting (once-daily oral dosing), selective PDE-5 inhibitor. In a human study, tadalafil decreased PAP but did not improve arterial oxygenation as sildenafil did.[77] In a study by Tay and colleagues,[78] use of tadalafil and sildenafil resulted in similar clinical improvement in people with idiopathic PH, suggesting that tadalafil could be used in place of sildenafil for improved compliance with once-daily dosing and potentially reducing the cost of treatment. Recently, Pepke-Zaba and colleagues[79] and Galie and colleagues[80] reported that there was improved health-related quality of life, improved exercise capacity, and reduced clinical worsening in people receiving once-a-day oral tadalafil for idiopathic PH. A single veterinary case study evaluating tadalafil in a dog with PAH showed a reduction in the estimated

PAP and clinical improvement.[81] The appeal of tadalafil as a treatment for PH in veterinary medicine is the once-a-day dosing as compared with the recommended every 8 hours dosing for sildenafil, and possible cost reductions.

Vardenafil (Levitra) is a longer-acting, once daily, selective PDE-5 inhibitor. When vardenafil was compared with sildenafil and tadalafil by Ghofrani and colleagues[77] in people with idiopathic PH, vardenafil produced a decrease in the PAP but did not improve arterial oxygenation and decreased the systemic vascular resistance to the same degree as the PVR. In a single long-term study in people receiving vardenafil for PAH, PAP was decreased, exercise capacity improved, and patients tolerated the medication well.[82] In rabbits, Toque and colleagues[83] demonstrated that vardenafil, and not sildenafil or tadalafil, had additional calcium channel blocking action in the pulmonary arteries. To date, there have been no published clinical veterinary investigations into the effects of vardenafil in dogs with PH.

Nitric oxide substrates

L-arginine is a substrate (available orally) for NO synthesis and a few studies have shown pulmonary vasodilatory effects in PH.[84–86] The potential mechanisms by which L-arginine works in PH is by augmenting endogenous NO production, reducing oxidative stress in the PA, and by promoting angiogenesis and increasing pulmonary vessel length, hence decreasing PVR.[86,87] A study by Souza-Silva and colleagues[88] demonstrated that L-arginine did increase NO levels, yet there was no additional attenuation in PAP when given in conjunction with sildenafil. There are no reported studies in veterinary medicine regarding the use of L-arginine in the syndrome of PH.

Calcium-sensitizing agents

Pimobendan and levosimendan are calcium-sensitizing agents and PDE-3 inhibitors. PDE-3 has activity at the level of large and small (resistance) PAs, whereas PDE-5 exerts its activity in primarily large pulmonary arteries. PDE-3 inhibitors promote PA vasodilation via enhancement of adrenergic relaxation. The dual action of PDE-3 inhibition and the positive inotropic effects of calcium sensitization may provide some attenuation of PH, especially in PH secondary to left-sided heart disease.[8,89–92] Recently, pimobendan has been used in dogs with PH associated with mitral valve disease, and there was a significant decrease in estimated PAPs and an improved quality of life in the short term.[35]

Nonselective Phosphodiesterase Inhibitors

The use of nonselective PDE inhibitors (3, 4, and 5), such as theophylline, have occasionally been recommended for the treatment of PH in dogs and people with little evidence of sustained improvement of PH.[93–95] Theophylline is a bronchodilator and a weak, nonselective PDE inhibitor. In people, the degree of PDE inhibition is very small at concentrations that are considered to be of therapeutic relevance for COPD.[93] Signs of clinical improvement in dogs with pulmonary hypertension may occur if the underlying etiology of the PH is COPD, and in this setting theophylline may prove beneficial.

The use of nonselective vasodilators/peripheral vasodilators such as calcium channel blockers (eg, diltiazem and amlodipine), hydralazine, angiotensin-converting enzyme (ACE) inhibitors, and nitroprusside may result in adverse side effects (eg, systemic hypotension) if used for the treatment of PH. Often these medications are given for afterload reduction with left-sided heart disease, yet blood pressure should be closely monitored. In people, there have been limited positive benefits seen with the use of calcium channel blockers (eg, diltiazem and nifedipine) for the treatment of PH.[96]

SUMMARY

Pulmonary hypertension has been recognized as a clinical syndrome for many years in veterinary medicine, but routine accurate clinical diagnosis in dogs was greatly enhanced by widespread use of echocardiography and Doppler echocardiography. In addition, effective medical therapy is now available to treat this often-devastating clinical complication of common chronic diseases, making accurate diagnosis even more important to patient longevity and quality of life.

REFERENCES

1. Kellum HB, Stepien RL. Sildenafil citrate therapy in 22 dogs with pulmonary hypertension. J Vet Intern Med 2007;21(6):1258–64.
2. Fleming E. Pulmonary hypertension. Compend Contin Educ Vet 2006;28:720–30.
3. Johnson L, Boon J, Orton EC. Clinical characteristics of 53 dogs with Doppler-derived evidence of pulmonary hypertension: 1992–1996. J Vet Intern Med 1999;13(5):440–7.
4. Bach JF, Rozanski EA, MacGregor J, et al. Retrospective evaluation of sildenafil citrate as a therapy for pulmonary hypertension in dogs. J Vet Intern Med 2006; 20(5):1132–5.
5. Schober KE, Baade H. Doppler echocardiographic prediction of pulmonary hypertension in West Highland white terriers with chronic pulmonary disease. J Vet Intern Med 2006;20(4):912–20.
6. Pyle RL, Abbott J, MacLean H. Pulmonary hypertension and cardiovascular sequelae in 54 dogs. Int J Appl Res Vet Med 2004;2(2):99.
7. Simonneau G, Galie N, Rubin LJ, et al. Clinical classification of pulmonary hypertension. J Am Coll Cardiol 2004;43(12 Suppl S):5S–12S.
8. Stepien RL. Pulmonary arterial hypertension secondary to chronic left-sided cardiac dysfunction in dogs. J Small Anim Pract 2009;50(Suppl 1):34–43.
9. LaRue MJ, Murtaugh RJ. Pulmonary thromboembolism in dogs: 47 cases (1986–1987). J Am Vet Med Assoc 1990;197(10):1368–72.
10. Johnson LR, Lappin MR, Baker DC. Pulmonary thromboembolism in 29 dogs: 1985–1995. J Vet Intern Med 1999;13(4):338–45.
11. Norris CR, Griffey SM, Samii VF. Pulmonary thromboembolism in cats: 29 cases (1987–1997). J Am Vet Med Assoc 1999;215(11):1650–4.
12. Zabka TS, Campbell FE, Wilson DW. Pulmonary arteriopathy and idiopathic pulmonary arterial hypertension in six dogs. Vet Pathol 2006;43(4):510–22.
13. Serres F, Chetboul V, Gouni V, et al. Diagnostic value of echo-Doppler and tissue Doppler imaging in dogs with pulmonary arterial hypertension. J Vet Intern Med 2007;21(6):1280–9.
14. Serres FJ, Chetboul V, Tissier R, et al. Doppler echocardiography-derived evidence of pulmonary arterial hypertension in dogs with degenerative mitral valve disease: 86 cases (2001–2005). J Am Vet Med Assoc 2006;229(11): 1772–8.
15. Sasaki Y, Kitagawa H, Hirano Y. Relationship between pulmonary arterial pressure and lesions in the pulmonary arteries and parenchyma, and cardiac valves in canine dirofilariasis. J Vet Med Sci 1992;54(4):739–44.
16. Russell NJ, Irwin PJ, Hopper BJ, et al. Acute necrotising pulmonary vasculitis and pulmonary hypertension in a juvenile dog. J Small Anim Pract 2008;49(7):349–55.

17. Rawlings CA, Farrell RL, Mahood RM. Morphologic changes in the lungs of cats experimentally infected with dirofilaria immitis. Response to aspirin. J Vet Intern Med 1990;4(6):292–300.
18. Rawlings CA, Tackett RL. Postadulticide pulmonary hypertension of canine heartworm disease: successful treatment with oxygen and failure of antihistamines. Am J Vet Res 1990;51(10):1565–9.
19. Pyle RL, Park RD, Alexander AF, et al. Patent ductus arteriosus with pulmonary hypertension in the dog. J Am Vet Med Assoc 1981;178(6):565–71.
20. Oswald GP, Orton EC. Patent ductus arteriosus and pulmonary hypertension in related Pembroke Welsh corgis. J Am Vet Med Assoc 1993;202(5):761–4.
21. Mitchell CW. The imaging diagnosis of pulmonary thromboembolism. Can Vet J 2009;50(2):199–202.
22. Johnson L. Diagnosis of pulmonary hypertension. Clin Tech Small Anim Pract 1999;14(4):231–6.
23. Hirano Y, Kitagawa H, Sasaki Y. Relationship between pulmonary arterial pressure and pulmonary thromboembolism associated with dead worms in canine heartworm disease. J Vet Med Sci 1992;54(5):897–904.
24. Grover RF, Johnson RL Jr, McCullough RG, et al. Pulmonary hypertension and pulmonary vascular reactivity in beagles at high altitude. J Appl Physiol 1988; 65(6):2632–40.
25. Glaus TM, Soldati G, Maurer R, et al. Clinical and pathological characterisation of primary pulmonary hypertension in a dog. Vet Rec 2004;154(25):786–9.
26. Glaus TM, Tomsa K, Hassig M, et al. Echocardiographic changes induced by moderate to marked hypobaric hypoxia in dogs. Vet Radiol Ultrasound 2004; 45(3):233–7.
27. Glaus TM, Hassig M, Baumgartner C, et al. Pulmonary hypertension induced in dogs by hypoxia at different high-altitude levels. Vet Res Commun 2003;27(8): 661–70.
28. Glaus TM, Hauser K, Hassig M, et al. Non-invasive measurement of the cardiovascular effects of chronic hypoxaemia on dogs living at moderately high altitude. Vet Rec 2003;152(26):800–3.
29. Glaus TM, Grenacher B, Koch D, et al. High altitude training of dogs results in elevated erythropoietin and endothelin-1 serum levels. Comp Biochem Physiol A Mol Integr Physiol 2004;138(3):355–61.
30. Gavaghan BJ, Lapointe JM, Thomas WP. Acute onset of pulmonary necrotising arteritis in a dog with a left-to-right patent ductus arteriosus. Aust Vet J 1998; 76(12):786–91.
31. Cote E, Ettinger SJ. Long-term clinical management of right-to-left ("reversed") patent ductus arteriosus in 3 dogs. J Vet Intern Med 2001;15(1):39–42.
32. Chiavegato D, Borgarelli M, D'Agnolo G, et al. Pulmonary hypertension in dogs with mitral regurgitation attributable to myxomatous valve disease. Vet Radiol Ultrasound 2009;50(3):253–8.
33. Chetboul V, Serres F, Tissier R, et al. Association of plasma N-terminal pro-B-type natriuretic peptide concentration with mitral regurgitation severity and outcome in dogs with asymptomatic degenerative mitral valve disease. J Vet Intern Med 2009;23(5):984–94.
34. Borgarelli M, Zini E, D'Agnolo G, et al. Comparison of primary mitral valve disease in German shepherd dogs and in small breeds. J Vet Cardiol 2004;6(2):27–34.
35. Atkinson KJ, Fine DM, Thombs LA, et al. Evaluation of pimobendan and N-terminal probrain natriuretic peptide in the treatment of pulmonary hypertension secondary to degenerative mitral valve disease in dogs. J Vet Intern Med 2009;23(6):1190–6.

36. Ware WB. Multiple congenital cardiac anomalies and Eisenmenger's syndrome in a dog. Compend Contin Educ Vet 1988;10(8):932.
37. Yuan JX, Rubin LJ. Pathogenesis of pulmonary arterial hypertension: the need for multiple hits. Circulation 2005;111(5):534–8.
38. Corcoran BM, Cobb M, Martin MW, et al. Chronic pulmonary disease in West Highland white terriers. Vet Rec 1999;144(22):611–6.
39. Toyoshima Y, Kanemoto I, Arai S, et al. A case of long-term sildenafil therapy in a young dog with pulmonary hypertension. J Vet Med Sci 2007;69(10):1073–5.
40. Chemla D, Castelain V, Herve P, et al. Haemodynamic evaluation of pulmonary hypertension. Eur Respir J 2002;20(5):1314–31.
41. Jardin F, Dubourg O, Bourdarias JP. Echocardiographic pattern of acute cor pulmonale. Chest 1997;111(1):209–17.
42. Fine DM, Declue AE, Reinero CR. Evaluation of circulating amino terminal-pro-B-type natriuretic peptide concentration in dogs with respiratory distress attributable to congestive heart failure or primary pulmonary disease. J Am Vet Med Assoc 2008;232(11):1674–9.
43. Leuchte HH, El Nounou M, Tuerpe JC, et al. N-terminal pro-brain natriuretic peptide and renal insufficiency as predictors of mortality in pulmonary hypertension. Chest 2007;131(2):402–9.
44. Andreassen AK, Wergeland R, Simonsen S, et al. N-terminal pro-B-type natriuretic peptide as an indicator of disease severity in a heterogeneous group of patients with chronic precapillary pulmonary hypertension. Am J Cardiol 2006; 98(4):525–9.
45. McLaughlin VV, Archer SL, Badesch DB, et al. ACCF/AHA 2009 expert consensus document on pulmonary hypertension: a report of the American College of Cardiology Foundation Task Force on Expert Consensus Documents and the American Heart Association: developed in collaboration with the American College of Chest Physicians, American Thoracic Society, Inc., and the Pulmonary Hypertension Association. Circulation 2009;119(16):2250–94.
46. Yock PG, Popp RL. Noninvasive estimation of right ventricular systolic pressure by Doppler ultrasound in patients with tricuspid regurgitation. Circulation 1984; 70(4):657–62.
47. Fisher MR, Forfia PR, Chamera E, et al. Accuracy of Doppler echocardiography in the hemodynamic assessment of pulmonary hypertension. Am J Respir Crit Care Med 2009;179(7):615–21.
48. Martin-Duran R, Larman M, Trugeda A, et al. Comparison of Doppler-determined elevated pulmonary arterial pressure with pressure measured at cardiac catheterization. Am J Cardiol 1986;57(10):859–63.
49. Uehara Y. An attempt to estimate the pulmonary artery pressure in dogs by means of pulsed Doppler echocardiography. J Vet Med Sci 1993;55(2):307–12.
50. Tei C, Dujardin KS, Hodge DO, et al. Doppler echocardiographic index for assessment of global right ventricular function. J Am Soc Echocardiogr 1996; 9(6):838–47.
51. Baumwart RD, Meurs KM, Bonagura JD. Tei index of myocardial performance applied to the right ventricle in normal dogs. J Vet Intern Med 2005;19(6):828–32.
52. Yeo TC, Dujardin KS, Tei C, et al. Value of a Doppler-derived index combining systolic and diastolic time intervals in predicting outcome in primary pulmonary hypertension. Am J Cardiol 1998;81(9):1157–61.
53. Champion HC, Michelakis ED, Hassoun PM. Comprehensive invasive and noninvasive approach to the right ventricle-pulmonary circulation unit: state of the art and clinical and research implications. Circulation 2009;120(11):992–1007.

54. Farber HW, Loscalzo J. Pulmonary arterial hypertension. N Engl J Med 2004; 351(16):1655–65.
55. Stewart DJ, Levy RD, Cernacek P, et al. Increased plasma endothelin-1 in pulmonary hypertension: marker or mediator of disease? Ann Intern Med 1991;114(6): 464–9.
56. Rubens C, Ewert R, Halank M, et al. Big endothelin-1 and endothelin-1 plasma levels are correlated with the severity of primary pulmonary hypertension. Chest 2001;120(5):1562–9.
57. Channick RN, Simonneau G, Sitbon O, et al. Effects of the dual endothelin-receptor antagonist bosentan in patients with pulmonary hypertension: a randomised placebo-controlled study. Lancet 2001;358(9288):1119–23.
58. Rubin LJ, Badesch DB, Barst RJ, et al. Bosentan therapy for pulmonary arterial hypertension. N Engl J Med 2002;346(12):896–903.
59. McLaughlin VV, Sitbon O, Badesch DB, et al. Survival with first-line bosentan in patients with primary pulmonary hypertension. Eur Respir J 2005;25(2):244–9.
60. Barst RJ, Rich S, Widlitz A, et al. Clinical efficacy of sitaxsentan, an endothelin-A receptor antagonist, in patients with pulmonary arterial hypertension: open-label pilot study. Chest 2002;121(6):1860–8.
61. Galie N, Badesch D, Oudiz R, et al. Ambrisentan therapy for pulmonary arterial hypertension. J Am Coll Cardiol 2005;46(3):529–35.
62. Barst RJ, Rubin LJ, Long WA, et al. A comparison of continuous intravenous epoprostenol (prostacyclin) with conventional therapy for primary pulmonary hypertension. The primary pulmonary hypertension study group. N Engl J Med 1996; 334(5):296–302.
63. Olschewski H, Simonneau G, Galie N, et al. Inhaled iloprost for severe pulmonary hypertension. N Engl J Med 2002;347(5):322–9.
64. Laliberte K, Arneson C, Jeffs R, et al. Pharmacokinetics and steady-state bioequivalence of treprostinil sodium (remodulin) administered by the intravenous and subcutaneous route to normal volunteers. J Cardiovasc Pharmacol 2004;44(2): 209–14.
65. McLaughlin VV, McGoon MD. Pulmonary arterial hypertension. Circulation 2006; 114(13):1417–31.
66. Michelakis ED, Tymchak W, Noga M, et al. Long-term treatment with oral sildenafil is safe and improves functional capacity and hemodynamics in patients with pulmonary arterial hypertension. Circulation 2003;108(17):2066–9.
67. Galie N, Ghofrani HA, Torbicki A, et al. Sildenafil citrate therapy for pulmonary arterial hypertension. N Engl J Med 2005;353(20):2148–57.
68. Humpl T, Reyes JT, Holtby H, et al. Beneficial effect of oral sildenafil therapy on childhood pulmonary arterial hypertension: twelve-month clinical trial of a single-drug, open-label, pilot study. Circulation 2005;111(24):3274–80.
69. Ghofrani HA, Wiedemann R, Rose F, et al. Sildenafil for treatment of lung fibrosis and pulmonary hypertension: a randomised controlled trial. Lancet 2002; 360(9337):895–900.
70. Hoeper MM, Welte T. Sildenafil citrate therapy for pulmonary arterial hypertension. N Engl J Med 2006;354(10):1091–3 [author reply: 1091–3].
71. Klinger JR, Thaker S, Houtchens J, et al. Pulmonary hemodynamic responses to brain natriuretic peptide and sildenafil in patients with pulmonary arterial hypertension. Chest 2006;129(2):417–25.
72. Gan CT, Holverda S, Marcus JT, et al. Right ventricular diastolic dysfunction and the acute effects of sildenafil in pulmonary hypertension patients. Chest 2007; 132(1):11–7.

73. van Wolferen SA, Boonstra A, Marcus JT, et al. Right ventricular reverse remodeling after sildenafil in pulmonary arterial hypertension. Heart 2006;92(12): 1860–1.

74. Takimoto E, Champion HC, Li M, et al. Chronic inhibition of cyclic GMP phosphodiesterase 5A prevents and reverses cardiac hypertrophy. Nat Med 2005;11(2): 214–22.

75. Rondelet B, Kerbaul F, Van Beneden R, et al. Signaling molecules in overcirculation-induced pulmonary hypertension in piglets: effects of sildenafil therapy. Circulation 2004;110(15):2220–5.

76. Borlaug BA, Melenovsky V, Marhin T, et al. Sildenafil inhibits beta-adrenergic-stimulated cardiac contractility in humans. Circulation 2005;112(17):2642–9.

77. Ghofrani HA, Voswinckel R, Reichenberger F, et al. Differences in hemodynamic and oxygenation responses to three different phosphodiesterase-5 inhibitors in patients with pulmonary arterial hypertension: a randomized prospective study. J Am Coll Cardiol 2004;44(7):1488–96.

78. Tay EL, Geok-Mui MK, Poh-Hoon MC, et al. Sustained benefit of tadalafil in patients with pulmonary arterial hypertension with prior response to sildenafil: a case series of 12 patients. Int J Cardiol 2008;125(3):416–7.

79. Pepke-Zaba J, Beardsworth A, Chan M, et al. Tadalafil therapy and health-related quality of life in pulmonary arterial hypertension. Curr Med Res Opin 2009;25(10): 2479–85.

80. Galie N, Brundage BH, Ghofrani HA, et al. Tadalafil therapy for pulmonary arterial hypertension. Circulation 2009;119(22):2894–903.

81. Serres F, Nicolle AP, Tissier R, et al. Efficacy of oral tadalafil, a new long-acting phosphodiesterase-5 inhibitor, for the short-term treatment of pulmonary arterial hypertension in a dog. J Vet Med A Physiol Pathol Clin Med 2006;53(3):129–33.

82. Jing ZC, Jiang X, Wu BX, et al. Vardenafil treatment for patients with pulmonary arterial hypertension: a multicentre, open-label study. Heart 2009;95(18):1531–6.

83. Toque HA, Teixeira CE, Priviero FB, et al. Vardenafil, but not sildenafil or tadalafil, has calcium-channel blocking activity in rabbit isolated pulmonary artery and human washed platelets. Br J Pharmacol 2008;154(4):787–96.

84. Mehta S, Stewart DJ, Langleben D, et al. Short-term pulmonary vasodilation with L-arginine in pulmonary hypertension. Circulation 1995;92(6):1539–45.

85. Fagan JM, Rex SE, Hayes-Licitra SA, et al. L-arginine reduces right heart hypertrophy in hypoxia-induced pulmonary hypertension. Biochem Biophys Res Commun 1999;254(1):100–3.

86. Howell K, Costello CM, Sands M, et al. L-arginine promotes angiogenesis in the chronically hypoxic lung: a novel mechanism ameliorating pulmonary hypertension. Am J Physiol Lung Cell Mol Physiol 2009;296(6):L1042–50.

87. Souza-Costa DC, Zerbini T, Metzger IF, et al. L-Arginine attenuates acute pulmonary embolism-induced oxidative stress and pulmonary hypertension. Nitric Oxide 2005;12(1):9–14.

88. Souza-Silva AR, Dias-Junior CA, Uzuelli JA, et al. Hemodynamic effects of combined sildenafil and L-arginine during acute pulmonary embolism-induced pulmonary hypertension. Eur J Pharmacol 2005;524(1–3):126–31.

89. Kerbaul F, Gariboldi V, Giorgi R, et al. Effects of levosimendan on acute pulmonary embolism-induced right ventricular failure. Crit Care Med 2007;35(8): 1948–54.

90. Kerbaul F, Rondelet B, Demester JP, et al. Effects of levosimendan versus dobutamine on pressure load-induced right ventricular failure. Crit Care Med 2006; 34(11):2814–9.

91. Nieminen MS, Akkila J, Hasenfuss G, et al. Hemodynamic and neurohumoral effects of continuous infusion of levosimendan in patients with congestive heart failure. J Am Coll Cardiol 2000;36(6):1903–12.
92. Fuentes VL. Use of pimobendan in the management of heart failure. Vet Clin North Am Small Anim Pract 2004;34(5):1145–55.
93. Barnes PJ. Theophylline: new perspectives for an old drug. Am J Respir Crit Care Med 2003;167(6):813–8.
94. Johnson L. Patient selection and therapeutics in pulmonary hypertension. The European College of Veterinary Internal Medicine-Companion Animals Congress Proceedings. Amsterdam (The Netherlands), 2006.
95. Matthay RA. Favorable cardiovascular effects of theophylline in COPD. Chest 1987;92(1 Suppl):22S–6S.
96. Sitbon O, Humbert M, Jagot JL, et al. Inhaled nitric oxide as a screening agent for safely identifying responders to oral calcium-channel blockers in primary pulmonary hypertension. Eur Respir J 1998;12:265.

Feline Arrhythmias: An Update

Etienne Côté, DVM

KEYWORDS

• Feline arrhythmias • Electrocardiography • Cat

In the cat, electrocardiography is indicated for assessing the rhythm of the heartbeat and identifying and monitoring the effect of certain systemic disorders on the heart. Basic information regarding feline electrocardiography is contained in several textbooks, and the reader is referred to these sources for background reading.[1–5] The following article aims to describe selected clinical advances in feline cardiac arrhythmias and electrocardiography from the past decade.

HYPERKALEMIA

Increased serum potassium concentrations are known to alter the electrical function of the heart in many species of animals. In the cat, this observation was made experimentally in 1839, decades before the invention of the electrocardiogram,[6] and subsequent work has refined these data. Under controlled experimental conditions, incremental increases in serum potassium concentration are associated with distinctive electrocardiographic (ECG) abnormalities. Briefly, the following relationships have been described: mild hyperkalemia (serum $[K^+]$ = 5.5–7.0 mEq/L) – peaking of the T wave, shortening of the QT interval; moderate hyperkalemia (serum $[K^+]$=7.1–8.5 mEq/L) – widening of the QRS complex, and prolongation of the PR interval, then loss of the P wave/atrial standstill; severe hyperkalemia (serum $[K^+]$= 8.6–12.0 mEq/L) – further widening of the QRS complex, progressing to QRS complexes and T waves indistinctly fusing into a sine-wave morphology; critical hyperkalemia (serum $[K^+]$> 12.0 mEq/L) – cardiac arrest (ventricular fibrillation and/or asystole).[1,6]

For many years, clinicians have observed that naturally occurring hyperkalemia in cats, whether caused by urethral obstruction (most commonly) or oliguric/anuric renal failure, reperfusion injury, or other causes, does not consistently produce the rigorously defined ECG changes described in the criteria listed earlier (Fig. 1).[6] A cat with a serum $[K^+]$ of 11 mEq/L may not have changes so severe as those suggested by these definitions, whereas a cat with a serum $[K^+]$ of 9 mEq/L may fibrillate fatally, for example. The explanation for this discrepancy likely lies in the difference between experimentally induced hyperkalemia (which gave rise to the categories of ECG

Department of Companion Animals, Atlantic Veterinary College, University of Prince Edward Island, 550 University Avenue, Charlottetown, PE, C1A 4P3, Canada

Vet Clin Small Anim 40 (2010) 643–650
doi:10.1016/j.cvsm.2010.04.002
0195-5616/10/$ – see front matter © 2010 Elsevier Inc. All rights reserved.

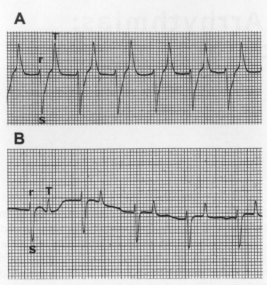

Fig. 1. Electrocardiograms from 2 cats with urethral obstruction and hyperkalemia. The serum K^+ concentration in both cats at the time of these tracings was 10.5 mEq/L. Both electrocardiograms show an absence of P waves consistent with atrial standstill, but there is a greater degree of QRS complex widening in (A) (140 milliseconds) and a taller, wider T wave versus 90 milliseconds in (B); normal ≤40 milliseconds. These findings indicate that serum potassium concentration alone does not account for all ECG changes observed in naturally hyperkalemic cats. Both tracings lead II: 25 mm/s; 10 mm=1 mV. A small amount of baseline fluctuation is present in (B) as a result of patient motion. (*From* the collection of the late Dr Brian Hill, *courtesy of* Dr Sherri Ihle, Atlantic Veterinary College, University of Prince Edward Island, Canada.)

changes based on serum $[K^+]$) and naturally occurring disease. As shown by Tag and Day[7] in 2008, cats with naturally occurring disorders that cause hyperkalemia vary widely with respect to their ECG abnormalities. In 22 hyperkalemic cats (serum $[K^+]$ >5.5 mEq/L), only 9 (41%) had ECG changes consistent with the level of hyperkalemia according to the criteria described earlier, and these cats were all severely hyperkalemic (serum $[K^+]$ >8.5 mEq/L). The heart rate of the severely hyperkalemic cats ranged from 102 to 240 beats/min. These results and the clinical reality from which they originate differ markedly from those observed after the deliberate infusion of large doses of "carbonate of potass" almost 200 years ago[6] or those obtained from multiple subsequent experiments.[8] Human clinical experience with naturally occurring hyperkalemia has likewise been at variance with traditional ECG criteria for similar reasons.[9] Therefore, criteria for assessing the severity of hyperkalemia in cats via electrocardiography do not seem to be valid in the clinical setting. The practical implications of these findings are that the electrocardiogram can and should be used for monitoring the cardiac rhythm in hyperkalemic cats, because other rhythm disturbances such as ventricular or supraventricular arrhythmias can occur and must be identified for appropriate management, but that direct analysis of a blood sample is preferable for diagnosis and monitoring of hyperkalemia.

Cats with diseases that cause hyperkalemia routinely have other systemic disturbances that may influence the effect of hyperkalemia on the heart. An important clinical correlate in feline medicine is hypocalcemia; a retrospective study of cats with naturally occurring urethral obstruction showed that 75% of these cats had ionized hypocalcemia.[10] Low circulating calcium concentrations compound the effect of hyperkalemia on myocardium by further decreasing the difference between resting membrane potential and action potential threshold.[11] Restoring this difference provides electrical stability to the myocardium and is the basis for treatment with intravenous calcium gluconate even although such treatment does not lower the potassium concentration. Therefore, optimal management of a hyperkalemic cat includes not only treatment of the potassium abnormality but rapid identification and correction of abnormalities involving other related and influential parameters (notably blood pH, lactate, and ionized calcium). When hypocalcemia is suspected (urethral obstruction) or proved, the notion that calcium gluconate administration should be reserved for the most serious cases of hyperkalemia is unsupported by evidence.

VENTRICULAR TACHYARRHYTHMIAS

Despite their prevalence in small animal practice, ventricular tachyarrhythmias (premature ventricular complexes, accelerated idioventricular rhythm, and ventricular tachycardia) remain poorly understood, and in the cat this lack of information is particularly severe. Nevertheless, some clinically useful information has emerged recently. A retrospective study of 106 cats with ventricular tachyarrhythmias identified that structural heart disease, consisting mainly of cardiomyopathies, was present in virtually all of them (102; 96%).[12] In contrast, the proportion of dogs at the same institution during the same time period that had arrhythmias and echocardiographically abnormal hearts was only 95 of 138 (69%) ($P = .001$). These results suggest that, compared with dogs, a greater proportion of cases of ventricular arrhythmias in cats is associated with underlying structural heart disease. An intriguing question to arise from these findings is whether ventricular tachyarrhythmias can be considered a marker for underlying structural heart disease in the cat; one implication would be the greater justification for further diagnostic testing, such as echocardiography, when a ventricular arrhythmia is identified incidentally in an overtly normal cat.

Treatment of ventricular tachyarrhythmias in cats remains challenging for many reasons, including the unproven survival benefit of antiarrhythmic therapy, the palliative nature of treatment, and the unpredictable occurrence of medication intolerance. In the absence of evidence, general guidelines for arrhythmia treatment in other species continue to be appropriate in feline cardiology. Thus, antiarrhythmic treatment should be considered when

- overt clinical signs can be shown to occur simultaneously with an arrhythmia, an association made easier by the greater availability of portable or implantable ECG monitors[13];
- treatment of concurrent precipitating or potentiating factors, including anemia, hypokalemia, and hyperthyroidism, has not significantly reduced the frequency of the arrhythmia (with or without overt clinical signs); or
- a sustained tachycardia persists at a rate that is considered likely to negatively affect hemodynamic stability. This rate is likely determined by many factors, and empirically, ventricular tachycardia at rates greater than 260 beats/min that persists despite treatment of underlying/concurrent causes (see earlier discussion) likely warrants antiarrhythmic treatment. This threshold is not supported by any clinical evidence and is used strictly as an approximate guideline.

Antiarrhythmic treatment may consist of lidocaine (0.25–1 mg/kg slow intravenously), sotalol (2 mg/kg by mouth every 12 hours), or other therapies, all of which are anecdotally supported but remain unproven in the cat. Monitoring parameters and potential adverse effects to be avoided include neurotoxicity manifesting as acute mental dullness, ataxia, and seizures (lidocaine) and worsening of syncope or onset of presyncope/lethargy with sotalol if the ventricular tachyarrhythmia coexists with intermittent bradycardia (eg, atrioventricular [AV] block), which may be worsened by the β-blocking activity of sotalol.

Bradycardias (mainly AV block) and tachycardias may occur independently, or together, in cats with hypertrophic cardiomyopathy (HCM) (**Fig. 2**). Because treatment of one of these rhythm disturbances might worsen the other, the importance of associating overt clinical signs such as syncope with the causative arrhythmia is reinforced, and ambulatory ECG monitoring may be particularly important. If ambulatory electrocardiography is not feasible, antiarrhythmic treatment may be detrimental. The risks of worsening a sporadic (and undocumented) bradycardia when treating a ventricular tachyarrhythmia, with drugs that result in βblockade such as sotalol, must be discussed with the owner.

AV BLOCK

Three important case series have been published recently that shed light on AV block in cats. Kellum and Stepien[14] identified third-degree AV block in 21 cats, and presented the following observations: in 6 of 21 (29%), the rhythm disturbance was an incidental finding, indicating that many cats tolerate third-degree AV block; median heart rate was 120 beats/min (range 80–140), suggesting that in some cases the ventricular escape rate may approximate the normal sinus heart rate of the cat and therefore that third-degree AV block may be underrecognized on physical examination in this species; and that the range of survival time was wide, from 1 to 2013 days (median 386), including 13 of 21 cats (62%) surviving for more than 1 year after the

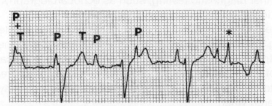

Fig. 2. Third-degree AV block in a 16-year-old female spayed domestic shorthaired cat with HCM. The P-P interval is regular, representing the normal, rhythmical depolarization of the sinoatrial node. The sinus rate is approximately 220 beats/min. There is complete failure of the atrial impulses to conduct to the ventricles, as indicated by the lack of a QRS complexes following each P wave at a fixed PR interval. Three predominantly negative, wide, bizarre QRS complexes are seen (ventricular escape beats), producing a ventricular rate of 145 beats/min. The fourth QRS complex (*asterisk*) is a completely different morphology than the first 3, and it occurs sooner than the ventricular escape rhythm (ie, it is premature). This is a premature ventricular contraction (PVC), which illustrates the dilemma of concurrent bradycardia (AV block) and tachycardia (PVC). Either bradycardia or tachycardia could explain the onset of syncope in this cat: a failure of the ventricular escape mechanism (causing prolonged bradycardia/asystole) or a rapid burst of ventricular tachycardia (compromising diastolic ventricular filling to such an extent as to cause hypotension), respectively. However, the required treatments would be diametrically opposite depending on which arrhythmia was responsible for the clinical signs. With concurrent bradycardia and tachycardia, a treatment option consists of beginning with pacemaker implantation to control the bradycardia, followed by medications to treat the ventricular tachyarrhythmia. Lead II: 50 mm/s, 20 mm/mV.

diagnosis regardless of treatment (a pacemaker was implanted in only 1 of 21 cats [5%]). These findings lend some support to a conservative approach in cases of third-degree AV block in cats, including the decision to withhold pacemaker implantation in cats in many cases. The clinical implication of Kellum and Stepien's study is that the traditionally touted advantages of pacemaker implantation for patients with third-degree AV block, including improved mentation and stamina as a result of increased cardiac output, reduced risk of sudden bradycardic death, and treatment of congestive heart failure when caused by a combination of structural heart disease and bradycardia, may in many cats legitimately be outweighed by the risk of complications, cost, drawbacks of concurrent structural heart disease such as cardiomyopathy, and fair prognosis even without treatment.

AV block was identified in 3 cats presenting with seizurelike episodes in a study by Penning and colleagues.[15] This important observation highlights an oversimplification that has been perpetuated for many years. It is common knowledge that seizures are disturbances of electrical activity in the brain triggered by an intra- or extracranial disturbance, are typically preceded by an aura, are characterized by tonic-clonic movements and possibly urination and defecation, and are followed by a postictal period of recovery to normal function. This traditional description is contrasted with an equally traditional characterization of syncope, according to which an episode consists of sudden collapse and loss of consciousness, atonic immobility, brief duration (<1 minute), and instantaneous recovery within seconds of return of consciousness. Although these broad features do apply to some patients, substantial overlap exists between categories with respect to clinical signs. Specifically, anoxic or anoxic-epileptic seizures can occur when deprivation of energy to the brain (eg, cardiac arrhythmia causing cerebral hypoperfusion) causes seizurelike activity or a true seizure, respectively.[15] This small but important case series, supported by references from human cardiovascular medicine that have identified up to 40% of patients previously believed to be epileptic as suffering from cardiovascular disease as the cause of their seizures, reinforces an important fact: cats with seizures, particularly if they have concurrent heart disease, may have a cardiovascular explanation for episodic clinical signs. All cats with unexplained seizures should have a cardiovascular examination consisting of physical examination, thoracic radiographs, echocardiogram, and electrocardiogram; and especially when structural heart disease is identified with these tests, ambulatory electrocardiography or prolonged telemetric ECG monitoring may be indicated preferably for as long a duration as is needed to obtain ECG data during an event (**Fig. 3**). The availability of small portable or implantable cardiac event recorders with an extended battery life makes this approach realistic.[13] Failing to obtain ambulatory ECG data poses a substantial risk: after routine laboratory tests, subsequent diagnostic steps for patients with unexplained seizures are usually dependent on general anesthesia (cerebrospinal fluid tap, computed tomography, magnetic resonance imaging), which, in addition to the liability resulting from unnecessary cost and delay in diagnosis, may miss the site of the lesion and place the patient with occult/intermittent arrhythmias at substantial risk of intraprocedural complications. Arrhythmic patients who survive the imaging procedure may furthermore be given antiseizure medications, to which they are unlikely to respond, instead of pacemaker implantation or other appropriate antiarrhythmic therapy.

An insight into the mechanisms behind AV block in cats may be found in a report by Liu and colleagues,[16] published in 1975. This seminal investigation identified histologic lesions associated with the intracardiac conduction system of 63 cats with cardiomyopathy. Findings included AV nodal degeneration and fibrosis in 55 and 56 cases (87%, 89%, respectively), and lesion(s) of the left bundle and right bundle in

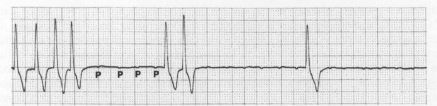

Fig. 3. Cardiac event recording of advanced second-degree AV block in a cat with recurrent seizurelike episodes. Initially, 3 sinus beats (150 beats/min, same rate as P waves) are seen, and the fourth beat is a premature complex. Then, consistent conduction through the AV node ceases; 4 P waves are blocked before 1 is conducted, and this sinus beat is immediately followed by another premature beat. After another period of block, 1 last sinus beat is seen. First-degree AV block is present during the sinus beats (PR interval = 160 milliseconds; normal = 40–90 milliseconds). After the last QRS complex on this tracing, a period of ventricular asystole lasting 26 seconds occurred (not shown), concurrent with collapse, loss of consciousness, and a brief episode of tonic-clonic activity in this cat followed by several minutes of disorientation and then further episodes. Pacemaker implantation was warranted but was not undertaken and a few hours after this tracing was obtained, the cat collapsed and died. Modified precordial lead (portable event monitor): 25 mm/s, 1 cm = 1 mV.

54 and 20 (86%, 32%, respectively) of cases. The latter finding may indicate the basis for the ECG left anterior fascicular block pattern that has since been reported in cats with HCM. More recently Kaneshige and colleagues[17] evaluated the hearts of 13 cats with HCM and concurrent third-degree AV block. Eight (62%) had a presenting complaint of syncope, 4 (31%) were lethargic, and in one the AV block was an incidental finding. In all cases, extensive fibrosis was observed in the branching portion of the AV bundle and in the left bundle branch. As previously noted by Liu and colleagues, the lesions of the left bundle branch were more severe than those of the right bundle branch. In contrast to Liu and colleagues' findings, the more proximal part of the His-Purkinje system (the AV node proper and the penetrating portion of the AV bundle) were less severely affected than the more distal branches. This observation could help to explain the minimal clinical response often observed with drugs intended to improve the activity of remaining, functional fibers in these structures, such as β-agonists, parasympatholytics, and methylxanthines, when the therapeutic target for these compounds is not the site of the most extensive lesions. The investigators hypothesized that this constellation of lesions may represent a combination of effects from natural aging and HCM.

HCM

HCM has long been known to be widely prevalent in cats. However, echocardiographic assessment of a population of seemingly healthy cats to identify cats with structural heart disease had not been undertaken until recently. In 2009, a study of overtly healthy cats revealed HCM in 16 of 103 cats, a prevalence of 16%.[18] This important prospective study in cats deserves repetition and confirmation; from the perspective of cardiac arrhythmias in the cat, the prevalence of HCM is important because a large proportion of cats with ventricular arrhythmias,[12] atrial fibrillation,[19] or AV block[14,15,17] have concurrent, and in the case of AV block, seemingly causative, HCM. Therefore, an understanding of the prevalence of HCM is likely to affect our understanding of the prevalence of cardiac arrhythmias in the cat, particularly when approximately one-quarter to one-third of cases of such arrhythmias are recognized as incidental findings, as with atrial fibrillation and third-degree AV block.

SUMMARY

Important and clinically useful information has emerged regarding feline arrhythmias in the last 5 years: the effect of hyperkalemia on the electrocardiogram is more accurately understood; structural heart diseases associated with ventricular tachyarrhythmias are better defined; AV block is more clearly characterized, clinically and pathologically; and the prevalence of HCM, the common denominator of many arrhythmias, has been quantified in the overtly healthy feline population for the first time. These elements of new information add to the foundation of knowledge that should be used as an ever-advancing starting point for further investigations in disturbances of the rhythm of the feline heartbeat.

REFERENCES

1. Tilley LP. Essentials of canine and feline electrocardiography. 3rd edition. Philadelphia: Lea & Febiger; 1993.
2. Fox PR, Harpster NK. Diagnosis and management of feline arrhythmias. In: Fox PR, Sisson DD, Moïse NS, editors. Textbook of canine and feline cardiology. 2nd edition. Philadelphia: Saunders; 1999. p. 386–99.
3. Côté E, Harpster NK. Feline arrhythmias. In: Bonagura JD, Twedt DC, editors. Kirk's current veterinary therapy XIV. St. Louis (MO): Elsevier; 2008. p. 731–9.
4. Harpster NK. Feline arrhythmias: diagnosis and management. In: Kirk RW, Bonagura JD, editors. Kirk's current veterinary therapy XI. Philadelphia: Saunders; 1992. p. 732–44.
5. Harpster NK. The cardiovascular system. In: Holzworth J, editor. Diseases of the cat: medicine and surgery. Philadelphia: Saunders; 1987. p. 820–933.
6. Norman BC, Côté E, Barrett KA. Wide-complex tachycardia associated with hyperkalemia in three cats. J Feline Med Surg 2006;8:372–8.
7. Tag TL, Day TK. Electrocardiographic assessment of hyperkalemia in dogs and cats. J Vet Emerg Crit Care 2008;18:61–7.
8. Ettinger PO, Regan TJ, Oldewurtel HA. Hyperkalemia, cardiac conduction, and the electrocardiogram: a review. Am Heart J 1974;88:360.
9. Parham WA, Mehdlrad AA, Biermann KM, et al. Hyperkalemia revisited. Tex Heart Inst J 2006;33:40–7.
10. Drobatz K, Hughes D. Concentration of ionized calcium in plasma from cats with urethral obstruction. J Am Vet Med Assoc 1997;211:1392–5.
11. DiBartola SP, Autran de Morais H. Disorders of potassium: hypokalemia and hyperkalemia. In: DiBartola SP, editor. Fluid, electrolyte, and acid-base disorders in small animal practice. 3rd edition. St. Louis (MO): Saunders; 2006. p. 91–121.
12. Côté E, Jaeger R. Ventricular tachyarrhythmias in 106 cats: associated structural cardiac disorders. J Vet Intern Med 2008;22:1444–6.
13. Ferasin L. Recurrent syncope associated with paroxysmal supraventricular tachycardia in a Devon Rex cat diagnosed by implantable loop recorder. J Feline Med Surg 2009;11:149–52.
14. Kellum HB, Stepien RL. Third-degree atrioventricular block in cats: 21 cases (1997–2004). J Vet Intern Med 2006;20:97–103.
15. Penning VA, Connolly DJ, Gajanayake I, et al. Seizure-like episodes in 3 cats with intermittent high-grade atrioventricular dysfunction. J Vet Intern Med 2009;23: 200–5.
16. Liu SK, Tilley LP, Tashjian RJ. Lesions of the conduction system in the cat with cardiomyopathy. Recent Adv Stud Cardiac Struct Metab 1975;10:681–93.

17. Kaneshige T, Machida N, Itoh H, et al. The anatomical basis of complete atrioventricular block in cats with hypertrophic cardiomyopathy. J Comp Pathol 2006;135: 25–31.
18. Paige CF, Abbott JA, Elvinger F, et al. Prevalence of cardiomyopathy in apparently healthy cats. J Am Vet Med Assoc 2009;234:1398–403.
19. Côté E, Harpster NK, Laste NJ, et al. Atrial fibrillation in cats: 50 cases (1979–2002). J Am Vet Med Assoc 2004;225:256–60.

Canine Degenerative Myxomatous Mitral Valve Disease: Natural History, Clinical Presentation and Therapy

Michele Borgarelli, DMV, PhD[a],*, Jens Haggstrom, DVM, PhD[b]

KEYWORDS

• Canine • Mitral valve • Myxomatous degeneration • Therapy

Chronic degenerative mitral valve disease as a result of myxomatous degeneration (MMVD) is the most common acquired cardiovascular disease in the dog representing 75% of all cardiovascular disease in this species.[1–3] Although the disease is more commonly diagnosed in small-breed dogs, it can also occur in large-breed dogs.[4,5] The prevalence of the disease has been correlated with the age and the breed. In some breeds, such as the cavalier King Charles spaniel, the prevalence of the disease in animals older than 10 years is greater than 90%.[6–9] Males are also reported to develop the disease at a younger age than females, which means that the prevalence at a given age is higher in males than in females.[2,3]

NATURAL HISTORY

Although MMVD is a common cause of left-sided congestive heart failure (CHF) in dogs, there are few studies documenting its natural history, and most of the known data on survival for the affected dogs come from clinical trials or retrospective studies.[10–16] The disease is characterized by a long preclinical period and many dogs affected die for other reasons and do not progress to CHF.[10,16] In 1 study including 558 dogs affected by MMVD at different stages of CHF, more than 70% of asymptomatic dogs were alive at the end of the follow-up period of 6.6 years (**Fig. 1**).[10] In another recent study, 82% of asymptomatic dogs were still asymptomatic

[a] Department of Clinical Sciences, Kansas State University, A-106 Mosier Hall, Manhattan, KS 66505, USA
[b] Department of Clinical Sciences, Swedish University of Agricultural Sciences, Box 7054, SE-750 07, Uppsala, Sweden
* Corresponding author.
E-mail address: mborgarelli@gmail.com

Vet Clin Small Anim 40 (2010) 651–663
doi:10.1016/j.cvsm.2010.03.008
0195-5616/10/$ – see front matter © 2010 Elsevier Inc. All rights reserved.

vetsmall.theclinics.com

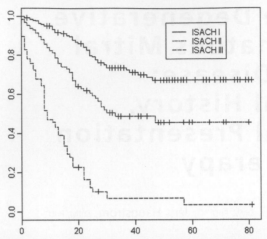

Fig. 1. Survival in 558 dogs with MMVD by heart failure classification according to the ISACHC. More than 60% of class I dogs were still alive at the end of the 70 months of observation period. Class ISACHC 2 dogs have 28 months median survival time. Class ISACHC 3 had a median survival time of 9 months. (*From* Borgarelli M, Savarino P, Crosara S, et al. Survival characteristics and prognostic variables of dogs with mitral regurgitation attributable to myxomatous valve disease. J Vet Intern Med 2008;22:123; with permission.)

at 12 months from inclusion in the study.[16] A study aimed at evaluating the efficacy of treatment with enalapril, an angiotensin-converting enzyme inhibitor (ACE-I), in delaying the onset of heart failure in asymptomatic dogs showed a median time free of CHF of 851 days for the treated group and 778 days for the placebo group.[17] Another study with the same aim but including only cavalier King Charles spaniels reached similar results.[11] These data provide some evidence that asymptomatic MMVD is a relatively benign condition similar to what has been reported in people.

For dogs that progress to CHF, survival time can be related to several factors including owner compliance in providing adequate care, treatment, cardiovascular complications such as pulmonary hypertension or rupture of chordae tendinae, and the presence of other concomitant diseases. In our study of survival in MMVD, dogs with moderate or severe CHF (classes 2 and 3 according to the International Small Animal Cardiac Health Council [ISACHC] classification) had median survival times of 33 and 9 months, respectively.[10] Estimates of survival time in CHF caused by MMVD can also be inferred from the existing clinical trial data. The Long-Term Investigation of Veterinary Enalapril (LIVE) and BENazepril in Canine Heart Disease (BENCH) trials compared enalapril and benazepril, respectively, with placebo in canine patients with heart failure caused by either MMVD or dilated cardiomyopathy. More recently, QUEST was designed to compare the efficacy of pimobendan to benazepril in dogs receiving background therapy for furosemide with or without digoxin; heart failure caused by MMVD was the primary inclusion criterion. In the QUEST trial, the median survival time for all dogs to reach the primary end point represented by sudden cardiac death, euthanasia as a consequence of the cardiac disease, or treatment failure, was about 6 months.[18] Survival time was similar for the group of dogs in LIVE that were treated with enalapril.[12] In the BENCH study the mean survival time for dogs receiving benazepril was about 14 months.[13] Differences in these studies can be related to differences in inclusion criteria and end points. The results of these studies suggest that dogs with moderate to severe CHF caused by MMVD can have relatively long survival with medical management.

DIAGNOSIS

Mitral valve regurgitation results in a systolic murmur that generally is heard best over the left cardiac apex. The diagnosis of MMVD can be suspected when this auscultatory finding is encountered in a patient of typical signalment. The intensity of the murmur has been correlated with the severity of MMVD in some studies.[19,20] In more severe cases, the murmur radiates toward the left heart base and to the right hemithorax as a consequence of left atrial and ventricular enlargement and in some patients, the concomitant presence of tricuspid regurgitation. In large-breed dogs the murmur may not correlate with the severity of the disease.[5] This difference might be because large-breed dogs affected by MMVD more commonly present with atrial fibrillation and myocardial failure; both these conditions can influence the intensity of the murmur. In the very early stage of the disease the only auscultatory finding may be the presence of a midsystolic click.[21] This sound is often intermittent and may be best heard using the diaphragm of the stethoscope. It is considered a reliable indicator of mitral valve prolapse (MVP) in people. The origin of the midsystolic click has been postulated to be caused by the tensing of redundant chordae tendinae and rapid deceleration of blood against the leaflets at maximum prolapse into the left atrium.[22]

Although the presence of a systolic left apical murmur in a typical breed is strongly suggestive of the presence of MMVD, echocardiographic confirmation of the diagnosis is required to exclude the presence of other cardiovascular diseases leading to mitral regurgitation, such as mitral valve dysplasia. The recently published American College of Veterinary Internal Medicine (ACVIM) consensus statement recommends that echocardiography should be performed to answer specific questions regarding the cause of the murmur of mitral regurgitation and presence of cardiac chamber enlargement in dogs with suspected MMVD.[23] The echocardiographic characteristics of MMVD include prolapse or thickening of 1 or both mitral valve leaflets (**Fig. 2**). MVP is characterized by an abnormal systolic displacement or bowing of the mitral valve leaflets from the left ventricle toward the left atrium. In dogs, some studies suggest that the right parasternal 4-chamber, long axis view is the gold standard view to identify the presence of MVP (**Fig. 3**A).[24] In people, the gold standard view to recognize MVP is a right parasternal long axis view that includes the left ventricular outflow tract (**Fig. 3**B). In people, the mitral valve has a saddle shape and reliance on other image

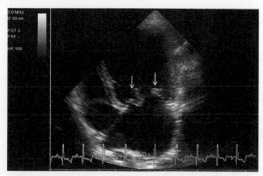

Fig. 2. Left apical 4-chamber view of a dog with MMVD. The arrows indicate the thick and irregular mitral valve leaflets.

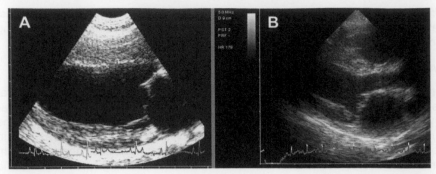

Fig. 3. MVP in 2 dogs. (*A*) Right parasternal 4-chamber view. The anterior mitral valve leaflet appears displaced toward the left atrium. (*B*) Right parasternal long axis view. There is a mild prolapse of the mid portion of the anterior mitral valve leaflet with the parachute appearance of the valve.

planes, such as the apical view, can overestimate the prevalence of MVP.[25] In dogs, the mitral valve can have 1 of 2 different annular geometries, either circular or elliptical, and this could influence the echocardiographic estimation of the MVP (Borgarelli, personal communication, ACVIM Forum, Montreal, 2009). According to these data, we suggest that the presence of MVP in dogs should be confirmed in at least 2 echocardiographic views.

Echocardiography can also provide important information concerning the severity of the disease, such as the degree of left atrial and left ventricular enlargement, the presence of systolic or diastolic dysfunction and the diagnosis of pulmonary hypertension.[26–29] Some echocardiographic variables may be useful to identify individuals at increased risk of progression of the disease. Among these variables, left atrial enlargement seems to represent the most reliable independent indicator. In our study, the risk of death from cardiac disease for dogs with a left atrium/aortic root ratio exceeding 1.7 was 2.1 times that of dogs with smaller atria (**Fig. 4**).[10] Also, in the QUEST study, left

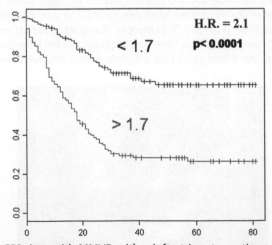

Fig. 4. Survival in 558 dogs with MMVD with a left atrium to aortic root ratio (La/Ao) less than 1.7 and in dogs with a LA/Ao greater than 1.7. Dogs without left atrial enlargement have a significantly longer survival time. OR, odds ratio.

atrial size was 1 of the independent predictors of outcome in dogs with symptomatic MMVD.[18]

The ACVIM consensus statement recommends thoracic radiography for all dogs with MMVD to assess the hemodynamic significance of the murmur and to obtain a baseline when the patient is asymptomatic.[23] Careful evaluation of thoracic radiographs may help in diagnosing concomitant primary respiratory diseases, such as tracheobronchial disease or lung tumors that may be the cause for the clinical signs, such as cough. Thoracic radiographs, together with physical examination, are also essential for monitoring dogs with MMVD. A recent study shows that radiographic assessment of left atrial size has higher interobserver agreement compared with assessment of left ventricular size in dogs with MMVD, and that left atrial size is most useful to assess the heart size and indirectly, the severity, of mitral regurgitation on radiographs.[30]

CLINICAL PRESENTATION AND TREATMENT

MMVD is a chronic disease in which the clinical presentation is variable; some patients remain completely asymptomatic, whereas others develop life-threatening pulmonary edema. The authors of the ACVIM consensus statement proposed a modification of a staging system that has been used to classify human patients with heart failure. In this schema, dogs are placed in 1 of 4 categories according to clinical status and risk factors for the development of MMVD (**Table 1**).[23] This classification introduces the concept of patients at risk for developing heart disease but that currently do not have a heart disease. Included in this category are dogs of breeds predisposed to MMVD including the cavalier King Charles spaniel and the dachshund. The recognition of this stage should encourage the veterinary community to develop appropriate screening programs and adopt measures intended to reduce the risk for an animal of developing the disease. For the purpose of this review, 3 categories of patients are considered: the asymptomatic, the coughing, and the dog with documented presence of CHF.

The Asymptomatic Dog (Stage B ACVIM Consensus)

This category includes dogs with MMVD that have not developed CHF. In our experience, this group represents most dogs presenting with MMVD. The minimum

Table 1		
Classification system for dogs affected by MMVD		
	Definition	
Stage A	Dogs at risk for developing MMVD that have no identifiable cardiac structural disorder (ie, Cavalier King Charles spaniel, dachsunds)	
Stage B1	Dogs with MMVD that have never developed clinical signs and have no radiographic or echocardiographic evidence of cardiac remodeling	
Stage B2	Dogs with MMVD that have never developed clinical signs but have radiographic or echocardiographic evidence of cardiac remodeling (ie, left-sided heart enlargement)	
Stage C	Dogs with MMVD and past or current clinical signs of heart failure associated with structural heart remodeling (dogs presenting heart failure for the first time may present severe clinical signs and may require hospitalization)	
Stage D	Dogs with end-stage MMVD and heart failure that is refractory to standard therapy (ie, furosemide, ACE-I, pimobendan ± spironolactone)	

Adapted from Atkins C, Bonagura J, Ettinger S, et al. Guidelines for the diagnosis and treatment of canine chronic valvular heart disease. J Vet Intern Med 2009;26:1142–50; with permission.

suggested database for these dogs includes a physical examination and thoracic radiographs. Echocardiography is recommended to confirm the diagnosis. The ACVIM consensus statement includes the suggestion that asymptomatic dogs can be further subdivided: dogs without radiographic or echocardiographic evidence of cardiac enlargement are in stage B1 and dogs with left atrial and ventricular enlargement are in stage B2. This subclassification emphasizes that asymptomatic dogs are a nonhomogeneous group that includes patients with very mild disease and others that have not developed CHF but have more advanced disease and are at risk for progression to CHF. The heterogeneity of this group of dogs may be an explanation for the conflicting data concerning neurohormonal activation presented in the veterinary literature for dogs with asymptomatic MMVD.[31–36] The recognition that asymptomatic dogs are a heterogeneous group underlines the importance of identifying risk factors for the development of CHF. Proposed risk factors for death or progression of MMVD include age, gender, intensity of heart murmur, degree of valve prolapse, severity of valve lesions, degree of mitral valve regurgitation, and left atrial enlargement.[6,37–39] A recent study suggests that a change in radiographic or echocardiographic cardiac dimensions observed between 2 different time points may be a more powerful predictor of outcome than the absolute value of the measurement.[40]

In people, brain natriuretic peptide (BNP) has been showed not only to be an excellent biomarker for identifying the presence of CHF but also for identifying patients that are at high risk of CHF or death.[41–43] A recent study conducted on 72 asymptomatic dogs with MMDV showed, in agreement with previous studies,[31] that the N-terminal fragment of proBNP (NT-proBNP) is correlated with the severity of mitral regurgitation. In this study a cutoff of 466 pmol/L had 80% sensitivity and 76% specificity for predicting 12-month progression (cardiac death or CHF).[16] Although these data seem very promising, further studies are needed to confirm the value of BNP in distinguishing, among asymptomatic dogs, those that will progress to CHF. In our opinion the evaluation of risk progression for these dogs should be based on evaluation of multiple parameters.

Treatment of dogs with asymptomatic MMVD has been the subject of controversy. The ACVIM consensus group did not recommend treating dogs with MMVD in stage B1 of the disease. The same group however did not reach a consensus for dogs with cardiac enlargement.[23] Two multicenter double-blinded studies evaluating the efficacy of enalapril on delaying the onset of CHF in dogs with MMVD without clinical signs have shown no significant effect of ACE-I therapy on the primary outcome variable, which was time from inclusion in the study to the onset of signs of CHF.[11,17] Another recently published study reported a possible benefit of early treatment with benazepril.[15] However, this was a retrospective case series, and studies of this type are invariably associated with systematic errors. Consequently, the results should be interpreted with caution. A prospective, randomized, multicenter double-blinded study involving a larger number of dogs would be necessary to confirm the results of this study.[44] In our opinion, the currently available data from clinical trials and the observation that only a relatively small percentage of dogs with asymptomatic disease progress to CHF or die as a consequence of the disease, do not support the early treatment with an ACE-I. However, it is possible, although not proved, that dogs with MMVD and severe cardiac enlargement, but not CHF, may benefit from medical treatment. The authors believe that asymptomatic cases should be individually evaluated and therapeutic decisions taken on a case-by-case basis. The available data concern only treatment with an ACE-I. Hitherto, no studies have been conducted with other classes of drugs, such as β-blockers, pimobendan, spironolactone, or amlodipine.

The Coughing Dog

The presence of cough and mitral valve murmur represents a challenging problem for the clinician. Cough as a consequence of pulmonary edema is a possible sign of CHF in dogs. However, cough is a general clinical sign of respiratory disease and its presence in a dog with a murmur should not be the reason for starting CHF treatment. Old small-breed dogs are commonly affected by tracheobronchial disease and by MMVD. In these patients, the cough is often the result of their primary respiratory disease and not heart disease. Thoracic radiographs should always be obtained in a coughing dog with a murmur typical for MMVD to determine if primary respiratory disease is the cause of the cough. This is also true for patients with a documented history of CHF that start to cough. In these patients the cough may be related to reasons other than worsening of CHF (**Fig. 5**). Cough in dogs with MMVD can also be related to compression of left mainstem bronchus by an enlarged left atrium. However, it has been suggested that this is more likely to occur in the presence of primary bronchomalacia.[45] Indeed, some unpublished data from our group seems to confirm this hypothesis. In a group of 68 dogs with MMVD at different stages, cough was not associated with the dimension of the left atrium or the presence of CHF. It was, however, associated with concomitant presence of tracheobronchial disease (Borgarelli, unpublished data, 2007). It is possible that coughing dogs with moderate to severe left atrial enlargement without evidence of CHF but with a primary tracheobronchial disease could benefit from treatments aimed at decreasing the left atrial volume, as the decrease in pressure on the main stem bronchus could decrease the stimulus for coughing. However, the types of drugs that have the potential to achieve this are all associated with potential adverse reactions. Furthermore, moderate to high doses of furosemide in dogs with tracheobronchial disease without CHF may not only dehydrate the dog but also worsen the cough as a consequence of drying the airways.

The Symptomatic Dog (Stage C ACVIM Consensus)

According to the ACVIM consensus statement, patients with stage C mitral valve disease are those with a documented cardiac structural abnormality and current or

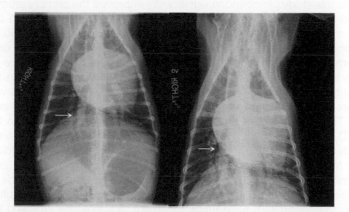

Fig. 5. Dorsoventral thoracic radiograph from a dog with severe MMVD. On the left, the radiograph shows a normally outlined right caudal bronchus (*arrow*). On the right, the same dog 1 month later. Radiographs were obtained because the owner was reporting the presence of cough. The arrow shows the presence of a collapsed right caudal main stem bronchus but no worsening of pulmonary venous congestion or presence of pulmonary edema.

previous clinical signs of CHF.[23] Management of these patients is based on administration of a combination of several drugs including diuretics, pimobendan, ACE-I, and others. Although no study has specifically addressed the question of efficacy of furosemide in dogs with MMVD, there is a general consensus that diuretics are essential for patients with CHF. Most dogs enrolled in the multicenter studies evaluating the efficacy of the ACE-I and pimobendan in symptomatic dogs with MMVD received concomitant treatment with furosemide.[12–14,18,46] In our opinion, the diagnosis of CHF should be reevaluated if it is possible to discontinue the furosemide administration in a patient without a reoccurrence of clinical signs. The dosage of furosemide should be adjusted to keep the patients free from clinical signs; the optimal dose likely being the lowest effective dose. Although the suggested mean dosage for these patients is 2 mg/kg by mouth every 12 hours, in our experience it could range from 0.5 mg/kg by mouth every 12 hours to 4 to 6 mg/kg by mouth every 8 hours. Dogs with refractory heart failure could also benefit from administration of 1 of the doses of the drug by subcutaneous injection. It has been shown in people that teaching the patients to adjust their furosemide dosage on the base of monitoring their weight and their clinical signs significantly reduces the number of hospitalizations and may be associated with prolonged survival.[47] The authors try to use this approach with the owners whenever possible. The use of an ACE-I together with furosemide in dogs with CHF caused by MMVD is based on evidence provided by several multicenter double-blind studies.[12–14,48] These studies, although recently the subject of criticism,[49] provide evidence that an ACE-I added to standard therapy improves quality of life and survival time in dogs with CHF caused by MMVD. ACE-I should be used at the dosage that has been shown to be effective in the clinical trials. There is no proven evidence that using ACE-I at dosages higher than the recommended dose presents any clinical advantage.

Two recent studies have shown that pimobendan improves survival and quality of life in dogs with MMVD and overt heart failure compared with standard treatment consisting of an ACE-I and furosemide. The first study was conducted as a blinded, randomized, positive-controlled, multicenter study and included 76 dogs. The study had a mandatory 56-day treatment period that was followed by optional long-term treatment. In this study pimobendan significantly improved the primary study variable represented by heart insufficiency score and also significantly improved survival.[46] One criticism of this study concerned concomitant treatment as only 56 dogs (31 in the pimobendan group and 25 in the standard treatment group) were on concurrent furosemide treatment, suggesting that the diagnosis of heart failure could be questioned in the remaining dogs. However, the results of a subanalysis of data provided only by dogs receiving concurrent furosemide were consistent with those of the entire dataset. Moreover, the long-term part of the study was conducted unblinded. The results of this study led to a larger study conducted on 260 dogs with MMVD and overt CHF. This was a prospective multicenter, randomized, single-blinded study and the primary end point was a composite of cardiac death, euthanasia for heart failure, or treatment failure. In this study treatment with pimobendan was associated with a significant improvement in survival time and this benefit persisted after adjusting for all baseline variables.[18] All dogs enrolled in this study were on concomitant furosemide treatment. It should be stressed that none of these studies addressed the possibility of an interaction between ACE-I and pimobendan; it is not known whether or not triple therapy consisting of furosemide, ACE-I, and pimobendan is superior to therapy consisting of pimobendan plus furosemide. The ACVIM consensus recommends that chronic management of stage C dogs includes all these drugs.[23]

Spironolactone has recently been approved in Europe for treatment of dogs with MMVD. A recent study shows that in dogs with moderate to severe MMVD spironolactone added to an ACE-I, furosemide ± digoxin treatment reduces the risk of cardiac death and the risk of severe worsening of CHF.[50] The dosage used in this clinical trial was 2 mg/kg every 24 hours and this dosage seems to have little diuretic effect in normal dogs.[51] One possible mechanism of action for spironolactone could be related to the antifibrotic effects of this drug that have been shown in experimental studies.[52,53] A recent study has shown that geriatric dogs affected by MMVD have intramyocardial arterial changes associated with area of fibrosis, so-called replacement fibrosis.[54] The exact role of these findings in the pathogenesis of MMVD is still to be clarified as is the possible antifibrotic effect of spironolactone in natural occurring disease in dogs. Positive effects of blocking aldosterone in dogs with heart failure with a specific antagonist such as spironolactone could also be related to the phenomenon of aldosterone escape[55,56] that can occur in dogs with severe CHF. It has been shown the aldosterone concentration can be increased in dogs with MMVD receiving furosemide and an ACE-I.[56] This phenomenon is dependent on the dose of furosemide and has been attributed to the fact that ACE inhibition does not completely block ACE activity. In dogs in particular, it has been speculated that other enzymes such as chymase can play a major role in producing angiotensin II.[1] The exact mechanism of action through which spironolactone exerts its possible benefits in improving outcome in dogs with MMVD needs further studies.

Other drugs frequently used for treatment of dogs with overt CHF caused by MMVD are digoxin and amlodipine. Digoxin is commonly used to treat dogs with concomitant atrial fibrillation to control the heart rate. There are no controlled studies in veterinary medicine evaluating digoxin, but it is general expert opinion that its administration could improve clinical signs of heart failure in dogs. In humans, relative to placebo, the effect of digoxin on mortality of ambulatory human patients with heart failure is neutral. However, this drug decreases rates of hospitalization and there may be subpopulations of patients with heart failure in which digoxin has a favorable effect on longevity.[57] Amlodipine at the dosage of 0.05 to 0.1 mg/kg every 12 hours is listed in the ACVIM consensus statement as a possible agent for those dogs with a more advanced stage of heart failure (stage D) to obtain a more effective reduction in afterload[23] and improve cardiac output. Arteriolar vasodilation associated with the use of this drug can lead to severe hypotension in these patients. Therefore, slow up-titration of amlodipine dosage with monitoring of blood pressure is recommended to avoid serious hypotension. In our experience, the use of this drug or other intravenous vasodilators, such as sodium nitroprusside, can be of some help for dogs with uncontrolled CHF that experience an acute episode of pulmonary edema.

In our experience, most dogs with heart failure caused by MMVD can be managed using a combination of furosemide, an ACE-I, pimobendan, and spironolactone. Treatment should be individualized for each patients and the goal is to keep the dogs free of clinical signs of CHF as long as possible.

SUMMARY

MMVD is a common condition in geriatric dogs. Most dogs affected are clinically asymptomatic for a long time. However, about 30% of these animals present a progression to heart failure and eventually die as a consequence of the disease. Left atrial enlargement, and particularly a change in left atrial size, seems to be the most reliable predictor of progression in some studies, however further studies are needed to clarify how to recognize asymptomatic patients at higher risk of developing heart failure. According to the published data on the natural history of the disease and the results of published studies evaluating the effect of early therapy on delaying the progression of the disease, it seems that no currently available treatment delays the onset of clinical signs of CHF. Although the ideal treatment of more severely affected dogs is probably surgical mitral valve repair or mitral valve replacement, this is not a currently available option. The results of several clinical trials together with clinical experience suggest that dogs with overt CHF can be managed with acceptable quality of life for a relatively long time period with medical treatment including furosemide, an ACE-I, pimobendan, and spironolactone.

REFERENCES

1. Haggstrom J, Hoglund K, Borgarelli M. An update on treatment and prognostic indicators in canine myxomatous mitral valve disease. J Small Anim Pract 2009;50(Suppl 1):25–33.
2. Haggstrom J, Kvart C, Pedersen HD. Acquired valvular heart disease. In: Ettinger SJ, Feldman EC, editors. Textbook of veterinary internal medicine. 6th edition. St. Louis (MO): Elsevier Saunders; 2005. p. 1022–39.
3. Sisson D, Kvart C, Darke P. Acquired valvular heart disease in dogs and cats. In: Fox PR, Sisson D, Moise NS, editors. Textbook of canine and feline cardiology. 2nd edition. Philadelphia: WB Saunders Company; 1999. p. 536–65.
4. Borgarelli M. Mitral valve insufficiency in large breed dogs [PhD thesis]. Grugliasco, Italy: Dept of Patologia Animale, University of Turin; 2004.
5. Borgarelli M, Zini E, D'Agnolo G, et al. Comparison of primary mitral valve disease in German Shepherd dogs and is small breeds. J Vet Cardiol 2004;6:25–31.
6. Haggstrom J, Hansson K, Kvart C, et al. Chronic valvular disease in the cavalier King Charles spaniels in Sweden. Vet Rec 1992;131:549–53.
7. Haggstrom J. Chronic valvular disease in Cavalier King Charles Spaniels: epidemiology, inheritance and pathophysiology [PhD thesis]. Uppsala, Sweden: Department of Physiology, Swedish University of Agricultural Sciences; 1996.
8. Pedersen HD, Lorentzen KA, Kristensen BO. Echocardiographic mitral valve prolapse in cavalier King Charles spaniels: epidemiology and prognostic significance for regurgitation. Vet Rec 1999;144:315–20.
9. Olsen LH, Fredholm M, Pedersen HD. Epidemiology and inheritance of mitral valve prolapse in dachshunds. J Vet Intern Med 1999;13:448–56.
10. Borgarelli M, Savarino P, Crosara S, et al. Survival characteristics and prognostic variables of dogs with mitral regurgitation attributable to myxomatous valve disease. J Vet Intern Med 2008;22:120–8.
11. Kvart C, Haggstrom J, Pedersen HD, et al. Efficacy of enalapril for prevention of congestive heart failure in dogs with myxomatous valve disease and asymptomatic mitral regurgitation. J Vet Intern Med 2002;16:80–8.
12. Ettinger SJ, Benitz AM, Ericsson GF, et al. Effects of enalapril maleate on survival of dogs with naturally acquired heart failure. The Long-Term Investigation of Veterinary Enalapril (LIVE) Study Group. J Am Vet Med Assoc 1998;213:1573–7.
13. The BENCH Study Group. The effect of benazepril on survival times and clinical signs of dogs with congestive heart failure: results of a multicenter, prospective, randomized, double-blinded, placebo-controlled, long-term clinical trial. J Vet Cardiol 1999;1:7–18.
14. Cove T. Controlled clinical evaluation of enalapril in dogs with heart failure: results of the Cooperative Veterinary Enalapril Study Group. The COVE Study Group. J Vet Intern Med 1995;9:243–52.

15. Pouchelon JL, Jamet N, Gouni V, et al. Effect of benazepril on survival and cardiac events in dogs with asymptomatic mitral valve disease: a retrospective study of 141 cases. J Vet Intern Med 2008;22:905–14.

16. Chetboul V, Serres F, Tissier R, et al. Association of plasma N-terminal pro-B-type natriuretic peptide concentration with mitral regurgitation severity and outcome in dogs with asymptomatic degenerative mitral valve disease. J Vet Intern Med 2009;23:984–94.

17. Atkins CE, Keene BW, Brown WA, et al. Results of the veterinary enalapril trial to prove reduction in onset of heart failure in dogs chronically treated with enalapril alone for compensated, naturally occurring mitral valve insufficiency. J Am Vet Med Assoc 2007;231:1061–9.

18. Haggstrom J, Boswood A, O'Grady M, et al. Effect of pimobendan or benazepril hydrochloride on survival times in dogs with congestive heart failure caused by naturally occurring myxomatous mitral valve disease: the QUEST study. J Vet Intern Med 2008;22:1124–35.

19. Ljungvall I, Ahlstrom C, Hoglund K, et al. Use of signal analysis of heart sounds and murmurs to assess severity of mitral valve regurgitation attributable to myxomatous mitral valve disease in dogs. Am J Vet Res 2009;70:604–13.

20. Haggstrom J, Kvart C, Hansson K. Heart sounds and murmurs: changes related to severity of chronic valvular disease in the Cavalier King Charles spaniel. J Vet Intern Med 1995;9:75–85.

21. Pedersen HD, Haggstrom J. Mitral valve prolapse in the dog: a model of mitral valve prolapse in man. Cardiovasc Res 2000;47:234–43.

22. Fontana ME. Mitral valve prolapse and floppy mitral valve: physical examination. In: Boudoulas HK, Wooley CF, editors. Mitral valve: floppy mitral valve, mitral valve prolapse, mitral valve regurgitation. Armonk (NY): Futura; 2000. p. 283–304.

23. Atkins C, Bonagura J, Ettinger S, et al. Guidelines for the diagnosis and treatment of canine chronic valvular heart disease. J Vet Intern Med 2009;26: 1142–50.

24. Pedersen HD, Kristensen B, Norby B, et al. Echocardiographic study of mitral valve prolapse in dachshunds. Zentralbl Veterinarmed A 1996;43:103–10.

25. Levine RA, Triulzi MO, Harrigan P, et al. The relationship of mitral annular shape to the diagnosis of mitral valve prolapse. Circulation 1987;75:756–67.

26. Borgarelli M, Tarducci A, Zanatta R, et al. Decreased systolic function and inadequate hypertrophy in large and small breed dogs with chronic mitral valve insufficiency. J Vet Intern Med 2007;21:61–7.

27. Bonagura JD, Schober KE. Can ventricular function be assessed by echocardiography in chronic canine mitral valve disease? J Small Anim Pract 2009; 50(Suppl 1):12–24.

28. Chiavegato D, Borgarelli M, D'Agnolo G, et al. Pulmonary hypertension in dogs with mitral regurgitation attributable to myxomatous valve disease. Vet Radiol Ultrasound 2009;50:253–8.

29. Stepien RL. Pulmonary arterial hypertension secondary to chronic left-sided cardiac dysfunction in dogs. J Small Anim Pract 2009;50(Suppl 1):34–43.

30. Hansson K, Haggstrom J, Kvart C, et al. Reader performance in radiographic diagnosis of signs of mitral regurgitation in cavalier King Charles spaniels. J Small Anim Pract 2009;50(Suppl 1):44–53.

31. Haggstrom J, Hansson K, Kvart C, et al. Relationship between different natriuretic peptides and severity of naturally acquired mitral regurgitation in dogs with chronic myxomatous valve disease. J Vet Cardiol 2000;2:7–16.

32. Moesgaard SG, Pedersen LG, Teerlink T, et al. Neurohormonal and circulatory effects of short-term treatment with enalapril and quinapril in dogs with asymptomatic mitral regurgitation. J Vet Intern Med 2005;19:712–9.

33. Pedersen HD. Effects of mild mitral valve insufficiency, sodium intake, and place of blood sampling on the renin-angiotensin system in dogs. Acta Vet Scand 1996; 37:109–18.

34. Dell'Italia LJ, Meng QC, Balcells E, et al. Increased ACE and chymase-like activity in cardiac tissue of dogs with chronic mitral regurgitation. Am J Physiol 1995;269:H2065–73.

35. Su X, Wei CC, Machida N, et al. Differential expression of angiotensin-converting enzyme and chymase in dogs with chronic mitral regurgitation. J Mol Cell Cardiol 1999;31:1033–45.

36. Fujii Y, Orito K, Muto M, et al. Modulation of the tissue renin-angiotensin-aldosterone system in dogs with chronic mild regurgitation through the mitral valve. Am J Vet Res 2007;68:1045–50.

37. Buchanan JW. Chronic valvular disease (endocardiosis) in dogs. Adv Vet Sci Comp Med 1977;21:75–106.

38. Olsen LH, Mow T, Koch J, et al. Heart rate variability in young, clinically healthy dachshunds: influence of sex, mitral valve prolapse status, sampling period and time of day. J Vet Cardiol 1999;1:7–16.

39. Olsen LH, Martinussen T, Pedersen HD. Early echocardiographic predictors of myxomatous mitral valve disease in dachshunds. Vet Rec 2003;152: 293–7.

40. Lord PF, Hansson K, Kvart C, et al. Rate of change of heart size before congestive heart failure in dogs with mitral regurgitation. J Small Anim Pract 2010;51: 210–8.

41. Campbell DJ. Can measurement of B-type natriuretic peptide levels improve cardiovascular disease prevention? Clin Exp Pharmacol Physiol 2008;35: 442–6.

42. de Lemos JA, Hildebrandt P. Amino-terminal Pro–B-type natriuretic peptides: testing in general populations. Am J Cardiol 2008;101(Suppl):16A–20A.

43. Hinderliter AL, Blumenthal JA, O'Conner C, et al. Independent prognostic value of echocardiography and N-terminal pro–B-type natriuretic peptide in patients with heart failure. Am Heart J 2008;156:1191–5.

44. Kittleson M, Rishniw M, Pion P, et al. Effect of benazepril on survival and cardiac events in dogs with asymptomatic mitral valve disease: a retrospective study of 141 cases. J Vet Intern Med 2009;23:953–4 [author reply: 955–6].

45. Ettinger S, Kantrowitz B. Disease of the trachea. In: Ettinger S, Feldman EC, editors. Textbook of veterinary internal medicine. 6th edition. St. Louis (MO): Elsevier Saunders; 2005. p. 1217–32.

46. Lombard CW, Jons O, Bussadori C. Clinical efficacy of pimobendan versus benazepril for the treatment of acquired atrioventricular valvular disease in dogs. J Am Anim Hosp Assoc 2006;42:249–61.

47. Gonseth J, Guallar-Castillon P, Banegas JR, et al. The effectiveness of disease management programmes in reducing hospital re-admission in older patients with heart failure: a systematic review and meta-analysis of published reports. Eur Heart J 2004;25:1570–95.

48. Improve T Acute and short-term hemodynamic, echocardiographic, and clinical effects of enalapril maleate in dogs with naturally acquired heart failure: results of the Invasive Multicenter PROspective Veterinary Evaluation of Enalapril study. The IMPROVE Study Group. J Vet Intern Med 1995;9:234–42.

49. Pion P, Rinshiw M. Canine chronic mitral valve disease - the search for the silver bullet. In: Proceedings of the ACVIM Forum. San Antonio (TX), June 4–7, 2008. p. 98–100.
50. Bernay F, Bland JM, Haggstrom J, et al. Efficacy of spironolactone on survival in dogs with naturally occurring mitral regurgitation caused by myxomatous mitral valve disease. J Vet Intern Med 2010;24:331–41.
51. Jeunesse E, Woehrle F, Schneider M, et al. Effect of spironolactone on diuresis and urine sodium and potassium excretion in healthy dogs. J Vet Cardiol 2007; 9:63–8.
52. Brilla CG, Matsubara LS, Weber KT. Antifibrotic effects of spironolactone in preventing myocardial fibrosis in systemic arterial hypertension. Am J Cardiol 1993; 71:12A–6A.
53. Miric G, Dallemagne C, Endre Z, et al. Reversal of cardiac and renal fibrosis by pirfenidone and spironolactone in streptozotocin-diabetic rats. Br J Pharmacol 2001;133:687–94.
54. Falk T, Jonsson L, Olsen LH, et al. Arteriosclerotic changes in the myocardium, lung, and kidney in dogs with chronic congestive heart failure and myxomatous mitral valve disease. Cardiovasc Pathol 2006;15:185–93.
55. Struthers AD. The clinical implications of aldosterone escape in congestive heart failure. Eur J Heart Fail 2004;6:539–45.
56. Ubaid-Girioli S, Ferreira-Melo SE, Souza LA, et al. Aldosterone escape with diuretic or angiotensin-converting enzyme inhibitor/angiotensin II receptor blocker combination therapy in patients with mild to moderate hypertension. J Clin Hypertens (Greenwich) 2007;9:770–4.
57. Ahmed A, Rich MW, Love TE, et al. Digoxin and reduction in mortality and hospitalization in heart failure: a comprehensive post hoc analysis of the DIG trial. Eur Heart J 2006;27:178–86.

Infective Endocarditis in Dogs: Diagnosis and Therapy

Kristin MacDonald, DVM, PhD

KEYWORDS

- Bacterial endocarditis • Bartonella • Echocardiography
- Congestive heart failure • Mitral regurgitation
- Aortic insufficiency

OVERVIEW

Infective Endocarditis (IE) is a deadly, difficult-to-diagnose disease caused by microbial invasion into the endothelium of heart valves or endocardium. Although the reported prevalence is low (0.09%–6.6%) in dogs presenting to a tertiary referral center, the true prevalence in the general population is likely to be highly underestimated because of the nebulous clinical signs and difficulty in diagnosis. IE in cats is extremely rare. Acute congestive heart failure is the most common pathophysiologic consequence of IE. Other sequelae include immune-mediated disease (glomerulonephritis, immune-mediated polyarthritis), thromboembolic disease, septic polyarthritis, and arrhythmias. The mitral and aortic valves are the most affected in small animals. The most common microbiologic causes include *Staphylococcus* spp, *Streptococcus* spp, and *Escherichia coli*. The most common cause of culture negative IE is *Bartonella*. IE is diagnosed by using a modified set of criteria including echocardiographic diagnosis of an oscillating vegetative lesion on a cardiac valve. Long-term treatment (8–12 weeks) is needed with broad-spectrum antibiotics, optimally including at least 1 week of intravenous antibiotics. Overall prognosis is poor, and survival depends on the type of valve that is infected. Dogs with IE of the aortic valve have a grave prognosis, with median survival time (MST) of 3 days compared with dogs with IE of the mitral valve that have significantly longer lives (MST 476 days).

This article reviews the key aspects of pathophysiology and sequelae, diagnosis using a modified criteria scheme, and appropriate treatment options for IE.

PATHOGENESIS OF IE

The normal endothelial surface of the heart and valves is naturally resistant to microbial invasion, but becomes susceptible when the surface is damaged. Formation of IE

VCA-The Animal Care Center of Sonoma, 6470 Redwood Drive, Rohnert Park, CA 94928, USA
E-mail address: macdoka@yahoo.com

Vet Clin Small Anim 40 (2010) 665–684
doi:10.1016/j.cvsm.2010.03.010
0195-5616/10/$ – see front matter © 2010 Elsevier Inc. All rights reserved.

is triggered by endothelial damage, followed by platelet-fibrin deposition that provides a milieu for bacterial colonization, and finally bacterial adherence to the coagulum (**Fig. 1**). Mechanical lesions (ie, subaortic stenosis or cardiac catheterization procedure) or inflammatory lesions can promote bacterial seeding within the endothelium.

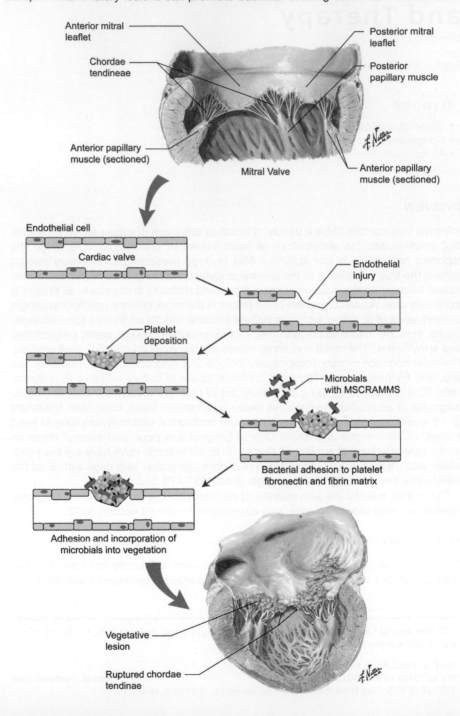

Anterior mitral leaflet

Posterior mitral leaflet

Chordae tendineae

Posterior papillary muscle

Anterior papillary muscle (sectioned)

Mitral Valve

Anterior papillary muscle (sectioned)

Endothelial cell

Cardiac valve

Endothelial injury

Platelet deposition

Microbials with MSCRAMMS

Bacterial adhesion to platelet fibronectin and fibrin matrix

Adhesion and incorporation of microbials into vegetation

Vegetative lesion

Ruptured chordae tendinae

Lesions of IE develop on the ventricular side of the aortic valve, and the atrial side of the mitral valve, in regions of the most significant blood flow injury (**Fig. 2**).[1] During disruption of the endothelium, extracellular matrix proteins, thromboplastin, and tissue factor trigger coagulation, and a coagulum forms on the damaged endothelium. This coagulum contains fibrinogen, fibrin, and platelet proteins, and avidly binds bacteria. Inflammation induces endothelial cell expression of integrins that bind bacteria and fibronectin to the exposed extracellular matrix. Fibronectin facilitates adherence of bacteria to the vegetation. Bacteremia must be present and the bacteria must be able to adhere to the coagulum for colonization to occur. This adherence is mediated by microbial surface components recognizing adhesive matrix molecules (MSCRAMMS) that are expressed on the surface of some bacteria. Organisms that commonly cause IE possess receptors for MSCRAMMS and have the greatest ability to adhere to damaged valves, including *Staphylococcus* spp and *Streptococcus* spp. These virulent bacteria can trigger tissue factor production and induce platelet aggregation, thereby building a larger vegetative lesion. *Streptococcus* spp produce surface glucans and dextran, which avidly bind to the coagulum on damaged valves. The fibrinous vegetative lesion shields bacteria from the blood stream and host defenses, and provides a formidable obstacle for antibiotic penetration (see **Fig. 2**). Extremely high concentrations of bacteria (10^9–10^{11} bacteria per gram of tissue) may accumulate within the vegetative lesion.[2] Bacteria also excrete enzymes that lead to destruction of valve tissue and rupture of chordae tendinae. Bacteria have also developed other mechanisms to evade the host. Although platelets release bactericidal proteins, most bacteria that cause IE are resistant to these proteins. Bacteria such as *Staphylococcus aureus* and *Bartonella* may become internalized within the endothelial cells and escape detection by the immune system. *Bartonella* also evade the immune system by colonizing red blood cells without causing hemolysis.

CAUSATIVE AGENTS

The most common causes of IE include *Staphylococcal* spp (*aureus*, *intermedius*, coagulase positive, and coagulase negative), *Streptococcus* spp (*canis*, *bovis*, and β-hemolytic), and *E coli* in order of frequency (**Table 1**). Less common bacterial isolates include *Pseudomonas*, *Erysipelothrix rhusiopathiae*, *Enterobacter*, *Pasteurella*, *Corynebacterium*, and *Proteus*. Rare causes of IE include *Bordetella avium*–like organism, *Erysipelothrix tonsillarum*, and *Actinomyces turicensis*.

IE CAUSED BY *BARTONELLA*

Bartonella has now been recognized as an important cause of culture-negative IE in people, and is more commonly screened for in dogs with systemic diseases including

---

Fig. 1. Pathogenesis of IE. A normal mitral valve (including leaflets and chordae tendinae) is represented (*top*) and a magnified view shows intact normal endothelium (*bottom*). The initiating step in development of IE is an injury to the endothelium, which exposes extracellular matrix proteins. A coagulum of platelets (*yellow*), fibrinogen, fibronectin, and fibrin develops. The fibronectin receptor (*blue*) on platelets and extracellular matrix proteins avidly bind bacteria that contain MSCRAMMS. The microorganism becomes embedded and incorporated into the vegetative lesion, and multiplies. The vegetative lesion may extend to chordae tendinae, opposing leaflet, or atrial endothelium, and may cause rupture of chordae tendinae. The end result is severe mitral regurgitation and congestive heart failure. (Netter Anatomy Illustration Collection, © Elsevier, Inc. All Rights Reserved. Labels revised with permission.)

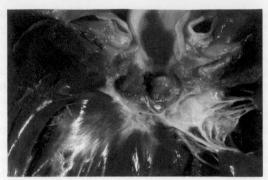

Fig. 2. Gross pathology of a dog with IE of the aortic valve. Vegetative lesions of the aortic valve appear as shaggy, thickened lesions (cauliflower-like appearance) that are also erosive to the underlying valve. This causes severe aortic insufficiency, which is a high-velocity jet that damages the endothelial surface of the interventricular septum and causes a fibrotic jet lesion. Subaortic stenosis is also seen as a fibrotic ring below the aortic cusp, which likely predisposed this dog to developing IE.

IE. In a recent case series of IE in 18 dogs living in Northern California, *Bartonella* was the most common causative agent in 28% of dogs, including 45% of dogs with negative blood cultures.[3] This may be an unusually high prevalence of IE caused by *Bartonella* compared with other parts of the country, but highlights the importance of testing for bartonellosis in dogs with IE. *Bartonella vinsonii* subsp *berkhoffii* is the most important species of *Bartonella* causing IE in dogs.[3,4] Other less common *Bartonella* species that cause IE in dogs include *B clarridgeiae*, *B washoensis*, *B quintana*, *B rochalimae*, *B clarridgeiae*–like, and *B koehlerae*.[5,6]

Bartonella primarily affects the aortic valve, and less commonly affects the mitral valve in dogs and causes unique valvular lesions characterized by fibrosis, mineralization, endothelial proliferation, and neovascularization.[7] *Bartonella* evades the immune system by colonizing red blood cells and endothelial cells, and also impairs the immune system by reducing the number of CD8+ lymphocytes and their cell adhesion

Table 1
Suggested criteria for diagnosis of IE in dogs

Major Criteria	Minor Criteria	Diagnosis
Positive echocardiogram	Fever	Definite
Vegetative, oscillating	Medium to large dog (>15 kg)	Pathology of valve
lesion	Subaortic stenosis	2 Major criteria
Erosive lesion	Thromboembolic disease	1 major and 2 minor
Abscess	Immune-mediated disease	Possible
New valvular insufficiency	Polyarthritis	1 major and 1 minor
>Mild AI in absence of	Glomerulonephritis	3 minor
subaortic stenosis or	Positive blood culture not	Rejected
annuloaortic ectasia	meeting major criteria	Firm alternative Dx
Positive blood culture	*Bartonella* serology ≥1:1024	Resolution <4 days of Rx
≥2 positive blood cultures		No pathologic evidence
≥3 with common skin		
contaminant		

Abbreviations: AI, aortic insufficiency. Dx, diagnosis. Rx, treatment.

From Bonagura JD, Twedt DC, editors. Current veterinary therapy XIV. St Louis: Saunders Elsevier; 2009. p. 786–91; with permission.

molecule expression, inhibition of monocyte phagocytosis, and impairment of B-cell antigen presentation within lymph nodes.[8] The clinical characteristics of dogs with IE due to *Bartonella* are no different to dogs with IE due to traditional bacteria. In the author's experience, dogs with IE due to traditional bacteria do not have coinfections with *Bartonella*.[3,7] Several epidemiologic studies have suggested that ticks and fleas may be vectors for *Bartonella*. Concurrent seroreactivity to *Anaplasma phagocytophilum*, *Ehrlichia canis*, or *Rickettsia rickettsii* is common in dogs with IE due to *Bartonella*, and titers should be submitted for tick-borne diseases in dogs that are seroreactive to *Bartonella* antigen.[3,9]

PREDISPOSING FACTORS

Presence of bacteremia and endothelial disruption are necessary for development of IE. The most common underlying cardiac defect in dogs with IE is subaortic stenosis, which creates turbulent blood flow and damage to the ventricular aspect of the aortic cusps.[10,11] No other cardiac diseases have been statistically shown to predispose dogs to IE.[11] Myxomatous valve degeneration is the most common heart disease in dogs, and occurs most commonly in small-breed aged dogs, who virtually never develop IE. Therefore, it is unlikely that myxomatous valve degeneration is a predisposing factor for development of IE. Common sources of bacteremia in dogs include diskospondylitis, prostatitis, pneumonia, urinary tract infection, pyoderma, periodontal disease, and long-term indwelling central venous catheters. The role of immunosuppression as a predisposing factor for IE is controversial. In a recent study of IE in dogs, only 1 of 18 dogs (5%) had been recently administered immunosuppressive therapy for treatment of pemphigus foliaceus.[3] However, an earlier study found that 17 of 45 dogs (38%) with IE received corticosteroids at some time during the course of disease.[12] Dental prophylaxis as a predisposing factor for development of IE in dogs has long been anecdotally touted as a clinical truth without any statistical evidence. A well-designed study has recently rejected the notion that dental prophylaxis predisposes dogs to develop IE, because it did not find any association between IE and dental procedures, oral surgical procedures, or oral infection in the preceding 3 months.[11] To echo this finding, the American Heart Association revised guidelines in 2007 for antibiotic dental prophylaxis to include only patients with prosthetic heart valve, a history of IE, certain forms of congenital heart disease, and valvulopathy after cardiac catheterization, and only before procedures that involve manipulation of gingival tissue or the periapical region of teeth.[13] Routine dental cleaning is excluded.

PATHOPHYSIOLOGY OF IE
Congestive Heart Failure

Congestive heart failure is the most common sequela of IE, and is the most common cause of death. Acute heart failure is a common feature of this rapidly progressive and virulent disease. IE of the aortic valve causes massive aortic insufficiency, which increases left ventricular end-diastolic volume and pressure. Similarly, IE of the mitral valve causes severe mitral regurgitation secondary to the large vegetative lesion causing a large gap in valve coaptation, rupture of chordae tendinae, and valvular erosion, which increases left ventricular end-diastolic pressure. Cardiogenic pulmonary edema develops once the left ventricular end-diastolic pressure (and pulmonary capillary wedge pressure) exceed 20 to 25 mm Hg.[14] Early edema formation occurs in the pulmonary interstitium, and appears as interstitial infiltrates in the perihilar region of the lungs. However, most cases of IE are rapid and severe, and cause fulminant pulmonary edema with alveolar flooding. Acute and fatal increase in the left ventricular diastolic pressure often occurs before the development of left atrial dilation. Pulmonary veins are typically distended despite the lack of marked cardiomegaly. If the animal is able to survive for weeks to months with severe aortic insufficiency, systolic myocardial failure develops secondary to marked increase in the left ventricular systolic wall stress. Chronic severe aortic insufficiency and mitral regurgitation secondary to IE cause volume overload to the left heart, and increased left ventricular end-diastolic diameter and left atrial diameter. Fractional shortening is often increased in dogs with chronic mitral regurgitation as long as the systolic function is preserved, but may normalize in dogs with secondary myocardial failure.

Immune-Mediated Disease

Patients with IE tend to develop high titers of antibodies against causative microorganisms, and there is continuous formation of circulating immune complexes.[15] Immune complexes consist of IgM, IgG, and C3 (complement). Factors such as rheumatoid factor may impair the ability of complement to solubilize immune complexes, and may lead to formation of large immune complexes. Extracardiac disease manifestations are caused by immune complex deposition and further complement activation and tissue destruction in the glomerular basement membrane, joint capsule, or dermis. Shortly after antibiotic therapy in people with IE, the circulating immune complexes are greatly reduced . Immune-mediated diseases including polyarthritis and glomerulonephritis are commonly seen in dogs with IE (75% and 36%, respectively).[3] Joint fluid analysis and culture should be performed in dogs with lameness to evaluate for immune-mediated polyarthritis or septic arthritis. Urine protein:creatinine ratio (UPC) should be evaluated in dogs with proteinuria to support the diagnosis of glomerulonephritis.

Thromboembolism

Thromboembolism (septic and aseptic) commonly occurs in 70% to 80% of dogs with IE examined at pathology.[3] Like people, dogs are more likely to suffer from thromboembolic disease with mitral valve IE.[16] In people, risk of thromboembolic disease is greatest with mitral valve IE, large mobile large vegetative lesions greater than 1 to 1.5 cm in size, or with increasing lesion size during antibiotic therapy.[17,18] Infarction of the kidneys and spleen are most common in dogs, followed by infarction of the myocardium, brain, and systemic arteries. Vascular encephalopathy occurs in approximately one-third of people with IE, and is uncommon in dogs. Recently a case series of 4 dogs with IE and vascular encephalopathy was described.[19] Thromboembolism most commonly occurs in the middle cerebral artery in both people and dogs, and results in brain ischemia and possible ischemic necrosis if persistent. A mycotic aneurysm is caused by a septic thromboembolus that lodges in a peripheral artery, often at a branch point, and causes destruction of the arterial wall and a localized, irreversible arterial dilatation. Mycotic aneurysms are often described in the cerebral vasculature of people with IE, which account for approximately 15% of neurologic complications.[2] The clinical syndrome in people ranges from a slow leak that produces only mild headache and meningeal irritation, to sudden intracranial hemorrhage and major neurologic deficits.

Other Uncommon Pathophysiologic Sequelae

Hypertrophic osteopathy is a rare sequela to IE in dogs.[20,21] Hypertrophic osteopathy is caused by increased blood flow to the extremities, triggering overgrowth of vascular connective tissue and subsequent fibrochondroid metaplasia and subperiosteal new bone formation. One potential mechanism of hypertrophic osteopathy associated with IE is that platelet clumps that detach from the vegetative endocardial lesion obstruct a peripheral artery. Platelets release platelet-derived growth factor, which increases vascular permeability and is chemotactic for neutrophils, monocytes, and fibroblasts. The end result is increased connective tissue and fibrochondroid metaplasia, starting in the metacarpals and metatarsals, and progressing proximally.

History and Presenting Complaint

Dogs with IE often have an ill-defined history of nonspecific signs of extracardiac systemic illness including lethargy, weakness, and weight loss. In a case series of 18 dogs, lameness was the most common presenting complaint in 44% of dogs diagnosed with IE.[3] Other common nonspecific signs include lethargy, anorexia, respiratory abnormalities, weakness, and collapse. Less common presenting complaints include neurologic abnormalities, vomiting, and epistaxis. An identifiable recent precipitating factor such as a surgical or dental procedure, catheterization, or trauma is usually absent. Dogs with *Bartonella* IE often have a history of ectoparasite infestation with fleas and ticks, and live in endemic areas for bartonellosis. Although widely expected, the pathognomonic history of a large-breed dog with a new murmur, fever, shifting leg lameness, and a predisposing factor for bacteremia is overemphasized and is not the norm. In a study of 18 dogs, less than half of the dogs diagnosed with IE had identifiable predisposing causes.[3] Fever may be masked by concomitant antibiotics or anti-inflammatory medications. Most dogs (80%) diagnosed with IE in one study were currently receiving antibiotics, with a majority (64%) receiving fluoroquinolones alone or in combination with other antibiotics.[3]

Signalment

Medium- to large-breed (median weight in one study was 35 kg, range 13–57 kg), middle-aged to older male dogs are most commonly affected with IE.[3] German Shepherd dogs were predisposed to develop IE in a postmortem study.[22]

Cardiovascular Examination

A murmur is ausculted in a majority of dogs with IE (89%–96%).[3,10] Presence of a new or changing (ie, increased intensity) murmur is the prototypical auscultation abnormality, but in one study only 41% of dogs with IE had a new murmur.[12] Mitral valve IE causes mitral regurgitation and a left apical systolic murmur, with the intensity roughly paralleling the severity of the regurgitation. Aortic valve IE causes aortic insufficiency, which is much more challenging to auscult. Aortic insufficiency creates a soft, diastolic murmur at the base of the heart, which can often be masked by increased respiratory noises or lack of experience. Often there is a systolic basilar ejection murmur in dogs with aortic IE, secondary to underlying subaortic stenosis, narrowed aortic lumen because of presence of a vegetative lesion, or increased stroke volume as a result of massive aortic insufficiency. A diastolic murmur is almost always present in conjunction with a systolic murmur (69%), and rarely alone (8%).[16] The combination of increased systolic turbulence at the aortic valve and diastolic leak in the aortic valve creates a "to-and-fro" murmur that may be confused with a continuous murmur of a patent ductus arteriosus. Clinical findings of a diastolic left basilar murmur and bounding femoral pulses should trigger a high level of suspicion of aortic valve IE, and further diagnostics should be immediately pursued as outlined later in this article. Bounding femoral arterial pulses occur in dogs with severe aortic insufficiency and reflect a widened pulse pressure caused by low diastolic pressure from the diastolic run-off of aortic insufficiency and potentially increased systolic pressure. Mucous membranes may appear injected in bacteremic, septic patients, or may appear pale in patients with low-output heart failure. Respiratory abnormalities including tachypnea, dyspnea, cough, or adventitious lung sounds are common, given the high frequency (50%) of heart failure in dogs with IE. Fever is often present (50%–74%), but may be episodic.

Other common physical examination abnormalities include lameness, joint pain, and swelling. In one study 57% of dogs were recumbent, reluctant to stand, and were stiff, lame, or weak.[16] Neurologic abnormalities are not uncommon (23% of dogs in one study) and include ataxia, deficits of conscious proprioception, obtundation, cranial nerve deficits, and vestibular signs.[16] Arterial thromboembolism occurs most frequently in the right thoracic limb or pelvic limbs and causes clinical abnormalities of cold extremities, cyanotic nail beds, pain and lameness, absence pulses, and firm musculature of the affected limb.

Electrocardiogram

Arrhythmias are present in 40% to 70% of dogs, and include in order of incidence ventricular arrhythmias, supraventricular tachycardia, third-degree atrioventricular block, and atrial fibrillation. The highest reported frequency of arrhythmias was seen in dogs with aortic IE, with 62% of dogs having ventricular arrhythmias.[10] Third-degree atrioventricular block may occur with periannular abscess formation secondary to aortic valve IE.[23]

Thoracic Radiographs

Cardiogenic pulmonary edema is present in almost half of patients, and is diagnosed by identification of perihilar to caudodorsal interstitial to alveolar pulmonary infiltrates. Acute congestive heart failure occurs in the absence of left atrial enlargement in 75% of cases of IE, which makes radiographic interpretation challenging (**Fig. 3**).[3] Often

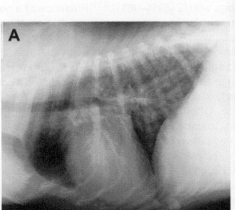
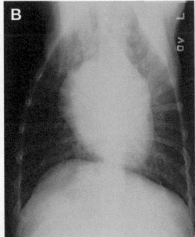

Fig. 3. Radiographs (A, B) of a dog with acute IE of the aortic valve. This dog presented for acute dyspnea, and thoracic radiographs show normal heart size and diffuse interstitial pulmonary infiltrates of the caudal lung lobes. Pulmonary veins were mildly distended. Because of the lack of cardiomegaly, there was debate whether the infiltrates were cardiogenic, and measurement of markedly elevated pulmonary capillary wedge pressure confirmed left heart failure as the cause of the infiltrates. This dog had acute aortic insufficiency from *Bartonella* IE of the aortic valve, causing acute cardiogenic pulmonary edema without overt cardiomegaly.

there is pulmonary venous distension despite unremarkable heart size. If the animal is able to survive long enough, left atrial dilation and left ventricular enlargement develop over weeks. Mitral and aortic IE equally lead to development of heart failure. Noncardiogenic pulmonary infiltrates including pneumonia or pulmonary hemorrhage are not uncommon, and occurred in approximately one-quarter of cases in one study.[3]

Clinicopathologic Abnormalities

The most common clinicopathologic abnormality is leukocytosis on a complete blood count, which occurred in 89% of dogs in a case series.[16] Typically there is a mature neutrophilia and monocytosis. Mild to severe thrombocytopenia is also commonly seen in more than half of all cases.[16] Anemia is common (52%) and is most often mild nonregenerative anemia. There is evidence of a procoagulable state in some dogs with IE, including an elevated D-dimer or fibrin degradation products in 87% of dogs in which they were measured, and hyperfibrinogenemia in 83% of dogs in which it was measured.[16] Serum chemistry often shows hypoalbuminemia (95% of dogs), elevated hepatic enzyme activity, and acidosis. Renal complications are commonly seen in at least half of dogs with IE, and may include prerenal or renal azotemia. Moderate to severe renal failure was present in approximately 33% of dogs in a case series.[3] Other significant abnormalities may include glomerulonephritis, pyelonephritis, and renal thrombosis. The most common abnormalities on urinalysis include cystitis (60% of dogs), proteinuria (50%–60%), and hematuria (18%–62%). A urine culture should always be obtained in an effort to identify a possible source of bacteremia and obtain a minimum inhibitory concentration (MIC) to guide appropriate antibiotic therapy. UPC is a necessary test in dogs with proteinuria to establish if there is excess protein loss from the kidneys, which may lead to a hypercoagulable state by loss of antithrombin III. An increased UPC ratio was present in 77% of dogs with IE, in which it was measured, and was moderate or severely elevated in 58% of these dogs.[16]

Joint Fluid Analysis

Arthrocentesis, cytologic analysis of joint fluid, and culture of the joint fluid are necessary in dogs with lameness or joint effusion. In a study of 71 dogs with IE, 35% of dogs had joint fluid analyzed, and 84% of these dogs had suppurative effusion.[16] Septic inflammation is less common than immune-mediated polyarthritis.

Diagnosis

Diagnosis of IE is challenging and elusive, and includes clinical abnormalities compatible with IE, blood culture, and echocardiographic evidence of characteristic oscillating vegetative lesions on a cardiac valve and valvular insufficiency. Definitive diagnosis of IE depends on identification of a vegetative or erosive lesion by echocardiography or by pathology. Because transthoracic echocardiography is relatively insensitive in humans for detection of IE, there is reliance on other major and minor criteria to determine a possible diagnosis.[15] In human medicine, the Modified Duke scoring system has been devised to quantify whether IE is unlikely or highly probable. Proposed veterinary criteria modeled on the human Modified Duke criteria may be useful to identify probable cases of IE in dogs (see **Table 1**)

Blood culture

Blood culture before treatment with antibiotics is an essential diagnostic tool to support the diagnosis of IE and to aid in proper selection of antimicrobial treatment. From different venous sites, 3 or 4 blood samples (5–10 mL each) should be aseptically collected at least 30 minutes to 1 hour apart and submitted for aerobic and anaerobic culture. Lysis centrifugation tubes (Isolator, Isostat microbial system, Wampole Laboratories, Cranbury, NJ, USA) may increase diagnostic yield. Adequate volumes of blood must be collected (if clinically appropriate based on patient size), because the concentration of bacteria in blood is very low (<5–10 bacteria/mL).[24] Bartonella is a fastidious organism that is rarely grown on culture medium, so routine culture is not recommended. Unfortunately, many patients (78% in one study) have been treated with antibiotics prior to blood culture, thus reducing the likelihood of a positive blood culture. Not surprisingly, there is a high incidence of negative blood cultures in dogs with IE, ranging from 60% to 70%.[3,10] In dogs already receiving antibiotics, collection of blood is ideally done during the trough level of the antibiotic. The most common bacterial isolates are Staphylococcus spp (aureus, intermedius, coagulase positive and coagulase negative), Streptococcus spp (canis, bovis, and β-hemolytic), and E coli (**Table 2**). Other lesser isolates include Pseudomonas, Erysipelothrix rhusiopathiae, Enterobacter, Pasteurella, Corynebacterium, Proteus, and rarely, Bordetella avium–like organism, Erysipelothrix tonsillarum, and Actinomyces turicensis.

Testing for Bartonella

Serologic testing for Bartonella spp is the main diagnostic method to determine if IE is highly likely to be caused by Bartonella. Because Bartonella is an extremely fastidious intracellular bacterium, it is rarely cultured from blood or body tissues even using specialized culture medium and long incubation periods. Therefore, diagnosis is limited to polymerase chain reaction (PCR) of the blood (fraught with false negatives) or cardiac valve on postmortem (gold standard), or probable cause is determined if there is a markedly elevated serologic titer against Bartonella. In one study, dogs with PCR evidence of Bartonella on infected heart valves were highly seroreactive to Bartonella spp, and all titers were greater than 1:1024.[3] There is cross-reactivity to different Bartonella species as well as to Chlamydia and Coxiella burnetii.

Based on the veterinary literature, high seroreactivity to Bartonella (>1:1024) may be an additional minor criterion for diagnosis of IE due to Bartonella in dogs (see **Table 1**). High seroreactivity to Bartonella spp has been recently proposed as a minor criterion for diagnosis of IE in people. A titer greater than 1:800 for IgG antibodies to Bartonella henselae or B quintana had a positive predictive value of 0.96 for detection of Bartonella infection in people with IE, and confirmed the diagnosis in 45 of 145 people (31%) with culture-negative IE with 100% sensitivity.[25] PCR on serum from people with confirmed IE due to Bartonella is relatively insensitive (58%) but specific (100%).[26]

Echocardiography

Echocardiography is the most important tool to diagnose IE. The pathognomonic lesion is a hyperechoic, oscillating, irregular-shaped (ie, shaggy) mass adherent to, yet distinct from, the endothelial cardiac surface (**Figs. 4** and **5**). The term "oscillating" means that the lesion is mobile with high-frequency movement independent from the underlying valve structure, and highly supports an echocardiographic diagnosis of vegetation. The mitral and aortic valves are almost exclusively affected in small animals. Erosive and minimally proliferative lesions are less uncommon and may be challenging to visualize. Valvular insufficiency of the affected valve is always present, and most often is moderate or severe (see **Figs. 4** and **5**). Valvular insufficiency is identified as a turbulent regurgitant jet on color flow Doppler investigation of the affected valve, including a retrograde systolic turbulent jet from the left ventricle into the left atrium with mitral regurgitation, or a turbulent jet arising from the aortic valve and leaking backward into the left ventricle in diastole with aortic insufficiency. Left atrial

Table 2
Common causative agents, typical antimicrobial sensitivity profiles, and treatment recommendations for dogs with IE

Causative Agent and Bacteremia Source	Typical Sensitivity Profile	Recommended Antibiotic
Staphylococcus intermedius Pyoderma	Usually sensitive	Acute: Timentin 50 mg/kg IV QID, or Enrofloxacin 10 mg/kg IV BID Chronic: Clavamox 20 mg/kg PO TID or Enrofloxacin 5–10 mg/kg PO BID × 6–8 wk
Staphylococcus aureus	Often resistant; if methicillin resistant, avoid β-lactams treatment	Individually dependent, evaluate MIC Acute: Amikacin or Vancomycin and Oxacillin, Nafcillin, or Cefazolin IV × 2 wk Chronic: If not methicillin resistant, high-dose first-generation cephalosporin PO 6–8 wk
Streptococcus canis Urogenital system, skin, respiratory tract	Usually sensitive	Acute: Ampicillin 20–40 mg/kg IV TID–QID or Ceftriaxone 20 mg/kg IV BID × 2 wk. If resistant, amikacin and high-dose penicillin Chronic: Amoxicillin or Clavamox PO 6–8 wk
Escherichia coli Gastrointestinal tract, peritonitis, urinary tract	Often resistant (β-lactamase), need extended MIC	Individually dependent, evaluate MIC Acute: Amikacin and/or Imipenem 10 mg/kg IV TID Chronic: Imipenem 10 mg/kg SQ TID 6–8 wk
Pseudomonas Chronic wounds, burns	Resistant, need extended MIC	Individually dependent, evaluate MIC Acute: Amikacin, Timentin, or Imipenem Chronic: Imipenem SQ or Clavamox PO
Bartonella Vector-borne disease	MIC not predictive of MBC	Acute: Amikacin 20 mg/kg IV × 1–2 wk, and Timentin 50 mg/kg IV QID × 1–2 wk Chronic: β-lactam PO × 6–8 wk or Doxycycline 5 mg/kg PO every 24 h × 6–8 wk or Azithromycin 5 mg/kg PO every 24 h × 7 d, then EOD
Culture negative	Unknown	Acute: Amikacin and Timentin IV × 1–2 wk Chronic: Clavamox 20 mg/kg TID × 6–8 wk and Enrofloxacin 5–10 mg/kg PO BID × 6–8 wk

Typical MIC profiles derived from UC Davis VMTH microbial service database of antimicrobial sensitivity of cultured microorganisms. Recommended antibiotics for particular bacteria were chosen based on greater than 90% sensitivity of the cultured isolates to the particular antibiotic.

Abbreviations: BID, twice a day; EOD, every other day; IV, intravenous; MBC, minimum bactericidal concentration; MIC, minimum inhibitory concentration; PO, by mouth; QID, 4 times a day; SQ, subcutaneous; TID, 3 times a day.

enlargement or eccentric hypertrophy of the left ventricle may not be present if the IE is acute in nature. A myocardial abscess may appear as a heterogeneous, thickened region or mass in the myocardium or annulus. A fistula or septal defect may be seen between 2 chambers if the abscess has ruptured.

Presence of moderate or severe aortic insufficiency on color flow Doppler should greatly raise the suspicion of aortic IE, and careful examination of the aortic cusps

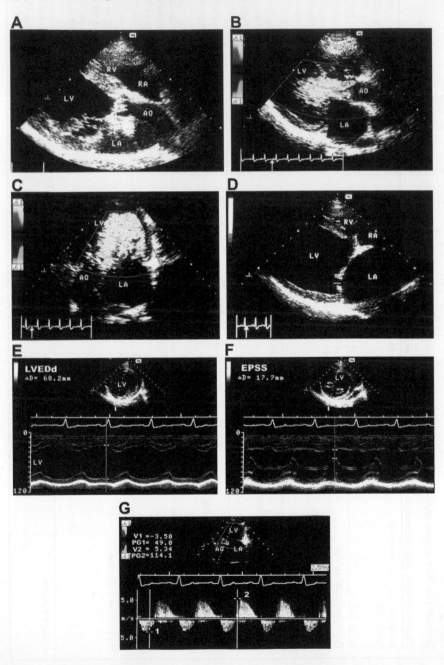

in several views is necessary. Subaortic stenosis is often present, and can be diagnosed by 2-dimensional evidence of fibrotic narrowing of the left ventricular outflow tract; severity may be determined by measurement of aortic blood flow velocity by continuous wave Doppler using the left apical 5-chamber view. Severity of aortic insufficiency may be estimated by the length of the insufficiency jet on color flow Doppler and the slope of the aortic insufficiency on continuous wave Doppler of the left apical 5-chamber view (ie, steep slope, severe aortic insufficiency) (**Fig. 4**). Chronic, severe aortic insufficiency leads to development of left ventricular eccentric hypertrophy, mild to moderate secondary myocardial failure, and left atrial dilation.

The main differential for echocardiographic diagnosis of IE of the mitral valve is myxomatous valve degeneration, which confers a dramatically better prognosis. Patient signalment is often helpful because dogs with marked myxomatous mitral valve degeneration are small breeds that rarely develop IE, and dogs with IE are medium to large breeds that do not commonly develop marked valvular thickening as a result of myxomatous valve degeneration. Large-breed dogs may develop myxomatous mitral valve degeneration, which is more subtle in structure with less proliferative valve thickening and minimal prolapse. Myxomatous valve degeneration appears in an echocardiograph as a thickened valve that often prolapses into the left atrium. Unlike IE, myxomatous valve degeneration does not cause an appearance of an oscillating shaggy mass–type lesion that moves independently from the endocardium.

Dogs with a high clinical suspicion of IE without characteristic lesions on transthoracic echocardiography should undergo transesophageal echocardiography to better evaluate the valve morphology, or transthoracic echocardiography should be repeated in a few days.

Treatment

Long-term bactericidal antibiotics are the cornerstone of therapy for IE. Empirical broad-spectrum antibiotic therapy is started while cultures are pending, and may be continued in cases with no identifiable pathogen. High serum concentration of

---

Fig. 4. (*A*) Echocardiogram of a dog with IE of the aortic valve. Using the right parasternal long-axis left ventricular outflow tract view, the aortic valve is visualized and is severely thickened with a hyperechoic, shaggy, oscillating mass lesion consistent with IE. (*B, C*) Color flow Doppler investigation of the aortic valve from the right parasternal long-axis left ventricular outflow tract view and the left apical 5-chamber view show severe aortic insufficiency, which is turbulent blood flow leaking back into the left ventricle from the aorta in diastole. (*From* MacDonald KA, Chomel BB, Kittleson M, et al. A prospective study of canine IE in northern California (1999–2001): emergence of Bartonella as a prevalent etiologic agent. J Vet Intern Med 2004;18:56–64; with permission.) (*D*) Severe aortic insufficiency causes a severe volume overload and eccentric hypertrophy of the left ventricle. (*E*) M-mode of the left ventricle shows severe left ventricular eccentric hypertrophy with a severely increased end-diastolic diameter (LVEDd) and mildly increased end-systolic diameter consistent with secondary myocardial failure. Fractional shortening was normal. (*F*) E-point to septal separation (EPSS) was markedly increased, which also indicates significant myocardial failure. (*G*) Continuous-wave Doppler measurement of the aortic blood flow velocity shows high-velocity turbulent systolic flow out of the aorta that is consistent with moderate subaortic stenosis (1), and high-velocity turbulent flow backward into the left ventricle during diastole (2) consistent with aortic insufficiency. The aortic insufficiency is severe, which leads to a rapid decrease in the aorta to left ventricular pressure gradient through diastole, which is visualized as a steep slope rather than a flat plateau of the aortic insufficiency jet. LA, left atrium; LV, left ventricle; AO, aorta; RA, right atrium; RV, right ventricle; V, velocity (m/s); PG, pressure gradient (mm Hg).

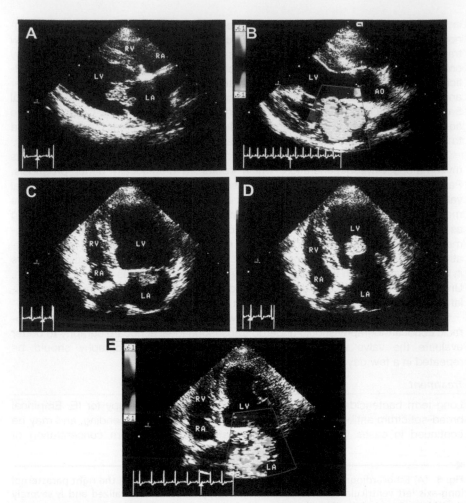

Fig. 5. (*A*) Echocardiogram of a dog with IE of the mitral valve. This right parasternal long-axis 4-chamber view shows a large, hyperechoic, vegetative lesion on the anterior mitral leaflet. (*B*) Color flow Doppler investigation of the mitral valve shows severe mitral regurgitation. (*C, D*) From the left apical 4-chamber view, the vegetative lesion is mobile (ie, oscillating), and prolapses into the left atrium during systole (*D*) and into the left ventricle during diastole (*C*). The left atrium is dilated secondary to severe mitral regurgitation. (*E*) Color flow Doppler of the mitral valve shows severe mitral regurgitation and a filling defect in the left atrium caused by the large vegetative lesion. LA, left atrium; LV, left ventricle; RA, right atrium; RV, right ventricle.

antibiotics with good tissue and intracellular penetrating properties are needed to penetrate within the vegetative lesion to kill the bacteria. Antibiotic doses used are typically on the high end of the range to achieve high blood levels. The optimal antibiotic treatment depends on culture of the microorganism and MIC of the antibiotics, which is often impossible as a result of previous antibiotic use. Common causative agents, their typical sensitivity profile, and therapeutic regimens are included in **Table 2**. Therapeutic recommendations were derived from the UC Davis VMTH microbial service database of antimicrobial sensitivity of microorganisms. Recommended antibiotics for particular bacteria were chosen based on sensitivity of greater than 90% of the cultured isolates to the particular antibiotic. However, general antibiotic sensitivities and resistance profiles may vary depending on the hospital, and may be more challenging in secondary or tertiary referral hospitals. There is significant resistance of many bacteria isolated from IE cases in the author's hospital to enrofloxacin and ampicillin, and they therefore cannot be recommended as an empirical, acute first line of defense when an MIC is unavailable. Patients should be supported with fluid therapy if aminoglycosides are given. Furosemide may potentiate nephrotoxicity of aminoglycosides, hence they are contraindicated in patients with congestive heart failure receiving diuretic therapy because furosemide may potentiate renal toxicity of aminoglycosides.

Intravenous antibiotic therapy for 1 to 2 weeks is necessary for acute aggressive treatment of IE. This therapy may be challenging (financially and emotionally for owners) as it involves long-term hospitalization and monitoring for this period of time. Placement of an indwelling long-term vascular access port is an option in these patients that ideally should be treated with intravenous antibiotics for several weeks. After the first 1 to 2 weeks of intravenous antibiotics, long-term oral antibiotics are needed for 6 to 8 weeks or longer. Some clinicians have suggested subcutaneous administration of antibiotics on an outpatient basis rather than oral antibiotics, but there is no clear advantage of subcutaneous antibiotic treatment over long-term oral antibiotic treatment with high bioavailability and blood levels. One exception is in the long-term treatment of resistant infections using imipenem administered subcutaneously after an initial 1- to 2-week course administered intravenously, although subcutaneous administration may cause discomfort with this drug.[27]

It is challenging to decide when long-term antibiotic therapy may be discontinued, because the affected valve often has residual thickening even with a sterile lesion. Serial monitoring of echocardiograms, and other parameters such as complete blood count, recheck urine or blood cultures (if previously positive), and body temperature are needed to follow the response to antibiotics. Lack of improvement in an oscillating vegetative lesion after the first week of antibiotic therapy in an animal without a previous bacterial isolate and MIC may indicate a more aggressive, resistant bacterium that may require switching antibiotics or adding additional antibiotics. During long-term therapy, the presence of an oscillating mass, recurrent fever, leukocytosis, or positive follow-up urine or blood cultures necessitates continued long-term therapy, possibly with a different antibiotic combination.

The superior antibiotic for treatment of *Bartonella* infections in dogs has not been defined, but acceptable choices include doxycycline, azithromycin, or fluoroquinolones. However, contrary to clinical experience, an in vitro study found that only gentamicin, and not ciprofloxacin, streptomycin, erythromycin, ampicillin, or doxycycline, exerted bactericidal activity against *Bartonella*.[28] Treatment with at least 2 weeks of aminoglycosides has been shown to improve survival in people with *Bartonella* IE.[29] In dogs with severe life-threatening IE due to *Bartonella*, aggressive treatment with aminoglycosides may be necessary, with careful monitoring of renal values and supportive intravenous fluid administration. In 24 dogs with various systemic manifestations secondary to bartonellosis, treatment with the following antibiotics resulted in clinical recovery and negative post-treatment titers: doxycycline, azithromycin, enrofloxacin, and amoxicillin/clavulanate.[30] Azithromycin achieves high intracellular concentrations and may be given with careful monitoring of the hepatic enzymes, as it may cause hepatotoxicity with long-term therapy.

At present, anticoagulant therapy is not recommended as a result of a trend in increased bleeding episodes and absence of benefit in vegetation resolution or reduced embolic events in humans with IE treated with aspirin.[15]

TREATMENT OF CONGESTIVE HEART FAILURE
Acute Heart Failure

Because of the often acute nature of IE, aggressive treatment of congestive heart failure is essential. These patients require 24-hour critical care and monitoring. High doses of parenteral furosemide (4–8 mg/kg intravenously every 1–4 hours or continuous-rate infusion of 1 mg/kg/h) are needed in the acute phase of fulminant pulmonary edema, and dose and frequency of administration should be rapidly tapered when respiratory rate and effort improve. A combination of positive inotropic therapy with dobutamine (5–10 μ/kg/min) and the potent balanced vasodilator nitroprusside (1–10 μg/kg/min) may be needed in dogs with refractory heart failure. Oxygen supplementation of 50% to 70% fractional inspired oxygen concentration for the first 12 hours, then reducing it to less than 50% helps increase arterial partial pressure of oxygen. In dogs with severe aortic insufficiency, acute afterload reduction with nitroprusside or hydralazine is indicated to lessen the severity of aortic insufficiency. Open heart surgery and valve replacement is a mainstay treatment for acute life-threatening IE in people, but is rarely done in dogs.[31]

Chronic Heart Failure

Once the dog has stabilized and pulmonary edema has been cleared by aggressive parenteral medications, multipharmacy long-term oral therapy may be started. Furosemide doses are often higher during the first week of chronic therapy and then tapered to the lowest effective dose. Typical initial furosemide doses may be 2 to 4 mg/kg orally three times a day, then tapered to twice a day. Pimobendan (0.25 mg/kg orally twice a day) is an inodilator that increases contractility and dilates systemic and pulmonary vasculature, and is an essential treatment for dogs with heart failure. In dogs with moderate or severe aortic insufficiency, addition of an arterial vasodilator (ie, afterload reducer) may lessen the severity of the aortic insufficiency. Afterload reduction is also necessary in dogs with severe or refractory heart failure secondary to mitral valve IE. Amlodipine (0.1–0.5 mg/kg orally every 24 hours to twice a day) is most effective and well-tolerated afterload reducer used for long-term oral therapy. Systolic blood pressure should be maintained less then 140 mm Hg (but >95 mm Hg), and 10 to 15 mm Hg lower than baseline blood pressure. Angiotensin-converting enzyme inhibitors are used for adjunctive heart failure therapy, and may be started once the dog is home and eating and drinking. Antiarrhythmic treatment may be necessary, especially if there are high-grade ventricular arrhythmias. A permanent pacemaker may be needed in dogs with third-degree atrioventricular block secondary to myocardial abscess spreading from aortic valve IE, although these patients are poor pacemaker candidates with a grave prognosis.

Follow-up

In patients with positive cultures (blood or urine), a repeat culture is recommended 1 week after starting antibiotic therapy and 2 weeks following termination of antibiotic therapy. An echocardiogram should be performed after 1 to 2 weeks of antibiotic treatment, in 4 to 6 weeks, and 2 weeks following termination of antibiotic therapy to assess size of vegetative lesion and severity of valvular insufficiency. Thoracic radiographs, blood pressure, and blood chemistry are needed to assess response to heart failure therapy and help tailor continued long-term therapy. In patients affected with *Bartonella*, repeat serology should be performed a month after initiation of treatment, and titers should be reduced. If titer values are persistently elevated, a different antibiotic may be needed.

Antibiotic Prophylaxis

Prophylactic perioperative antibiotics such as β-lactam or cephalosporin are indicated in dogs with subaortic stenosis, and may be indicated in other congenital heart diseases such as pulmonic stenosis or tetralogy of Fallot. Antibiotics should be given 1 hour before surgery or dentistry and 6 hours after the procedure. Clindamycin may be useful as a prophylactic antibiotic for dental procedures. The American Heart Association revised guidelines in 2007 for more stringent use of antibiotic dental prophylaxis to include only patients with prosthetic heart valve, a history of IE, certain forms of congenital heart disease, or valvulopathy after cardiac catheterization, and only before procedures that involve manipulation of gingival tissue or the periapical region of teeth, and not for routine dental cleaning.[13] Often veterinarians are saddled with the fear of risking a fatal disease versus empirical prophylactic antibiotics. However, even in human medicine the data are insufficient to substantiate efficacy of antibiotics in preventing endocarditis in patients undergoing dental procedures.[32] Likewise, there is no evidence that dogs with myxomatous valve degeneration have an increased risk of IE, or evidence of an association between a recent dental procedure and development of IE.[11] Therefore, the use of prophylactic antibiotics prior to dental procedures for dogs with myxomatous valve degeneration is controversial and needs to be reevaluated.

Prognosis

Dogs with aortic IE have a grave prognosis, and in one study median survival was only 3 days compared with a median survival of 476 days for dogs with mitral valve IE (**Fig. 6**).[3]

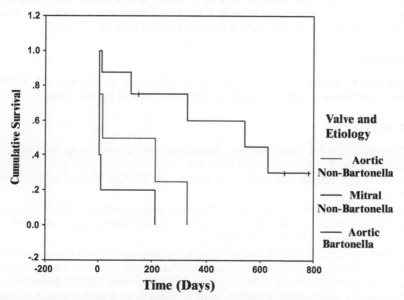

Fig. 6. Survival curve of 18 dogs diagnosed with IE with IE. Kaplan-Meier curve of the mitral and aortic valves.[3] Dogs with mitral valve endocarditis (*black line*) lived longer than dogs with aortic endocarditis from traditional bacteria (*red line*) (*P* = .004) or *Bartonella* (*black line*) (*P* = .002) (median survival time: mitral: 540 days; aortic: *Bartonella*, 3 days; non-*Bartonella*, 14 days). (*From* MacDonald KA, Chomel BB, Kittleson M, et al. A prospective study of canine IE in northern California (1999–2001): emergence of Bartonella as a prevalent etiologic agent. J Vet Intern Med 2004;18:56–64; with permission.)

Likewise, dogs with *Bartonella* IE have short survival times because the aortic valve is almost exclusively affected. Another case series of dogs with aortic IE reported similar outcomes, including 33% mortality in the first week and 92% mortality within 5 months of diagnosis.[10] Other risk factors for early cardiovascular death include glucocorticoid administration before treatment, presence of thrombocytopenia, high serum creatinine concentration, renal complications, and thromboembolic disease.[12,16] Short-term death is often a result of congestive heart failure or sudden death. Likewise, the presence of congestive heart failure has the greatest impact on poor prognosis in people with IE. Other causes of death within the first week of treatment in dogs with IE include renal failure, pulmonary hemorrhage, and severe neurologic disease.

SUMMARY

IE is an uncommon, deadly, and elusive disease to diagnose in dogs. IE primarily affects the mitral and aortic valves, and leads to severe valvular insufficiency and congestive heart failure. Other severe clinical sequelae include thromboembolism, immune-mediated disease (ie, immune-mediated polyarthritis and glomerulonephritis), arrhythmia, renal disease, and cerebral vasculopathy. The most common causative agents include *Staphylococcus* spp, *Streptococcus* spp, *E coli*, *Bartonella*, and *Pseudomonas*. Diagnosis is made by identification of a vegetative valvular lesion and valvular insufficiency on echocardiogram, and may be supported by other clinicopathologic abnormalities. Blood and urine cultures are needed to identify the offending microbial organism, although most cases are culture negative. Aggressive treatment with long-term broad-spectrum antibiotics is needed, ideally including 1 to 2 weeks of intravenous antibiotics followed by 6 to 8 weeks of oral antibiotics. Prognosis is grave for dogs with aortic valve IE, with a MST of 3 days in one study, and poor to fair in dogs with mitral valve IE, with a median survival time of 476 days.

ACKNOWLEDGMENTS

Thank you to Valerie Wiebe, PharmD (Pharmacy) for assistance with antibiotic recommendations and Barbara Byrne, DVM (Microbiology) for MIC data.

REFERENCES

1. Miller MW, Fox PR, Saunders AB. Pathologic and clinical features of infectious endocarditis. J Vet Cardiol 2004;6:35–43.
2. Bashore TM, Cabell C, Fowler V Jr. Update on IE. Curr Probl Cardiol 2006;31: 274–352.
3. MacDonald KA, Chomel BB, Kittleson M, et al. A prospective study of canine IE in northern California (1999-2001): emergence of *Bartonella* as a prevalent etiologic agent. J Vet Intern Med 2004;18:56–64.
4. Breitschwerdt EB, Atkins CE, Brown TT, et al. *Bartonella vinsonii* subsp. *berkhoffii* and related members of the alpha subdivision of the Proteobacteria in dogs with cardiac arrhythmias, endocarditis, or myocarditis. J Clin Microbiol 1999;37:3618–26.
5. Chomel BB, Kasten RW, Williams C, et al. *Bartonella endocarditis*: a pathology shared by animal reservoirs and patients. Ann N Y Acad Sci 2009;1166:120–6.
6. Ohad DG, Morick D, Avidor B, et al. Molecular detection of *Bartonella henselae* and *Bartonella koehlerae* from aortic valves of Boxer dogs with IE. Vet Microbiol 2010;141(1–2):182–5.
7. Pesavento PA, Chomel BB, Kasten RW, et al. Pathology of *Bartonella endocarditis* in six dogs. Vet Pathol 2005;42:370–3.

8. Pappalardo BL, Brown TT, Tompkins M, et al. Immunopathology of *Bartonella vinsonii* (berkhoffii) in experimentally infected dogs. Vet Immunol Immunopathol 2001;83:125–47.

9. Breitschwerdt EB, Hegarty BC, Hancock SI. Sequential evaluation of dogs naturally infected with *Ehrlichia canis*, *Ehrlichia chaffeensis*, *Ehrlichia equi*, *Ehrlichia ewingii*, or *Bartonella vinsonii*. J Clin Microbiol 1998;36:2645–51.

10. Sisson D, Thomas WP. Endocarditis of the aortic valve in the dog. J Am Vet Med Assoc 1984;184:570–7.

11. Peddle GD, Drobatz KJ, Harvey CE, et al. Association of periodontal disease, oral procedures, and other clinical findings with bacterial endocarditis in dogs. J Am Vet Med Assoc 2009;234:100–7.

12. Calvert CA. Valvular bacterial endocarditis in the dog. J Am Vet Med Assoc 1982; 180:1080–4.

13. Wilson W, Taubert KA, Gewitz M, et al. Prevention of IE: guidelines from the American Heart Association: a guideline from the American Heart Association Rheumatic Fever, Endocarditis, and Kawasaki Disease Committee, Council on Cardiovascular Disease in the Young, and the Council on Clinical Cardiology, Council on Cardiovascular Surgery and Anesthesia, and the Quality of Care and Outcomes Research Interdisciplinary Working Group. Circulation 2007; 116:1736–54.

14. Guyton AC, Lindsey AW. Effect of elevated left atrial pressure and decreased plasma protein concentration on the development of pulmonary edema. Circ Res 1959;7:649–57.

15. Baddour LM, Wilson WR, Bayer AS, et al. IE: diagnosis, antimicrobial therapy, and management of complications: a statement for healthcare professionals from the Committee on Rheumatic Fever, Endocarditis, and Kawasaki Disease, Council on Cardiovascular Disease in the Young, and the Councils on Clinical Cardiology, Stroke, and Cardiovascular Surgery and Anesthesia, American Heart Association: endorsed by the Infectious Diseases Society of America. Circulation 2005;111:e394–434.

16. Sykes JE, Kittleson MD, Chomel BB, et al. Clinicopathologic findings and outcome in dogs with IE: 71 cases (1992-2005). J Am Vet Med Assoc 2006; 228:1735–47.

17. Mugge A, Daniel WG, Frank G, et al. Echocardiography in IE: reassessment of prognostic implications of vegetation size determined by the transthoracic and the transesophageal approach. J Am Coll Cardiol 1989;14:631–8.

18. Macarie C, Iliuta L, Savulescu C, et al. Echocardiographic predictors of embolic events in IE. Kardiol Pol 2004;60:535–40.

19. Cook LB, Coates JR, Dewey CW, et al. Vascular encephalopathy associated with bacterial endocarditis in four dogs. J Am Anim Hosp Assoc 2005;41:252–8.

20. Dunn ME, Blond L, Letard D, et al. Hypertrophic osteopathy associated with IE in an adult boxer dog. J Small Anim Pract 2007;48:99–103.

21. Vulgamott JC, Clark RG. Arterial hypertension and hypertrophic pulmonary osteopathy associated with aortic valvular endocarditis in a dog. J Am Vet Med Assoc 1980;177:243–6.

22. Anderson CA, Dubielzig RR. Vegetative endocarditis in dogs. J Am Anim Hosp Assoc 1984;20:149–52.

23. Chomel BB, Mac Donald KA, Kasten RW, et al. Aortic valve endocarditis in a dog due to *Bartonella clarridgeiae*. J Clin Microbiol 2001;39:3548–54.

24. Peddle G, Sleeper MM. Canine bacterial endocarditis: a review. J Am Anim Hosp Assoc 2007;43:258–63.

25. Fournier PE, Mainardi JL, Raoult D. Value of microimmunofluorescence for diagnosis and follow-up of *Bartonella endocarditis*. Clin Diagn Lab Immunol 2002;9: 795–801.

26. Zeaiter Z, Fournier PE, Greub G, et al. Diagnosis of *Bartonella endocarditis* by a real-time nested PCR assay using serum. J Clin Microbiol 2003;41:919–25.

27. Barker CW, Zhang W, Sanchez S, et al. Pharmacokinetics of imipenem in dogs. Am J Vet Res 2003;64:694–9.

28. Rolain JM, Maurin M, Raoult D. Bactericidal effect of antibiotics on *Bartonella* and *Brucella* spp.: clinical implications. J Antimicrob Chemother 2000;46:811–4.

29. Raoult D, Fournier PE, Vandenesch F, et al. Outcome and treatment of *Bartonella endocarditis*. Arch Intern Med 2003;163:226–30.

30. Breitschwerdt EB, Blann KR, Stebbins ME, et al. Clinicopathological abnormalities and treatment response in 24 dogs seroreactive to *Bartonella vinsonii (berkhoffii)* antigens. J Am Anim Hosp Assoc 2004;40:92–101.

31. Arai S, Wright BD, Miyake Y, et al. Heterotopic implantation of a porcine bioprosthetic heart valve in a dog with aortic valve endocarditis. J Am Vet Med Assoc 2007;231:727–30.

32. Kim A, Keys T. IE prophylaxis before dental procedures: new guidelines spark controversy. Cleve Clin J Med 2008;75:89–92.

Feline Hypertrophic Cardiomyopathy: An Update

Jonathan A. Abbott, DVM

KEYWORDS

• Feline • Hypertrophic cardiomyopathy
• Feline myocardial disease

INTRODUCTION/HISTORICAL PERSPECTIVE

Recently proposed classifications of human cardiomyopathies have emphasized the etiology or molecular basis of myocardial disease.[1,2] Although the cause of a few specific breed-associated feline cardiomyopathies has been determined, feline myocardial disease remains largely idiopathic.[3,4] Accordingly, morphopathologic/functional designations remain valid. Given that premise, cardiomyopathy can be defined as a heart muscle disease that is associated with dysfunction.[5] Hypertrophic cardiomyopathy (HCM) is a disorder in which myocardial hypertrophy develops in the absence of hemodynamic load or metabolic cause; it is morphologically characterized by hypertrophy of a non-dilated ventricle.[6–8] Feline HCM is a diagnosis of exclusion that is valid when hypertrophy is echocardiographically evident in the absence of disorders such as systemic hypertension or hyperthyroidism.

The recognition of cardiomyopathies, and specifically HCM, is recent. The clinical characteristics of the entity that has become known as HCM were first described in human patients during the late 1950s.[9] The recognition of feline HCM occurred somewhat later. The association between feline cardiac disease and the occurrence of systemic arterial thromboembolism was reported by Holzworth, but early reports of thromboembolic phenomena do not specifically relate these events to heart muscle disease.[10,11] In 1970, Liu[12] retrospectively evaluated the postmortem features of acquired feline diseases that had resulted in congestive heart failure. Characteristic pathologic findings of advanced feline HCM, including left ventricular hypertrophy (LVH); left ventricular fibrosis; and left atrial dilation, were described but the term cardiomyopathy was not used. The use of the term cardiomyopathy in reference to feline heart disease seems to have first appeared in 1973.[13] Later publications, including an issue of this periodical from 1976, refer to feline cardiomyopathy and propose classifications of

Department of Small Animal Clinical Sciences, Virginia-Maryland Regional College of Veterinary Medicine, Virginia Polytechnic Institute and State University, Duck Pond Drive, Blacksburg, VA 24061-0442, USA
E-mail address: abbottj@vt.edu

Vet Clin Small Anim 40 (2010) 685–700
doi:10.1016/j.cvsm.2010.04.004
0195-5616/10/$ – see front matter © 2010 Elsevier Inc. All rights reserved.

this entity.[14] Tilley and Liu proposed the possibility that feline HCM might represent a model of the human disease in 1980, and the echocardiographic features of feline myocardial disease were defined later during that decade.[15,16]

ETIOPATHOGENESIS

It is now established that HCM in human beings is a genetic disease.[8,17] Several hundred distinct genetic mutations have been associated with HCM; genetic testing together with pedigree analyses have demonstrated that these mutations are casually related to the HCM phenotype.[18–20] Although exceptions have recently been identified, causative mutations primarily affect genes that encode proteins that are incorporated into the contractile elements, or sarcomeres, of the myocyte.[21]

Among feline patients, familial occurrence of HCM has been observed in mix-breed, Persian and American shorthair cats, and a mutation responsible for HCM in Maine coon cats has been identified.[3,22–24] The occurrence of HCM in Maine coon cats lacking this mutation has been reported, suggesting that other causative mutations exist in the gene pool of this breed or that there is a nongenetic cause of HCM in some Maine coon cats. A genetic mutation associated with HCM in ragdoll cats also has been recently identified.[4] Although other etiologic factors cannot be excluded, available evidence suggests that feline HCM probably has a genetic basis.

The precise mechanism by which genetic mutations lead to the development of hypertrophy has not been established. It is thought that altered sarcomeric proteins are responsible for myofiber dysfunction. Indeed, there are data acquired from in vitro investigations that provide evidence of diminished contractile function in HCM despite the finding that most affected patients have normal or enhanced ventricular emptying.[25,26] Why impaired systolic myocardial function should result in compensatory hypertrophy has not yet been determined. Activation of signaling pathways associated with trophic factors, such as angiotensin II, aldosterone, and insulin-like growth factor, may ultimately be responsible for the development of hypertrophy.[27,28]

In human beings with HCM, the phenotypic expression of causative mutations is highly diverse. The pathogenic potential of the various mutations is variable, but other factors also determine the consequences of abnormal genotype. Indeed, family members that share a causative mutation may differ markedly in clinical outcome and severity of myocardial hypertrophy.[20] It is likely that variable genetic expressivity observed in human HCM is related to factors that include the pathogenic heterogeneity of causative mutations; the presence of genetic co-modifiers; and epigenetic influences, possibly including the environment.[20] It is possible that feline HCM shares these features and, despite considerable progress, more complete characterization of this disease will therefore present challenges.

EPIDEMIOLOGY

Population characteristics of feline HCM have been retrospectively evaluated.[29,30] A sex predisposition for males is consistent and the mean age at diagnosis is close to 6 years.[29–31] Despite the fact that these data were obtained from referral populations, a substantive proportion, between 33% and 55%, were subclinical (asymptomatic) when the disease was identified.[29–31] One of these investigations identified the administration of corticosteroids as a historical antecedent to the development of heart failure.[30] The association between administration of glucocorticoids and development of heart failure in cats was also addressed in a separate retrospective investigation.[32] The design of the latter study does not allow conclusions regarding causality, but evidence was provided demonstrating that the development of heart failure associated with glucocorticoid administrations is a distinct clinical entity; specifically, patients that survive acute decompensation may have improved survival relative to cats that have not received glucocorticoids.[32]

Disease prevalence and identification of physical findings that represent markers of disease have been the focus of recent investigations.[33–36] Most studies have used a cross-sectional or retrospective study design, and therefore inferences regarding the causes of HCM are limited. However, prevalence (the instantaneous disease burden of a population) is potentially useful because it provides an a priori or pretest probability of disease in specific populations. This information has clinical relevance because it has a bearing on potential value of diagnostic screening and the interpretation of diagnostic tests.

The prevalence of cardiac murmurs in a sample of 103 cats recruited for participation in a blood donor program in New England was reported to be 21%.[33] Cats included in this investigation were between 1 and 9 years of age and, in the opinion of the pet owner, healthy. Murmurs were generally of low intensity and, in some cats, the intensity of murmurs varied in association with changes in heart rate. Quantitative echocardiographic variables were not reported but left ventricular hypertrophy or equivocal septal hypertrophy was identified in six of the seven cats that were echocardiographically examined. Systemic arterial blood pressure was not reported so it is possible that hypertrophy identified during this study was associated with systemic disease and did not reflect HCM.

Of 42 healthy purebred Maine coon cats subject to screening examinations in Scandinavia, only one had a cardiac murmur.[34] And indeed, this murmur was thought to be associated with pregnancy because it was not identified during reexamination performed after queening. Echocardiographic evidence of LVH was detected in 9.5% of these 42 cats. Reported follow-up data for some of these cats provide indirect evidence that noncardiac disorders were not responsible for the finding of LVH but blood pressure was not determined. Two cats that did not have LVH had echocardiographic evidence of systolic anterior motion of the mitral valve (SAM) suggesting an incipient or variant form of HCM. When these cats were included in the affected group, the prevalence of echocardiographic findings compatible with HCM was 14.3%.

Echocardiographic data obtained during pre-breeding evaluation of purebred cats thought to be at risk for heritable heart disease have also been retrospectively evaluated.[35] Of 144 cats, the majority were Maine coon cats but sphinx, British shorthair, Bengal, and Norwegian forest cats were also represented. Physical examination findings were not reported but echocardiographic evidence of HCM was detected in 8.3% of the cohort. In a recent investigation, the results of which have been presented in abstract form but not yet published, 34% of 199 apparently healthy cats had murmurs during at least one examination. Of cats with murmurs that were subject to echocardiographic examination, 50% had left ventricular hypertrophy.[37]

The author and colleagues recently reported the results of a community-based echocardiographic survey of apparently healthy cats.[36] One hundred three healthy cats were recruited from the pet-owning population of a veterinary college in the Southeastern United States. The echocardiographer was unaware of the physical findings and subjects with noncardiac disorders, including systemic hypertension and hyperthyroidism, were excluded. Of 103 cats, 16% had cardiac murmurs while at rest, during routine auscultatory examination. Dynamic auscultation was also performed during this study; the prevalence of murmurs in cats subject to a provocative maneuver that consisted of lifting the cat quickly in the air, was 27%. Of cats that had a murmur during dynamic auscultation, 46% did not have a murmur during routine auscultation. HCM was echocardiographically identified in 15% of the study population, but of cats with HCM, only 33% had heart murmurs.

The echocardiographic criteria used for diagnosis of HCM in this study are relevant to interpretation of the results. Two-dimensional echocardiography, not M-mode, was exclusively used for evaluation of ventricular wall thickness. Systematic quantitative assessment of wall thickness was made in short- and long-axis images. HCM was identified when any region of the left ventricular wall was equal to or exceeded 6 mm at end diastole. This method is apt to be more sensitive than the use of M-mode echocardiography for identification of hypertrophy. The majority of affected cats had mild and segmental hypertrophy and none had atrial enlargement. The diagnostic criteria used in this study were based on those that have been used for identification of HCM in humans and similar to those used in a published veterinary investigation.[31,38] The prevalence was seemingly high, but it is consistent with current understanding, as it is now accepted that HCM in humans is a disease that has a broad spectrum of phenotypic expression, occurs in a subclinical form, and is not inevitably associated with progression and poor outcome. To place the findings in perspective, the prevalence of HCM characterized by diffuse hypertrophy or marked SAM was 4%.

The various reported estimates of murmur and disease prevalence likely differ because of geographic variability and differences in methodology. However, it is clear that cardiac murmurs are often detected in apparently healthy cats, that murmurs in cats vary in intensity in association with environmental stimuli, and that the finding of a cardiac murmur is not consistently associated with echocardiographic abnormalities. The prevalence of mild, subclinical HCM in cats is probably close to 15%. HCM is the most common genetic heart disease in humans and has a reported prevalence of 0.2%.[38] Based on available data, the prevalence of HCM in cats is considerably higher, but this is credible if it is accepted that clinical signs are not the inevitable consequence of this disease. In humans, clinically evident HCM is rare.[8,39,40] In contrast, feline HCM is the disease most commonly responsible for heart failure in this species. In clinical studies that have evaluated biomarkers in feline subjects with respiratory distress, more than 50% of subjects with heart failure had HCM.[41,42] When echocardiographic case records are considered independent of clinical signs, HCM is identified in approximately 30% of patients.[43]

PATHOPHYSIOLOGY OF HYPERTROPHIC CARDIOMYOPATHY
Diastolic Dysfunction

It has generally been accepted that diastolic dysfunction is the pathophysiologic mechanism that is primarily responsible for the clinical manifestations of HCM. That systolic function contributes prominently to cardiac performance is readily evident but the importance of diastolic function is less obvious. Diastolic function (the ability of the ventricle to fill at low pressure) is complex but depends on the energy-dependent process of myocardial relaxation and mechanical properties of the ventricle that determine chamber stiffness. In most patients with HCM, global systolic performance is normal or hyperdynamic but delayed myocardial relaxation and diminished ventricular compliance potentially result in elevated filling pressures when ventricular volumes are normal or small.[43] Rises in ventricular filling pressures can result in pulmonary venous congestion and edema. Chronic elevation of ventricular filling pressures contributes atrial enlargement.

Dynamic Left Ventricular Outflow Tract Obstruction

The phenomenon of dynamic left ventricular outflow tract (LVOT) obstruction (LVOTO) has generated considerable interest and has been a subject of debate. Usually dynamic, as opposed to fixed or anatomic, obstruction of left ventricular outflow results from systolic motion of the mitral valve leaflets toward the interventricular septum (IVS).[17,31] Because the IVS represents the anterior boundary of the subvalvular LVOT and because of the parallel anatomic arrangement of left ventricular inflow and outflow, the displaced leaflets cause a mechanical impediment to ventricular ejection. As a consequence, a systolic pressure gradient develops across the LVOT. Mitral valve regurgitation usually accompanies SAM because the abnormal orientation of the valve apparatus results in incomplete leaflet apposition during systole (**Fig. 1**). The cause of SAM has been the subject of considerable speculation. The notion that SAM was a result of the Venturi effect was initially favored.[44] Venturi forces develop when narrowing of a conduit results in the acceleration of flow and the development of a pressure gradient. In the context of HCM, the development of lower systolic pressures distal to the site of leaflet-septal apposition results in lift, or Venturi, forces that act perpendicular to flow, pulling the mitral leaflets toward the septum. More recently it has been recognized that SAM may begin in early systole, even before ejection, at a time when Venturi forces are apt to be negligible.[45] Current evidence suggests that the hydrodynamic pushing force, or drag, is primarily responsible for anterior movement of the leaflets.[44] Abnormal geometry of the mitral valve apparatus, with or without structural abnormalities, likely plays a predisposing role. In fact, in a canine model, experimental displacement of the left ventricular papillary muscles toward the geometric center of the ventricle results

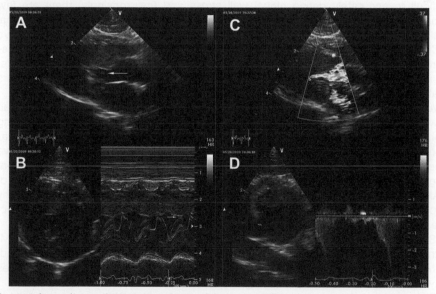

Fig. 1. Echocardiographic images obtained from a cat with hypertrophic cardiomyopathy. Left ventricular outflow tract obstruction and mitral valve regurgitation caused by systolic anterior motion of the mitral valve are evident. (*A*) Systolic right parasternal long-axis image that includes the left ventricular outflow. Arrow indicates point of mitral leaflet-septal contact. (*B*) M-mode image of the mitral valve. Arrow indicates point of mitral leaflet-septal contact. (*C*) Systolic right parasternal long-axis image that includes the left ventricular outflow with superimposed color Doppler map; there is caudally detected jet of mitral valve regurgitation. Disturbed flow is evident within the subvalvular left ventricular outflow tract. (*D*) Continuous-wave Doppler spectrogram of the left ventricular outflow tract. The peak velocity exceeds 3 ms/s. There is late-systolic acceleration, which provides evidence of dynamic obstruction.

in SAM.[46] It is probable that the cause of SAM is multifactorial. Abnormalities of the mitral apparatus that result in chordal laxity together with hyperdynamic systolic performance result in a substrate in which drag forces cause anterior displacement of the mitral valve leaflets. SAM is not an intrinsic feature of HCM and has been observed in other clinical and experimental scenarios in which there is absolute or relative redundancy of the mitral leaflets or chordae in the setting of hyperdynamic systolic performance.[47] Therefore, echocardiographic identification of SAM is not necessarily a specific echocardiographic marker of feline HCM but in most cases, it is finding that is highly suggestive of the diagnosis. It is clinically relevant that the tendency to develop SAM is load dependent and highly labile. Decreases in preload and afterload, and increases in contractile state can all induce or augment SAM in susceptible individuals. As a result, the pressure gradient and resulting heart murmur associated with SAM can vary markedly during brief time intervals.

The clinical importance of SAM has been debated, and indeed whether or not SAM results in actual obstruction was once questioned.[48] It is now accepted that SAM not only results in a systolic pressure gradient across the LVOT but also causes an impediment to ventricular ejection.[8] The pathophysiologic consequences of this obstruction are reported to include increased wall stress.[8,49] Wall stress, or the tension borne by the ventricle, is determined by intracavitary pressure, chamber volume, and wall thickness; it is directly proportional to the first two factors and inversely related to the last. The prevalence of asymmetrical ventricular geometry in patients with HCM makes it difficult to accurately define global wall stress and unsurprisingly, there are few reported, relevant data. However, in one study of human patients with HCM, global wall stress was not different when patients with obstructive and nonobstructive HCM were compared.[50] It is relevant that the supraphysiologic intraventricular pressures in HCM develop during late systole. During this phase of the cardiac cycle, ventricular wall thickness and radius are high and low, respectively, which are factors that limit the development of high wall stress.

As increase in wall thickness can serve to normalize wall stress, and therefore, even if wall stress is not increased in patients with HCM, the pressure gradient resulting from SAM might be an additional stimulus for hypertrophy. Indeed there are observational data obtained from cohorts of human subjects with obstructive HCM who have been subject to surgical treatment that decreases systolic pressure gradient that suggest regression of hypertrophy.[51] Still, it is difficult to reconcile the notion of SAM as a cause of hypertrophy with the prevalence of asymmetric septal hypertrophy in people with HCM. Presumably, if SAM were the cause of hypertrophy it would affect the free wall and septum equally.[50]

Structural and functional coronary artery abnormalities are associated with HCM. Intramural coronary arteries are narrowed because of medial hypertrophy and, although there are inconsistencies in the published literature, perfusion abnormalities have been associated with pressure gradients across the LVOT.[52–55]

The presence of dynamic LVOTO in human patients with HCM has been associated with poor outcome and particularly with sudden unexpected death.[49] This association, however, has been questioned.[56] The risk for poor outcome reported in one influential publication was not statistically related to magnitude of pressure gradient. Instead, it was simply the presence of obstruction at rest (treated as a yes/no binary variable) that was associated with poor outcome.[49] When this is considered in light of the marked lability of pressure gradient in human HCM (a day-to-day change of as much as 32 mmHg can apparently reflect random variation) and the prevalence of LVOTO in human beings that are subject to provocations, including exercise, it raises questions regarding the association between LVOTO and poor prognosis.[56–59]

Ultimately, uncertainty persists. SAM is undoubtedly the cause of LVOTO obstruction and mitral valve regurgitation, abnormalities that may be responsible for rises in filling pressures, altered coronary perfusion, and therefore perhaps the development of myocardial fibrosis. Furthermore, in human beings, clinical signs that are not responsive to medical therapy and are associated with LVOTO are successfully treated by surgery.[8] Still, it is possible that resting obstruction is a confounding variable that is associated with malignant phenotype but is not the proximate cause of mortality. Although inherently limited by the retrospective nature of the observations, it is interesting that SAM in feline patients has been associated with better rather than worse survival.[30,31] In the cat, the effect of obstruction on clinically relevant end points, including morbidity and mortality, is unclear and the suitability of SAM as therapeutic target can therefore be debated.

CLINICAL PRESENTATION

Feline HCM is usually identified when auscultatory findings, such as arrhythmias, gallop sounds, or murmurs, are incidentally detected during routine veterinary examinations or when clinical signs result from heart failure or embolism.[29,30] In a few affected cats, sudden unexpected death is the first clinical manifestation of the disease. Respiratory distress related to pulmonary edema or sometimes, pleural effusion, is the most common clinical manifestation of heart failure in feline HCM. Clinical signs of feline heart failure typically have a sudden onset and, in contrast to canine patients with heart failure, cough is rarely observed. In some cats with heart failure, clinical signs of low cardiac output, including hypothermia and pre-renal azotemia are observed. In cats, tachycardia is not consistently associated with heart failure and in some cases, bradycardia is evident.

Murmurs in patients with HCM have been associated with SAM, which results in LVOTO and mitral regurgitation (MR), as well as with MR caused by hypertrophic remodeling and distortion of the mitral apparatus.[43] It appears that murmurs in cats with or without cardiomyopathy are commonly associated with dynamic and labile phenomena. Fairly often, the intensities of murmurs heard in cats vary from moment to moment. The lability of SAM no doubt accounts for this observation in some cats. Additionally, dynamic right ventricular outflow tract obstruction has been identified as a cause of murmurs in healthy cats and cats with noncardiac disease.[60] In an echocardiographic survey of apparently healthy cats, the prevalence of cardiac murmurs was 16%, of which only 31% had echocardiographically identified structural heart disease.[36] However, the Doppler finding of late-systolic acceleration of either right or left ventricular outflow in apparently healthy cats was statistically associated with the finding of a murmur independent of the presence of structural heart disease. Some cats had late-systolic acceleration that was anatomically localized to the proximal LVOT. Dynamic mid-LVOT obstruction perhaps related to sympathetic activation, but not obviously associated with HCM, may therefore cause murmurs in some cats that do not have structural cardiac disease. The statistical association between murmurs and late-systolic acceleration of ventricular ejection was stronger when provoked murmurs were included in the analysis.[36] Auscultation and echocardiography were performed by different examiners at different times so the association is not necessarily causal, but it is plausible that sympathetic activation causes dynamic outflow tract obstruction that explains some apparently physiologic feline murmurs.

Echocardiography

Feline HCM has been echocardiographically defined by end-diastolic measurements of ventricular wall thickness that equal or exceed 6 mm.[31] Hypertrophy is commonly asymmetric and in Maine coon cats with HCM, it is often the left ventricular posterior wall and papillary muscles that are most affected.[61] Ejection phase indices of left ventricular systolic performance such as %fractional shortening are usually normal or reflect hyperdynamic ventricular emptying. Left atrial size in cats with HCM is generally greater than in healthy cats, but left atrial enlargement is not an intrinsic feature of the disease nor required for its diagnosis.[62] However, left atrial size is a surrogate measure of hemodynamic burden and left atrial enlargement has been associated with poor outcome in people and cats with HCM.[30,63] Furthermore, left atrial enlargement is a clinically important finding and is almost always present when clinical signs of respiratory distress result from feline myocardial disease. As previously described, SAM is commonly identified in cats with HCM and associated with SAM are Doppler findings of a labile, late-systolic pressure gradient across the LVOT and usually concurrent MR.

Progressive decline in systolic myocardial function is observed in some affected cats and presumably this is caused by ischemia related to small vessel disease or LVOTO.[64] Feline myocardial disease sometimes defies simple classification even after echocardiographic examination. Indeed, some examples of unclassified cardiomyopathy may represent progression of long-standing HCM. Restrictive cardiomyopathy (RCM) is generally considered to be a distinct disorder, which is characterized by atrial enlargement in association with normal, or nearly normal, ventricular wall thickness. Although some forms of RCM may represent the sequela of endomyocardial fibrosis, it is interesting that a restrictive phenotype has been documented in people who have sarcomeric mutations that are known to result in HCM.[65]

Early echocardiographic descriptions suggested that outflow tract obstruction was infrequently observed in feline HCM.[16] However, more recent data suggest that the prevalence is as high as 67%.[31] This figure is considerably higher than that reported from humans in which approximately 30% of the those affected manifested LVOT obstruction at rest.[59] However, current data suggest that the classification of obstructive and non-obstructive HCM may represent a false dichotomy. When human subjects with HCM are echocardiographically evaluated immediately after exercise or after provocations known to induce LVOTO, the proportion of those subjects that have obstruction exceeds 60%.[59,66,67] It is clear that the phenomenon of SAM is labile and highly dependent on functional state. The high prevalence of SAM in cats might reflect sympathetic activation associated with a "white-coat effect" in hospitalized cats; in a sense all echocardiographic examinations of non-sedated cats are performed in a state that is analogous to that immediately after exercise.

SCREENING FOR HCM

Recent interest in the epidemiology of feline heart disease raises questions regarding screening for this disease. The cost-benefit ratio of screening for clinically occult disease is favorable if an affordable test can identify a disease that is serious and treatable. Feline HCM, in its severe form, is undoubtedly serious and is clearly an important cause of morbidity and mortality in cats. Unfortunately, there is little known of the natural history of feline HCM; the rate at which subclinical HCM progresses to a clinical stage and indeed, the proportion of subclinically affected patients that ultimately develop clinical signs is not known. There is also little known regarding the efficacy of treatment for HCM. Several therapeutic strategies intended to prevent the development of congestion and the occurrence of embolism have been employed but none systematically evaluated. For purebred cats with a known or presumed genetic basis for HCM, screening can be justified because genetic counseling might reduce the prevalence of disease in specific populations. The question of screening for HCM might also be relevant for populations subject to elective procedures, such as dental cleaning, that require anesthesia.

In apparently healthy cats, auscultation is an insensitive diagnostic marker of HCM, meaning that few cats with subclinical HCM have murmurs. The positive predictive value of a test (the proportion of individuals that have the disease among those that have a positive test) is dependent on the prevalence of the disease. If the prevalence of subclinical HCM is close to 15%, the positive predictive value of a murmur in apparently healthy cats is only 31%. The negative predictive value of a cardiac murmur might be more diagnostically useful; it can be anticipated that 87% of cats that do not have murmurs do not have cardiomyopathy. In practical terms, echocardiographic examination of outwardly healthy cats with heart murmurs is advisable, but it should be recognized that many murmurs are apt to represent false positives; that is, echocardiographic examination prompted by identification of a cardiac murmur will disclose a sizable proportion of cats that are free of structural cardiac disease.

Echocardiographic screening, without regard to physical findings, for HCM can be justified in populations subject to the development of familial HCM. Otherwise, the cost of the examination might be excessive given the prevalence of the disease and the lack of proven therapies. In the absence of a hypothetical and flawless molecular or genetic test, there is no definitive, gold-standard test for HCM. Even postmortem examination is likely to have diagnostic limitations given the interindividual variability in cardiac mass among normal cats; the potential subjectivity of the examination; and the fact that histologic abnormalities, such as myofiber disarray, are not necessarily diffuse.[68] Although the sensitivity and specificity of echocardiography for diagnosis of HCM has not been evaluated, echocardiographic examination is, for all intents and purposes, the gold standard. Even then, the accuracy of echocardiographic identification of HCM depends on not only technical factors, including the experience of the examiner, but also on the cut point of wall thickness that is used as the diagnostic criterion. Many, but not all, clinical investigations of feline HCM have used an end-diastolic wall thickness equal to or exceeding 6 mm as the primary diagnostic criterion.[30,31,61] Provided metabolic and hemodynamic causes of hypertrophy are excluded, this dimension (6 mm) likely represents a specific, but not necessarily sensitive, marker of HCM. In fact, reference intervals defined by published normative echocardiographic data have upper limits that are generally less than 5.5 mm and less than 5 mm for two.[43] The feline study that included the largest number of subjects suggests that 95% of healthy cats have septal and free wall dimensions that are less than 5.6 mm.[69] Although it is not generally taken into account, end-diastolic ventricular wall thickness is weakly related to body weight, which might be relevant to the evaluation of exceptionally heavy cats. The results of studies of healthy Maine coon cats, a breed which tends to have a large body size, refute this because unaffected individuals of this breed have end-diastolic measurements of wall thickness that are similar to mixed-breed cats.[70] Indeed, statistical analysis of echocardiographic data obtained during screening examinations of Maine coon cats suggests that 6 mm might be overly conservative as a marker of ventricular hypertrophy. Evaluation of jackknife distances, which statistically identify extreme observations or outliers, suggested the possibility that a measurement of wall thickness that exceeds 5 mm is outside the normal range.[34]

Biomarkers, specifically B-type natriuretic peptide (BNP), have been evaluated as screening strategies and this subject is more completely addressed in another article by David J. Connolly elsewhere in this issue. Although differences in criteria used to define the severity of HCM make the data difficult to interpret, the sensitivity of raised BNP for the identification of subclinical HCM may be as high as 94% or even

100%.[71–73] However, sensitivity (the proportion of patients with the disease that have a positive test) is an intrinsic feature of the test. In contrast, positive predictive value is highly dependent on disease prevalence. Because of the dependence on prevalence, even a test with 95% sensitivity and 95% specificity has only a 77% positive predictive value when prevalence is 15%. Because of this and other factors, the suitability of BNP measurement as a screening test is uncertain at this time.[74]

THERAPY
Subclinical HCM

Optimally, it would be possible to identify patients that have a subclinical form of HCM that is destined to worsen and to intervene in a way that would slow or prevent progression of disease. Unfortunately, there is little known of the natural history of feline HCM and as yet no published evidence that medical therapy can alter the course of subclinical disease. The use of beta-blockers, such as atenolol, is often advocated particularly in patients that have resting LVOTO, but the efficacy of this intervention has not been determined. In cats, a causal relationship between LVOTO and poor outcome has not been established, and as noted, retrospectively evaluated case series have associated LVOTO with improved outcome in cats.[30,31] However, the latter argument must be viewed with circumspection. Cases of HCM associated with LVOTO generally have murmurs and therefore are apt to be identified when patients are subclinical. Furthermore, if progression to clinical disease is associated with a decrease in systolic myocardial function, a notion for which there is some evidence, cross-sectional or retrospective studies might associate poor outcome with lack of LVOTO.[75] The role of LVOTO is presently inconclusive. However, there is evidence that beta-blockade may hasten the recurrence of pulmonary edema in cats that have developed heart failure caused by HCM or RCM and, in the absence of evidence to the contrary, this raises the possibility that beta-blockade might harm cats with subclinical disease.[76] The occurrence of pulmonary edema caused by HCM is an objective marker that is a suitable inclusion criterion for clinical trials but it is a factor without an established relationship to characteristics that might predispose patients with HCM to adverse outcome in response to beta-blockade. If beta-blockade does indeed harm cats that have developed edema, the absence of data makes it impossible to determine precisely when, during the natural history of HCM, patients are at risk for these adverse effects.

Because there are data that suggest a role for abnormal response to hormones in the pathogenesis of HCM, the possibility that neuroendocrine modulating drugs might favorably affect the natural history of the disease has been investigated.[77,78] Evidence obtained from studies of transgenic mice suggests that aldosterone may be relevant to the pathogenesis of HCM insofar as spironolactone attenuates the development of myocardial fibrosis and myofiber disarray.[28] Based on these experimental findings, there may be a role for the use of spironolactone in cats with cardiac disease. However, relative to placebo, 4-months therapy with oral spironolactone did not alter echocardiographic indices of diastolic function in a colony of Maine coon cats with HCM.[79] The same group also evaluated the effect of angiotensin-converting enzyme inhibition.[77] Maine coon cats with HCM but without heart failure were randomly assigned to receive placebo or ramipril. Evidence that the circulating renin angiotensin system was suppressed was presented, but despite this, echocardiographic and magnetic resonance indices of myocardial mass and diastolic function were unaffected. Given the genetic heterogeneity that probably exists in feline HCM, it is possible that these agents or others might slow progression of HCM in other breeds of cats. And of course, it is possible that longer duration of therapy and the evaluation of clinically relevant outcome measures, such as time to onset of heart failure or mortality, might have disclosed benefit. At this time, however, evidence that medical therapy favorably alters the course of subclinical feline HCM is lacking.

Heart Failure

Other than furosemide, for which efficacy is assumed, there are no medical interventions that have demonstrated efficacy in the management of feline heart failure. Attempts to improve diastolic function have been made through interventions that are thought to speed myocardial relaxation or slow heart rate. Diltiazem is a calcium channel blocker that has been widely used in the therapy of feline HCM. The effect of diltiazem on heart rate is modest.[80] However, there is evidence to suggest that this drug has a positive lusitropic effect; that is, it improves ventricular filling through a salutary effect on myocardial relaxation.[81] The presumed favorable effects of beta-blockers on diastolic function are primarily indirect and result from decreases in heart rate. In an open-label clinical trial, the effects of diltiazem, propranolol, and verapamil on cats with pulmonary edema caused by HCM were compared. Of the three, diltiazem was the most efficacious.[81] However, this trial did not include a negative control in the form of a placebo group. Ace inhibition has also been used in the management of heart failure due to feline HCM.[82] These drugs are apparently safe and the concern that vasodilation due to ACE inhibition might result in adverse effects related to worsening LVOTO may not be valid.[82] However, conclusive evidence of efficacy is lacking.

The results of a multicenter, randomized, placebo-controlled trial that had been designed to evaluate the relative efficacy of atenolol, diltiazem, and enalapril in feline patients with congestive heart failure caused by HCM or RCM have been presented at a national meeting, but not yet published.[76] The primary outcome variable was time until recurrence of congestive signs and none of the agents was superior to placebo in this regard. Patients that received enalapril remained in the trial longer than those receiving the alternatives, although this result was not statistically significant. Patients receiving atenolol fared less well than did those in the placebo group.[83] The finding that atenolol may harm cats with pulmonary edema was possibly unexpected but is consistent with the result of the only comparable study in which administration of propranolol was associated with decreased survival.[81] Based on the results of the aforementioned randomized clinical trial,[76] the use of enalapril together with furosemide seems a reasonable approach to the management of feline patients with congestive heart failure caused by diastolic dysfunction.

PROGNOSIS/NATURAL HISTORY

Survival data obtained from retrospective evaluation of teaching hospital records have been reported by two groups of investigators.[29,30] Survival times for the entire study samples were similar for both studies and were close to 700 days. Median survival times of 92 days and 563 days were reported for patients with heart failure. The retrospective nature of the studies makes it difficult to interpret these differences but it seems that patients with heart failure in general, fare poorly. However, both groups of investigators reported median survival for subclinical HCM that was in excess of 3 years.[29,30]

Much of the early clinical literature that relates to HCM in human beings originated from a small number of tertiary, HCM centers and was therefore subject to referral bias. This bias contributed to the notion that HCM was generally associated with an ominous prognosis.[8] It is now recognized that human HCM is a disorder that exhibits a broad spectrum of severity. In fact, in a recent review, human HCM was described as a "relatively benign disease"; the finding that survival times of non-selected cohorts are similar to those of the general population supports this view.[20] Little is known of the natural history of feline HCM. However, it is possible that referral bias has similarly shaped perception of this disease and it may be that the feline disorder is also characterized by genetic heterogeneity and a broad spectrum of phenotypic expression that includes mild, non-progressive disease and lethal variants that cause congestive failure, embolism, and death.

REFERENCES

1. Maron BJ, Towbin JA, Thiene G, et al. Contemporary definitions and classification of the cardiomyopathies: an American Heart Association Scientific Statement from the Council on Clinical Cardiology, Heart Failure and Transplantation Committee; Quality of Care and Outcomes Research and Functional Genomics and Translational Biology Interdisciplinary Working Groups; and Council on Epidemiology and Prevention. Circulation 2006;113:1807–16.
2. Thiene G, Corrado D, Basso C. Cardiomyopathies: is it time for a molecular classification? Eur Heart J 2004;25:1772–5.
3. Meurs KM, Sanchez X, David RM, et al. A cardiac myosin binding protein C mutation in the Maine Coon cat with familial hypertrophic cardiomyopathy. Hum Mol Genet 2005;14:3587–93.
4. Meurs KM, Norgard MM, Ederer MM, et al. A substitution mutation in the myosin binding protein C gene in ragdoll hypertrophic cardiomyopathy. Genomics 2007; 90:261–4.
5. Richardson P, McKenna W, Bristow M, et al. Report of the 1995 World Health Organization/International Society and Federation of Cardiology Task Force on the Definition and Classification of cardiomyopathies. Circulation 1996;93: 841–2.
6. Maron BJ, McKenna WJ, Elliott P, et al. Hypertrophic cardiomyopathy. JAMA 1999;282:2302–3.
7. Maron BJ, Epstein SE. Hypertrophic cardiomyopathy: a discussion of nomenclature. Am J Cardiol 1979;43:1242–4.
8. Maron BJ, McKenna WJ, Danielson GK, et al. ACC/ESC Clinical expert document on hypertrophic cardiomyopathy: a report of American College of Cardiology Foundation Task Force on Clinical Expert Consensus Documents and European Society of Cardiology Committee for Practice Guidelines. J Am Coll Cardiol 2003;42:1687–713.
9. Roberts WC. Fifty years of hypertrophic cardiomyopathy. Am J Cardiol 2009;103: 431–4.
10. Buchanan J, Baker G, Hill J. Aortic embolism in cats: prevalence, surgical treatment and electrocardiography. Vet Rec 1966;79:496–506.
11. Holzworth J. University of Pennsylvania Veterinary Extension Quarterly. 1958;151:101.
12. Liu SK. Acquired cardiac lesions leading to congestive heart failure in the cat. Am J Vet Res 1970;31:2071–88.
13. Harpster N. Acquired heart disease in the cat. In: 40th Annual Meeting of the American Animal Hospital Association. San Antonio (TX), April 8–13, 1973. Southbend (IN): American Animal Hospital Association. p. 118.
14. Tilley L. Feline cardiology. Vet Clin North Am 1976;6:415–32.

15. Liu SK, Tilley LP. Animal models of primary myocardial diseases. Yale J Biol Med 1980;53:191–211.
16. Moise NS, Dietze AE, Mezza LE, et al. Echocardiography, electrocardiography, and radiography of cats with dilatation cardiomyopathy, hypertrophic cardiomyopathy, and hyperthyroidism. Am J Vet Res 1986;47:1476–86.
17. Maron BJ. Hypertrophic cardiomyopathy: a systematic review. JAMA 2002;287: 1308–20.
18. Jarcho JA, McKenna W, Pare JA, et al. Mapping a gene for familial hypertrophic cardiomyopathy to chromosome 14q1. N Engl J Med 1989;321:1372–8.
19. Geisterfer-Lowrance AAT, Kass S, Tanigawa G, et al. A molecular basis for familial hypertrophic cardiomyopathy: a [beta] cardiac myosin heavy chain gene missense mutation. Cell 1990;62:999–1006.
20. Marian AJ. Hypertrophic cardiomyopathy: from genetics to treatment. Eur J Clin Invest 2010;40:360–9.
21. Bos JM, Ommen SR, Ackerman MJ. Genetics of hypertrophic cardiomyopathy: one, two, or more diseases? Curr Opin Cardiol 2007;22:193–9.
22. Kraus MS, Calvert CA, Jacobs GJ. Hypertrophic cardiomyopathy in a litter of five mixed-breed cats. J Am Anim Hosp Assoc 1999;35:293–6.
23. Marin L, VandeWoude S, Boon J, et al. Left ventricular hypertrophy in a closed colony of Persian cats [abstract]. J Vet Intern Med 1994;8:143.
24. Meurs KM, Kittleson MD, Towbin J, et al. Familial systolic anterior motion of the mitral valve and/or hypertrophic cardiomyopathy is apparently inherited as an autosomal dominant trait in a family of American shorthair cats. J Vet Intern Med 1997;11:138.
25. Nicol RL, Frey N, Olson EN. From the sarcomere to the nucleus: role of genetics and signaling in structural heart disease. Annu Rev Genomics Hum Genet 2000; 1:179–223.
26. Tardiff J. Sarcomeric proteins and familial hypertrophic cardiomyopathy: linking mutations in structural proteins to complex cardiovascular phenotypes. Heart Fail Rev 2005;10:237–48.
27. Roberts R, Sigwart U. Current concepts of the pathogenesis and treatment of hypertrophic cardiomyopathy. Circulation 2005;112:293–6.
28. Tsybouleva N, Zhang L, Chen S, et al. Aldosterone, through novel signaling proteins, is a fundamental molecular bridge between the genetic defect and the cardiac phenotype of hypertrophic cardiomyopathy. Circulation 2004;109: 1284–91.
29. Atkins CE, Gallo AM, Kurzman ID, et al. Risk factors, clinical signs, and survival in cats with a clinical diagnosis of idiopathic hypertrophic cardiomyopathy: 74 cases (1985–1989). J Am Vet Med Assoc 1992;201:613–8.
30. Rush JE, Freeman LM, Fenollosa NK, et al. Population and survival characteristics of cats with hypertrophic cardiomyopathy: 260 cases (1990–1999). J Am Vet Med Assoc 2002;220:202–7.
31. Fox PR, Liu S-K, Maron BJ. Echocardiographic assessment of spontaneously occurring feline hypertrophic cardiomyopathy: an animal model of human disease. Circulation 1995;92:2645–51.
32. Smith SA, Tobias AH, Fine DM, et al. Corticosteroid-associated congestive heart failure in 12 cats. Int J Appl Res Vet Med 2004;2:159–70.
33. Cote E, Manning AM, Emerson D, et al. Assessment of the prevalence of heart murmurs in overtly healthy cats. J Am Vet Med Assoc 2004;225:384–8.
34. Gundler S, Tidholm A, Haggstrom J. Prevalence of myocardial hypertrophy in a population of asymptomatic Swedish Maine coon cats. Acta Vet Scand 2008;50:22.

35. Riesen SC, Kovacevic A, Lombard CW, et al. Echocardiographic screening of purebred cats: an overview from 2002 to 2005. Schweiz Arch Tierheilkd 2007; 149:73–6.
36. Paige CF, Abbott JA, Pyle RL, et al. Prevalence of cardiomyopathy in apparently healthy cats. J Am Vet Med Assoc 2009;234:1398–403.
37. Wagner T, Luis Fuentes V, McDermott N, et al. Association between cardiac murmurs and left ventricular hypertrophy in 199 healthy adult cats. J Vet Intern Med 2009;23:1332 [abstract #29].
38. Maron BJ, Gardin JM, Flack JM, et al. Prevalence of hypertrophic cardiomyopathy in a general population of young adults. Echocardiographic analysis of 4111 subjects in the CARDIA Study. Coronary Artery Risk Development in (Young) Adults. Circulation 1995;92:785–9.
39. Goda A, Yamashita T, Suzuki S, et al. Prevalence and prognosis of patients with heart failure in Tokyo: a prospective cohort of Shinken Database 2004–5. Int Heart J 2009;50:609–25.
40. Maron BJ, Peterson EE, Maron MS, et al. Prevalence of hypertrophic cardiomyopathy in an outpatient population referred for echocardiographic study. Am J Cardiol 1994;73:577–80.
41. Connolly DJ, Soares Magalhaes RJ, Fuentes VL, et al. Assessment of the diagnostic accuracy of circulating natriuretic peptide concentrations to distinguish between cats with cardiac and non-cardiac causes of respiratory distress. J Vet Cardiol 2009;11:S41–50.
42. Fox PR, Oyama MA, Reynolds C, et al. Utility of plasma N-terminal pro-brain natriuretic peptide (NT-proBNP) to distinguish between congestive heart failure and non-cardiac causes of acute dyspnea in cats. J Vet Cardiol 2009;11:S51–61.
43. Fox P. Feline cardiomyopathies. In: Fox PR, Sisson D, Moise NS, editors. Textbook of canine and feline cardiology: principles and practice. 2nd edition. Philadelphia: WB Saunders Co; 1999. p. 621–78.
44. Sherrid MV. Pathophysiology and treatment of hypertrophic cardiomyopathy. Prog Cardiovasc Dis 2006;49:123–51.
45. Sherrid MV, Gunsburg DZ, Moldenhauer S, et al. Systolic anterior motion begins at low left ventricular outflow tract velocity in obstructive hypertrophic cardiomyopathy. J Am Coll Cardiol 2000;36:1344–54.
46. Levine RA, Vlahakes GJ, Lefebvre X, et al. Papillary muscle displacement causes systolic anterior motion of the mitral valve. Experimental validation and insights into the mechanism of subaortic obstruction. Circulation 1995;91:1189–95.
47. Paige CF, Abbott JA, Pyle RL. Systolic anterior motion of the mitral valve associated with right ventricular systolic hypertension in 9 dogs. J Vet Cardiol 2007;9: 9–14.
48. Maron BJ, Maron MS, Wigle ED, et al. The 50-year history, controversy, and clinical implications of left ventricular outflow tract obstruction in hypertrophic cardiomyopathy: from idiopathic hypertrophic subaortic stenosis to hypertrophic cardiomyopathy. J Am Coll Cardiol 2009;54:191–200.
49. Maron MS, Olivotto I, Betocchi S, et al. Effect of left ventricular outflow tract obstruction on clinical outcome in hypertrophic cardiomyopathy. N Engl J Med 2003;348:295–303.
50. Blanksma PK. Is regional wall stress a stimulus for myocardial hypertrophy in hypertrophic cardiomyopathy? Z Kardiol 1987;76(Suppl 3):57–60.
51. Deb SJ, Schaff HV, Dearani JA, et al. Septal myectomy results in regression of left ventricular hypertrophy in patients with hypertrophic obstructive cardiomyopathy. Ann Thorac Surg 2004;78:2118–22.

52. Knaapen P, Germans T, Camici PG, et al. Determinants of coronary microvascular dysfunction in symptomatic hypertrophic cardiomyopathy. Am J Physiol Heart Circ Physiol 2008;294:H986–993.

53. Celik S, Dagdeviren B, Yildirim A, et al. Comparison of coronary flow velocities between patients with obstructive and nonobstructive type hypertrophic cardiomyopathy: noninvasive assessment by Transthoracic Doppler Echocardiography. Echocardiography 2005;22:1–7.

54. Maron MS, Olivotto I, Maron BJ, et al. The case for myocardial ischemia in hypertrophic cardiomyopathy. J Am Coll Cardiol 2009;54:866–75.

55. Liu SK, Roberts WC, Maron BJ. Comparison of morphologic findings in spontaneously occurring hypertrophic cardiomyopathy in humans, cats and dogs. Am J Cardiol 1993;72:944–51.

56. Efthimiadis GK, Parcharidou DG, Giannakoulas G, et al. Left ventricular outflow tract obstruction as a risk factor for sudden cardiac death in hypertrophic cardiomyopathy. Am J Cardiol 2009;104:695–9.

57. Kizilbash AM, Heinle SK, Grayburn PA. Spontaneous variability of left ventricular outflow tract gradient in hypertrophic obstructive cardiomyopathy. Circulation 1998;97:461–6.

58. Geske JB, Sorajja P, Ommen SR, et al. Left ventricular outflow tract gradient variability in hypertrophic cardiomyopathy. Clin Cardiol 2009;32:397–402.

59. Maron MS, Olivotto I, Zenovich AG, et al. Hypertrophic cardiomyopathy is predominantly a disease of left ventricular outflow tract obstruction. Circulation 2006;114:2232–9.

60. Rishniw M, Thomas WP. Dynamic right ventricular outflow obstruction: a new cause of systolic murmurs in cats. J Vet Intern Med 2002;16:547–52.

61. Kittleson MD, Meurs KM, Munro MJ, et al. Familial hypertrophic cardiomyopathy in Maine coon cats: an animal model of human disease. Circulation 1999;99: 3172–80.

62. Abbott JA, MacLean HN. Two-dimensional echocardiographic assessment of the feline left atrium. J Vet Intern Med 2006;20:111–9.

63. Nistri S, Olivotto I, Betocchi S, et al. Prognostic significance of left atrial size in patients with hypertrophic cardiomyopathy (from the Italian registry for hypertrophic cardiomyopathy). Am J Cardiol 2006;98:960 5.

64. Fox PR. Hypertrophic cardiomyopathy. Clinical and pathologic correlates. J Vet Cardiol 2003;5:39–45.

65. Kubo T, Gimeno JR, Bahl A, et al. Prevalence, clinical significance, and genetic basis of hypertrophic cardiomyopathy with restrictive phenotype. J Am Coll Cardiol 2007;49:2419–26.

66. Nishimura RA, Ommen SR. Hypertrophic cardiomyopathy: the search for obstruction. Circulation 2006;114:2200–2.

67. Shah JS, Esteban MT, Thaman R, et al. Prevalence of exercise-induced left ventricular outflow tract obstruction in symptomatic patients with non-obstructive hypertrophic cardiomyopathy. Heart 2008;94:1288–94.

68. Liu S-K, Maron BJ, Tilley LP. Feline hypertrophic cardiomyopathy: gross anatomic and quantitative histologic features. Am J Pathol 1981;102:388–95.

69. Sisson DD, Knight DH, Helinski C, et al. Plasma taurine concentrations and M mode echocardiographic measures in healthy cats and in cats with dilated cardiomyopathy. J Vet Intern Med 1991;5:232–8.

70. Drourr L, Lefbom BK, Rosenthal SL, et al. Measurement of M-mode echocardiographic parameters in healthy adult Maine Coon cats. J Am Vet Med Assoc 2005; 226:734–7.

71. Connolly DJ, Soares Magalhaes RJ, Syme HM, et al. Circulating natriuretic peptides in cats with heart disease. J Vet Intern Med 2008;22:96–105.
72. Wess G, Daisenberger P, Hirschberger J, et al. The utility of NT-proBNP to detect early stages of hypertrophic cardiomyopathy in cats and to differentiate disease stages. J Vet Intern Med 2009;23:687 [abstract 9].
73. Fox PR, Oyama MA, MacDonald KA, et al. Assessment of NT proBNP concentration in asymptomatic cats with cardiomyopathy. J Vet Intern Med 2008;22:759 [abstract 191].
74. Hsu A, Kittleson MD, Paling A, Investigation into the use of plasma NT-proBNP concentration to screen for feline hypertrophic cardiomyopathy. J Vet Cardiol 2009;11(Suppl 1):S63–70.
75. Baty CJ, Malarkey DE, Atkins CE, et al. Natural history of hypertrophic cardiomyopathy and aortic thromboembolism in a family of domestic shorthair cats. J Vet Intern Med 2001;15:595–9.
76. Fox PR. Prospective, double-blinded, multicenter evaluation of chronic therapies for feline diastolic heart failure: interim analysis [abstract]. J Vet Intern Med 2003; 17:398.
77. MacDonald KA, Kittleson MD, Larson RF, et al. The effect of ramipril on left ventricular mass, myocardial fibrosis, diastolic function, and plasma neurohormones in Maine Coon cats with familial hypertrophic cardiomyopathy without heart failure. J Vet Intern Med 2006;20:1093–105.
78. Amberger CN, Glardon O, Glaus T, et al. Effects of benazepril in the treatment of feline hypertrophic cardiomyopathy: results of a prospective, open-label, multicenter clinical trial. J Vet Cardiol 1999;1:19–26.
79. MacDonald KA, Kittleson MD, Kass PH. Effect of spironolactone on diastolic function and left ventricular mass in Maine Coon cats with familial hypertrophic cardiomyopathy. J Vet Intern Med 2008;22:335–41.
80. Johnson LM, Atkins CE, Keene BW, et al. Pharmacokinetic and pharmacodynamic properties of conventional and CD-formulated diltiazem in cats. J Vet Intern Med 1996;10(5):316–20.
81. Bright JM, Golden AL, Gompf RE, et al. Evaluation of the calcium channel-blocking agents diltiazem and verapamil for treatment of feline hypertrophic cardiomyopathy. J Vet Intern Med 1991;5:272–82.
82. Rush JE, Freeman LM, Brown DJ, et al. The use of enalapril in the treatment of feline hypertrophic cardiomyopathy. J Am Anim Hosp Assoc 1998;34:38–41.
83. Fox PR. Newest developments: feline heart disease and management. In: Proceedings of the North American Veterinary Conference. Orlando (FL), January 17–21, 2004. Gainesville (FL): Eastern States Veterinary Association. p. 133–5.

Genetics of Cardiac Disease in the Small Animal Patient

Kathryn M. Meurs, DVM, PhD*

KEYWORDS

- Familial • Mutation • Cardiomyopathy
- Congenital heart disease

Common Genetic Terminology

Genotype: The genetic makeup of an individual
Heterozygous: Having 2 different forms of a gene for a specific trait or disease
Homozygous: Having 2 identical forms of a gene for a specific trait or disease
Penetrance: The likelihood that a given gene will result in disease; *incomplete penetrance* suggests that it is less than 100%
Phenotype: The observable characteristics of an individual resulting from the interaction of the animal's genetic makeup and the environment
Polygenic: A disease or trait caused by 2 or more genes.

There is increasing evidence that many forms of congenital and acquired cardiovascular disease in small animal patients are of familial origin.[1–18] The large number of familial diseases in domestic purebred animals is thought to be associated with the desire to breed related animals to maintain a specific appearance and the selection of animals from a small group of popular founders (founder effect).[19]

Clinicians can use knowledge that a particular trait or disease may be inherited to provide guidance to owners and animal breeders to reduce the frequency of the trait. Even if the molecular cause is not known, identification of a pattern of inheritance and information on clinical screening can be useful for a breeder trying to make breeding decisions. Common forms of inheritance for veterinary diseases include autosomal recessive, autosomal dominant, X-linked recessive, and polygenic (**Table 1**).

AUTOSOMAL RECESSIVE

Autosomal recessive traits are those carried on an autosomal chromosome. These traits are clinically unapparent unless both copies of the individual's gene have the

Department of Veterinary Clinical Sciences, College of Veterinary Medicine, Washington State University, Pullman, WA 99164, USA
* Corresponding author.
E-mail address: Meurs@vetmed.wsu.edu

Vet Clin Small Anim 40 (2010) 701–715
doi:10.1016/j.cvsm.2010.03.006
0195-5616/10/$ – see front matter © 2010 Published by Elsevier Inc.

vetsmall.theclinics.com

Table 1
Patterns of inheritance of common cardiovascular diseases

Disease	Breed	Mode of Inheritance
Arrhythmogenic right ventricular cardiomyopathy	Boxers	Autosomal dominant with varied penetrance[1]
Atrial septal defect	Poodle	Unknown[2]
Degenerative valve disease	Dachshund	Polygenic[3]
Degenerative valve disease	Cavalier King Charles Spaniel	Polygenic[4]
Dilated cardiomyopathy	Doberman pinscher	Autosomal dominant[5]
Dilated cardiomyopathy	Great Dane	X-linked[6]
Dilated cardiomyopathy	Irish Wolfhound	Autosomal recessive with sex-specific alleles[7]
Dilated cardiomyopathy	Newfoundland	Autosomal dominant with incomplete penetrance[8]
Dilated cardiomyopathy	Portuguese water dog	Autosomal recessive[9]
Hypertrophic cardiomyopathy	Maine Coon	Autosomal dominant[10]
Hypertrophic cardiomyopathy	Ragdoll	Unknown[11]
Patent ductus arteriosus	Poodle	Polygenic[12]
Pulmonic stenosis	Beagle	Polygenic[13]
Tetralogy of Fallot	Keeshond	Polygenic[14]
Tricuspid valve dysplasia	Labrador retriever	Autosomal dominant[15]
Subvalvular aortic stenosis	Newfoundland	Polygenic[16]
Ventricular septal defect	Beagle	Autosomal recessive[17]
Ventricular septal defect	English Springer Spaniel	Autosomal dominant[18]

mutation. Evaluation of pedigrees of affected animals should identify the following pattern: the disease should appear to "skip" a generation (parents do not show the phenotype) and males and females should equally show the phenotype. A common observation is that the mating of 2 individuals that appear normal produces approximately 25% of offspring with the affected phenotype and 75% that do not demonstrate the trait. This outcome suggests that the 2 parents are silent carriers of a recessive trait. If both parents show the trait, all offspring should show the trait.

AUTOSOMAL DOMINANT

Autosomal dominant traits are those carried on autosomal chromosomes that are clinically evident even when one gene copy has a mutation. Evaluation of pedigrees of affected animals should identify the following pattern: males and females should equally show the trait and every affected individual should have at least one affected parent. Animals that show the phenotype will be either heterozygotes or homozygotes. Heterozygotes will produce approximately 50% affected offspring and homozygotes should produce 100% affected offspring.

X-LINKED

X-linked traits are caused by a gene(s) carried on the X chromosome. These traits are most commonly recessive. Therefore, affected males almost always show the phenotype (trait) because they only have one X chromosome. Because females have two X chromosomes, they may be silent carriers if they have the mutant copy of the gene on only one of their X chromosomes; they will show the phenotype if both X chromosomes have the mutant copy of the gene. Evaluation of pedigrees of affected animals should identify the following pattern: more affected males than females, an affected male crossed with a normal female should produce silent (unaffected) females. Silent carrier females have a 50% chance of passing the trait on to male offspring. Affected females are the result of a cross between a silent carrier female and an affected male, and should be uncommon.

POLYGENIC

Many forms of inherited heart disease in veterinary medicine have been characterized as polygenic.[3,4,12-14,16] Polygenic traits are those that require 2 or more genes working together to develop a specific trait. Polygenic traits are particularly difficult traits for both clinicians and geneticists. It may take years to identify all of the genes that work together to develop and influence the severity of the trait, therefore development of molecular tests may be very difficult. In addition, the lack of knowledge of the individual genes also makes it very difficult to develop specific breeding recommendations.

GENETIC PENETRANCE

Genetic penetrance and expressivity are phenomena that determine the proportion of genetically affected individuals that express a trait and the extent to which a trait is demonstrated in the individual. Many genetic diseases are inherited with variability in penetrance and expressivity. If a trait has incomplete penetrance it means that less than 100% of individuals with a causative mutation will show the trait. Variable expressivity of a trait results in a spectrum of phenotypic expression so that some individuals are more severely affected than others. For example, some Maine Coon cats with the Maine Coon hypertrophic cardiomyopathy mutation may have significant ventricular hypertrophy and develop congestive heart failure, whereas litter mates with the same mutation may not even ever show the disease. The mutation exhibits incomplete penetrance and variable expressivity. The mechanisms for the phenomena of variable expressivity and incomplete disease penetrance are poorly understood even in human genetics. It is possible that environmental or genetic factors may have an impact on a particular mutation.

Penetrance and genetic expressivity are important considerations in the development of breeding guidelines. It is very important that pet owners and pet breeders understand that not all individuals that carry a genetic mutation or are the offspring of affected parents will show the disease, or will show it with the same severity. These individuals are certainly at increased risk of disease but are not guaranteed to develop disease.

MAKING BREEDING RECOMMENDATIONS

At this time, a molecular genetic basis has not been determined for the majority of inherited cardiovascular disease in veterinary medicine. However, if the pattern of inheritance has been determined for a trait, clinicians may be able to provide some guidance for pet breeders. In some cases, a molecular cause has been identified and genetic testing is possible. How this information is used requires careful development of screening guidelines by clinicians to determine the type of test, the interpretation of the test, frequency of the tests, and criteria for inclusion and exclusion of breeding animals. It is important that as clinical and genetic screening guidelines are developed, it will become increasingly easy to identify which animals are at risk of developing disease or passing the disease forward to future generations. It may seem desirable to develop very strict guidelines to remove all at-risk animals from the breeding program, but this should be strongly discouraged. Most pure breeds have a closed, fairly small gene pool. If aggressive removal of too many animals from a breed's breeding population occurs because of the presence of certain risk factors, it could have a detrimental impact on the breed. As the number of available breeding animals becomes smaller it will necessitate some degree of inbreeding. The problem will get worse as additional genetic defects in other systems (eyes, hips, and so forth) are identified and animals are removed for additional genetic reasons. Therefore, screening information on individual animals should be used to make educated decisions based on many factors, including presence of a heterozygous or homozygous mutation (if known), mode of inheritance, severity of disease in parents, disease penetrance, and size of population. Aggressive removal of borderline animals may need to be discouraged.

INHERITED CONGENITAL HEART DISEASE
Feline Congenital Heart Disease

Congenital heart disease in the cat is fairly rare, and specific breed predispositions have not been observed for most defects.

Endomyocardial Fibrosis

Endomyocardial fibrosis is a rare feline congenital heart disease characterized by left atrial and ventricular dilation with severe endocardial thickening. Endomyocardial fibrosis has been shown to be inherited in the Siamese and Burmese breeds as well as in a colony of domestic short-hair cats. The mode of inheritance is not known.[20–22]

Canine Congenital Heart Disease

Many forms of congenital disease in the dog are inherited in at least some breeds; however, it should be remembered that occasionally developmental (not inherited) defects can occur. A defect that occurs in a breed in which there is not a known breed predisposition, or in a family with no known history of that form of defect, is not necessarily inherited.

Atrial Septal Defect

Atrial septal defect (ASD) is not a common canine congenital heart defect, but it has been associated with a strong breed predisposition in several breeds including Boxers, Doberman pinschers, Samoyeds, and most recently Standard Poodles.[2,23,24] Pedigree evaluation demonstrating the familial nature of the disease has been performed in the Standard Poodle and less extensively in the Doberman pinscher.[2,24]

The ASD in the Standard Poodle is an ostium secundum defect. Initial pedigree evaluation suggests that it is most likely an autosomal dominant trait because it appears without skipping a generation, but this cannot be definitively concluded given the dogs evaluated so far.[2] The Doberman pinscher also appears to have an ostium secundum defect, and the pattern of inheritance has not yet been determined.[24]

The genetics of the ASD even in human beings is poorly understood. However, because transcription factor genes play a role in the septogenesis of the heart, they have become important candidates for evaluation.[25] At this time 2 transcription factors have been implicated in the development of familial ostium secundum ASDs in humans, GATA4 and NKC2.5.[25] The GATA4 gene has now been evaluated in both the Standard Poodle and the Doberman, and causative mutations were not identified.[2,24]

Clinical screening for the ASD can include auscultation for the presence of a heart murmur. However, in some dogs with an ASD a heart murmur is not identified. Therefore, an echocardiogram with Doppler is the most sensitive and specific screening test at this time.[2]

At this time the pattern of inheritance is not definitive, but an autosomal dominant trait seems most likely. For autosomal dominant traits, breeding of affected individuals is generally not recommended. If a dog is homozygous it would certainly pass on the trait. If a dog is heterozygous, it would have a 50% chance of passing on the trait and a 50% chance of not passing on the trait. Therefore, unaffected offspring of affected dogs that have been carefully cleared of the defect by echocardiography should be allowable for breeding because silent carriers should not exist (they did not inherit the trait). In addition, with an autosomal dominant trait all affected dogs should have at least one affected parent. Therefore, it is recommended that all parents of affected dogs be carefully evaluated with echocardiography to ensure that they do not have a small ASD that is not detectable on physical examination.

Patent Ductus Arteriosus

The patent ductus arteriosus (PDA) has been demonstrated to be inherited in the Poodle.[12] Inheritance was suggested to most likely be polygenic (at least 2 genes contribute to the development of the trait). Inheritance of the PDA in other canine breeds has not been well studied but is certainly possible and perhaps likely, as several canine breeds are strongly predisposed to PDA.

Clinical screening should include cardiac auscultation for a continuous murmur at the left base of the heart. Most dogs with a PDA have a fairly identifiable heart murmur and are likely to be detectable by physical examination. However, if a particular family of dogs has a high prevalence of PDAs, it may be valuable to have closely related family members evaluated with Doppler echocardiography even if they do not have a heart murmur. It is possible that some breeding animals may have a small PDA with very soft murmur that has been missed and that they are passing on the defect.

Until the pattern of inheritance is better understood, breeding of Poodles with PDAs cannot be recommended. However, because the genetics appear to be polygenic as opposed to a simple mendelian trait, there is no clear reason to remove the parents of an affected puppy from a breeding program. The parents should be carefully screened for the defect with Doppler echocardiography. If they do not have the defect, it may be reasonable to continue to use the dogs in a breeding program. The parents should not be bred to each other again or to closely related dogs. Echocardiography may not detect the presence of a nonpatent ductal structure—the aortic diverticulum—which is thought to be the forme fruste of hereditary PDA. Therefore, if a particular dog has a history of producing puppies with this defect, it should be removed from use as a breeding animal even if it has been echocardiographically cleared. Inheritance of the PDA in other dog breeds has not been well studied. However, it would seem reasonable to apply the recommendations for the poodle for other breeds that may have familial PDA until further study is completed.

Pulmonic Stenosis

There are several breeds of dogs shown to have an increased prevalence of valvular pulmonic stenosis (PS) including Scottish terriers, wire-haired terriers, miniature schnauzers, and beagles, among others.[23] The only breed in which the inheritable form has been well studied is the beagle.[13] In the beagle the pattern of inheritance is thought to be polygenic, and a specific genetic mutation has not been identified.

Clinical screening should include cardiac auscultation for a systolic left basilar murmur. If a heart murmur is heard, echocardiography should be performed to confirm the etiology and severity of the defect.

Because the PS is believed to be polygenic at least in the beagle, breeding recommendations are similar to those stated for PDA.

Subvalvular Aortic Stenosis

Subvalvular aortic stenosis (SAS) has been demonstrated to be inherited in the Newfoundland breed.[16] The strong prevalence of the defect in additional breeds including the Golden Retriever and Rottweiler among others would suggest that it is inherited in these breeds as well, although it has not been thoroughly studied. In the Newfoundland, inheritance has been described as polygenic.[16]

Clinical screening should include cardiac auscultation for a systolic left basilar murmur. Some breed organizations also require Doppler echocardiography of the left ventricular outflow track even if a heart murmur is not heard. Current clearance criteria from the American College of Veterinary Internal Medicine (ACVIM) Registry of Cardiac Health (http://www.archcertify.org/faqs.html) are the following. Dogs without a murmur may be considered clear of SAS. Dogs with a left ventricular outflow track velocity (LVOT) less than 1.9 m/s in the absence of either structural abnormalities of the LVOT or abrupt acceleration within the LVOT can be considered normal. Dogs with an LVOT velocity between 1.9 and 2.4 m/s in the absence of structural abnormalities of the LVOT or abrupt acceleration within the LVOT are categorized as "uncertain," and dogs with structural abnormalities of the LVOT or abrupt acceleration within the LVOT or a velocity greater than 2.4 m/s are considered to be affected.

Because SAS is believed to be polygenic at least in the Newfoundland, breeding recommendations are similar to those stated for the PDA. The parents of an affected puppy should be carefully evaluated and echoed even if they do not have a heart murmur. It is particularly difficult to advise owners of dogs who are determined to be in the "uncertain" category. It is possible that these dogs may have a mild variant if SAS and could be at risk of passing on this trait, but this is not known. Careful discussion of possible risks of using the animal as well as the dog's positive attributes that may be desirable to keep in a breeding line should occur. In some cases it may be reasonable to try a test breeding of a dog in an uncertain category to a clear dog to see if affected puppies are produced.

Tetralogy of Fallot

Familial tetralogy of Fallot (TOF) has been extensively studied in the Keeshond breed by Patterson and colleagues.[14] In the Keeshond breed, the TOF is characterized by a spectrum of defects from subclinical defects to the complete, severe TOF.[14] TOF has been determined to be a polygenic defect.[14] Recent molecular work by the same group identified genetic linkage to 3 different canine chromosomes.[26] The investigators suggested that genes at each of these 3 chromosomal regions act together to cause the development of the TOF.[26] In human beings, zinc finger protein multitype 2 (ZFPM2), a modulator of GATA transcription factor, has been implicated in the development of conotruncal defects. Recent molecular evaluation of the ZFPM2 gene in several minia-ture schnauzers and Sapsaree dogs with TOF did not identify a causative mutation.[27]

Clinical screening for dogs at risk of TOF should include an echocardiogram to diag-nose and to determine the severity of the defect.

Because the TOF is believed to be polygenic at least in the Keeshond, breeding recommendations are similar to those stated for PDA.

Tricuspid Valve Malformation/Dysplasia

Tricuspid valve malformation/dysplasia (TVD) is a heritable disease in the Labrador retriever.[15,28] One study suggested that it was inherited as an autosomal dominant trait with reduced penetrance and is genetically linked to an area on canine chromo-some 9.[15] A specific genetic mutation has not been identified.

Clinical screening should include cardiac auscultation and possibly also echocardi-ography, as some affected dogs do not have heart murmurs. Echocardiographic criteria for TVD are not well defined but might include thickening and redundancy of the valve leaflets, abnormal adherence of the septal leaflet to the interventricular septum, and presence of a large, fused right ventricular papillary muscle rather than normal, small, discrete muscles.

Because there is some evidence that TVD is an autosomal dominant trait, breeding of affected dogs is not recommended. Breeding recommendations are similar to those stated for ASD, another autosomal dominant trait.

Ventricular Septal Defect

Breed predispositions for the ventricular septal defect (VSD) have been reported in Lakeland Terriers, West Highland White Terriers, English Springer Spaniels, and Basset hounds, among others.[23] It has been reported to be inherited in beagles and English Springer Spaniels.[17,18] In the beagle, the VSD has been reported to be an autosomal recessive trait.[17] In the English Springer Spaniel, the VSD has been suggested to be an autosomal dominant trait with incomplete penetrance, or possibly a polygenic trait.[18]

Screening for familial VSDs should include physical examination. Most individuals with a VSD have a cardiac murmur. However, spontaneous closure of membranous VSD occasionally occurs due to adherence of elements of the tricuspid valve appa-ratus to the interventricular septum. That this has occurred can sometimes be surmised from the echocardiographic appearance of the septum. Therefore, echocar-diography is indicated for screening of populations at risk.

In the beagle, the VSD has been suggested to be an autosomal recessive trait.[17] In the case of an autosomal recessive trait, 2 copies of the genetic mutation are needed to be able to show the trait. Silent carriers exist because dogs that only have one copy of the trait may pass the gene on, but will not show the trait. The risk of an individual inheriting the mutation from both parents and having clinical evidence of the trait can generally be decreased by outbreeding and not breeding to related dogs, because this should decrease the risk of inadvertently breeding 2 dogs that have the same genetic mutation. In the English Springer Spaniel the VSD has been suggested to be auto-somal dominant. Breeding recommendations would be similar to those stated for ASD, another autosomal dominant defect.

ACQUIRED HEART DISEASE
Feline Hypertrophic Cardiomyopathy

Hypertrophic cardiomyopathy (HCM) is an inherited disease in the Maine Coon and Ragdoll cat breeds.[10,11] In addition, it has been observed to be familial in at least one family of mixed-breed cats.[29] It has been suggested to be inherited in other cat breeds including the Norwegian Forest Cat, Siberian, Sphynx, and Bengals, among others, although these breeds have not been well studied.

In the Maine Coon, HCM is inherited as autosomal dominant trait.[10] A genetic mutation has been identified in the myosin binding protein C (MYBPC3) gene.[30] Myosin binding protein C is an important cardiac sarcomeric protein and has been associated with the development of familial HCM in human beings as well.[31] In the Maine Coon cat, the mutation is a single base-pair change that changes the structure of myosin binding protein C and alters its ability to interact with other contractile proteins.

The Maine Coon mutation seems to be quite breed specific. It does not appear to be associated with familial HCM in other breeds of cats. The mutation is inherited with incomplete penetrance and variable expressivity, meaning that not all cats with the mutation will show the disease or will show the same severity of the disease. Cats that are homozygous for the mutation appear to be more likely to show the disease and perhaps have a more severe form.[30,32]

However, it would seem that not all Maine Coon cats with HCM have this mutation. In people there are now more than 400 reported HCM mutations.[31] Therefore, it is likely that there is more than 1 mutation in the Maine Coon cat as well.[30] Because the Maine Coon mutation is not the only cause for HCM in the Maine Coon, genetic screening has not replaced the need for annual clinical screening by echocardiography. Current ACVIM Cardiac Health Registry (http://www.archcertify.org/faqs.html) guidelines for clinical screening of HCM include the following: cats that have a diastolic left ventricular free wall (LVPWD) and diastolic interventricular septal wall (IVSD) thickness less than 5.5 mm are considered normal. Cats that have focal or diffuse LVPWD and/or IVSD wall thickness measuring 5.5 to 6.0 mm and without LV dilation are considered to be equivocal, and cats that have focal (segmental) or diffuse LVPWD and/or IVSD wall thickness greater than 6.0 mm at end-diastole, without LV dilation, and in absence of systemic hypertension, hyperthyroidism, or acromegaly, are considered affected.

Mutation screening can now be used to determine if a Maine Coon has the known HCM mutation. If a cat is positive for the mutation, one should carefully consider continued use as a breeding animal. It appears that approximately 30% of all Maine Coon cats tested for the mutation at Washington State University are positive for the mutation. Due to the high prevalence of the mutation in this breed, it would seem to be unwise to recommend that all cats with the mutation be removed from the breeding programs because altering the gene pool by 30% could increase the prevalence of other genetically determined disorders. Recommendations might be to remove cats that are homozygous for the mutation from the breeding pool. Heterozygous cats should be evaluated by echocardiography. If they do not show signs of hypertrophy it may suggest that they have low disease penetrance. If the cat has many other positive breed attributes and is disease negative at time of breeding, it could possibly be bred to a mutation-negative cat. The offspring of that mating should be screened, and if possible, a mutation-negative kitten with desirable traits selected to replace the mutation-positive parent in the breeding pool. Over a few generations this will decrease the prevalence of the disease mutation in the population, hopefully without greatly altering the gene pool. Disease-negative but mutation-positive cats should be evaluated annually for the presence of disease, and removed from use if they develop the disease.

Ragdoll Cardiomyopathy

A substitution mutation has also been identified in the myosin binding protein C gene in the Ragdoll cat.[11] However, the Ragdoll mutation is different from the Maine Coon mutation and is located in a different region of the gene. Because these 2 mutations are from such different locations in the gene, it is extremely unlikely that the Maine Coon and Ragdoll mutations were inherited from a common ancestor.

The mode of inheritance of this mutation in the Ragdoll cat has not been identified. In the Ragdoll, homozygous cats appear to be very severely affected with development of heart failure and thromboembolic episodes often before 2 years of age. Heterozygous cats appear to have a much more mild form of the disease that may include only mild papillary muscle hypertrophy.

The Ragdoll mutation also appears to be bred specific to the Ragdoll and has not been identified in other breeds of cats. Although there is no evidence as yet that there is more than one mutation in the Ragdoll, annual clinical screening is still recommended. Echocardiographic criteria for clinical clearance should be the same as indicated for Maine Coons.

At this time, approximately 20% of all Ragdolls tested at Washington State University have the Ragdoll mutation. Therefore, removal of all breeding animals form the gene pool is not without possible detriment to the breed. Breeding recommendations for interpretation and use of the Ragdoll test are the same as described for the Maine Coon.

ADULT-ONSET DISEASE IN THE DOG
Arrhythmogenic Right Ventricular Cardiomyopathy in the Boxer

Arrhythmogenic right ventricular cardiomyopathy (ARVC) is a familial disease in the boxer, and appears to be inherited as an autosomal dominant trait with incomplete penetrance.[1] An 8–base-pair deletion associated with the development of canine ARVC has been identified in an untranslated region of a desmosomal gene. Homozygous dogs appear to have a more severe form of the disease, with a statistically greater number of ventricular premature complexes (VPCs) per 24 hours than heterozygous.[33] It is not yet known if this is the only causative mutation for canine ARVC; therefore, clinical screening is still recommended.

Because ARVC presents as an electrical abnormality more often than one of myocardial dysfunction, clinical screening efforts should be based on annual Holter monitoring as well as annual echocardiography. Unfortunately, clear criteria for the diagnosis of occult ARVC do not exist. However, dogs that are symptomatic (syncope, heart failure) or have evidence of ventricular tachycardia on a Holter should not be used for breeding. In addition, dogs that have more than 100 left bundle branch block morphology VPCs per 24 hours are probably affected.

Genetic testing can now be performed for the ARVC mutation. It is not yet known what percentage of Boxers have the ARVC mutation, but it is likely to be high enough such that removal of all dogs with the mutation from the breeding pool could have a deleterious impact on the breed. It should be remembered that this is a disease of incomplete penetrance and variable expressivity. Therefore, not all affected dogs will ever develop clinical signs and many may live a normal life span. It is likely that there are multiple factors that may influence which dogs become symptomatic for the disease. Therefore, dogs that are positive heterozygous for the mutation should be carefully evaluated for signs of disease (Holter monitor and possibly an echocardiogram). Adult dogs that do not show signs of disease and that have other positive breed attributes could be bred to mutation-negative dogs. These may be dogs that have reduced penetrance. Puppies may be screened for the mutation and over a few generations, mutation-negative puppies may be selected to replace the mutation-positive parent and gradually decrease the number of mutation-positive dogs in the population. Boxers that are homozygous for the mutation should probably not be used for breeding. Boxers have more significant disease and because this is an autosomal dominant trait, they will certainly pass on the mutation.

Dilated Cardiomyopathy

Dilated cardiomyopathy (DCM) has now been shown to be inherited in several breeds of dogs including Doberman pinschers, Great Danes, Newfoundlands, Irish wolfhounds, and Portuguese Water dogs.[5–9] In human beings, the disease has been shown to be inherited in at least 20% to 40% of cases, and causative mutations have been identified in 24 genes.[34]

Doberman pinscher

Dilated cardiomyopathy in the Doberman pinscher appears to be inherited as an autosomal dominant trait with incomplete penetrance.[5] Several genes known to cause the human form of the disease have been evaluated in the Doberman pinscher including desmin, delta-sarcoglycan, phospholamban, actin, lamin A/C, MYH7, troponin T, troponin C, and the CSRP3 gene.[35–39] A causative mutation has not been identified.

Because a genetic mutation has not been identified, clinical screening on an annual basis is strongly recommended. Screening should include both echocardiography and ambulatory electrocardiography (Holter monitoring).[40,41] Owners should be advised that because this is an adult-onset disease with variability in the age of onset, screening tests should be performed annually.

Because this is an autosomal dominant trait, breeding of affected individuals is generally not recommended. If a dog is homozygous it would certainly pass on the trait. If a dog is heterozygous, it would have a 50% chance of passing on the trait and a 50% chance of not passing on the trait. Therefore, unaffected offspring of affected dogs that have been carefully cleared of the disease annually by echocardiography and Holter should be allowable for breeding because silent carriers should not exist. In addition, with an autosomal dominant trait all affected dogs should have at least one affected parent. Therefore, it is recommended that all parents of affected dogs be carefully evaluated with echocardiography and Holter monitoring.

Great Dane

Dilated cardiomyopathy (DCM) in the Great Dane is a familial disease.[6] In one study affected male dogs were overrepresented, suggesting an X-linked pattern of inheritance.[16] A recent study that evaluated the molecular aspects of the disease identified a difference in RNA expression for 2 cardiac transcripts, calstabin 2 and triadin.[42] Both calstabin and triadin are regulatory components of the cardiac ryanodine receptor. These findings may indicate that Great Dane DCM is associated with alterations of cellular calcium handling.[42]

Common clinical findings include a left apical systolic murmur and the presence of atrial fibrillation. Some Great Danes may develop atrial fibrillation first, before the presence of a heart murmur or ventricular dilation. Therefore, Great Danes with atrial fibrillation may be dogs with early DCM. However, some large breeds dogs also develop lone atrial fibrillation, which does not appear to have a relationship to DCM, thus not all dogs with atrial fibrillation will develop DCM.

If Great Dane DCM is an X-linked trait, sons of affected females should develop the disease because they inherit their X chromosome from their mother. Daughters of these affected male dogs are likely to be silent carriers because they will inherit one abnormal X chromosome from their father. Sons of affected male dogs should not develop DCM because they do not inherit any X chromosomes from their father.

Irish wolfhound

Dilated cardiomyopathy appears to be a familial disorder with an autosomal recessive mode of transmission, with sex-specific alleles in the Irish wolfhound. Male dogs appear to be overrepresented and often develop disease at an earlier age.[43] Molecular studies have focused on genetic markers on the X chromosome as well as the tafazzin gene, titin-cap, actin-alpha, cysteine- and glycine-rich protein 3, desmin, phospholambam, sarcoglycan-delta, and tropomodulin genes. A causative mutation has not been identified.[43–45]

Atrial fibrillation appears to frequently precede the development of a heart murmur and clinical signs.[46,47] Therefore, identification of atrial fibrillation may be an early sign. Annual screening with at least physical examination, electrocardiogram, and echocardiogram may be warranted. Additional electrocardiographic abnormalities have occasionally been described, including ventricular premature complexes and left anterior fascicular block patterns.

In the case of an autosomal recessive trait, 2 copies of the genetic mutation are needed to be able to show the trait. Silent carriers exist because dogs that only have one copy of the trait may pass the gene on, but will not show the trait. The risk of an individual inheriting the mutation from both parents and having clinical evidence of the trait can generally be decreased by outbreeding and not breeding to related dogs because this should decrease the risk of inadvertently breeding 2 dogs that have the same genetic mutation.

Newfoundland

Familial adult-onset DCM without a gender predisposition has been reported in the Newfoundland.[8] An autosomal dominant mode of inheritance with incomplete penetrance related to age has been suggested.[48] Common presenting complaints included dyspnea and ascites. Only a small percentage of dogs had an auscultable heart murmur,[8] but many dogs had atrial fibrillation.

Annual evaluation with a physical examination, echocardiogram, and electrocardiogram are warranted for screening.

Breeding recommendations are similar to those stated for the Doberman pinscher, another breed with an autosomal dominant form of DCM.

Portuguese Water dog

A juvenile form of familial DCM has been reported in the Portuguese Water dog. It is thought to be inherited as an autosomal recessive trait that is linked to a region on canine chromosome 8.[9] Affected puppies were from seemingly unaffected parents and typically died between 2 and 32 weeks of age, from sudden collapse and death without any preceding signs or congestive heart failure.[49] Echocardiography may detect this juvenile form of DCM 1 to 4 weeks before clinical signs.[9]

A test for a genetic marker highly associated with this disease is available through PennGen, http://research.vet.upenn.edu/penngen. Because this is a recessive trait, dogs that have 2 copies of the mutation are most likely to develop the disease. Silent carriers exist because dogs that only have one copy of the trait may pass the gene on, but will not show the trait. The risk of an individual inheriting the mutation from both parents and having clinical evidence of the trait can generally be decreased by outbreeding and not breeding to related dogs.

VALVULAR DISEASE
Valvular Disease in the Cavalier King Charles Spaniel

Chronic valvular disease (CVD) is a common finding in the Cavalier King Charles Spaniel. It has been suggested to be an inherited polygenic trait.[4,50] The offspring of parents with early onset or high-intensity murmurs were more likely to have developed a murmur by the age of 5 years than the offspring of nonmurmur parents.[4,50] Therefore, parental CVD status is an important factor influencing the probability of heart murmurs and their intensity in offspring.[4]

Current recommendations for clinical screening include annual evaluation for a heart murmur consistent with CVD. The ACVIM Cardiac Health Registry (http://www.archcertify.org/faqs.html) recommendations for breeding screening are the following: if auscultation does not detect a murmur or a click, the patient can be considered to be clear of disease at that time. If a heart murmur or click is present, the dog can still be considered clear if echocardiography does not detect CVD. If a typical murmur of valvular insufficiency is present, CVD can be diagnosed based on auscultation or echocardiography.

Ideally, affected dogs should not be bred; however, based on the high prevalence of CVD within the breed it may sometimes be necessary to breed affected dogs. Given the relationship of disease to severity of parents, it would be ideal to breed the most mildly affected to clear dogs that are offspring of parents that developed mild disease relatively late in life.

Mitral Valve Prolapse in the Dachshund

Mitral valve prolapse (MVP) has been found to be inherited in the dachshund, and the mode of inheritance is believed to be polygenic.[3] Parental severity was positively correlated to severity of MVP in offspring. However, gender may serve as a modifying influence because male dogs did appear to progress faster than females. Coat type was found to be related to the presence and severity of MVP, with long-haired dogs having more severe disease than short and wire haired.

Evaluation by auscultation appears to be a reasonable screening method for the presence of MVP.

Breeding recommendations would be similar to those suggested for other polygenic traits.

SUMMARY

Many forms of cardiovascular disease in the small animal patient are of an inherited etiology. Although the exact molecular cause is only known in a small percentage of diseases, understanding the mode of inheritance may provide important insight for the pet-owning population. Development of screening programs to reduce the prevalence of certain heart diseases in a population should be undertaken carefully, as aggressive exclusion of too many breeding animals because they have a higher risk of disease or mild disease could have a negative impact on the breed as a whole.

REFERENCES

1. Meurs KM, Spier AW, Miller MW, et al. Familial ventricular arrhythmias in Boxers. J Vet Intern Med 1999;13:437–9.
2. Gordon SG, Meurs KM. ASD in standard poodles: an update. In: Proceedings of the 26th Annual Veterinary Medical Forum. Dallas (TX), 2008. p. 121–2.
3. Olsen LH, Fredholm M, Pedersen HD. Epidemiology and inheritance of mitral valve prolapsed in Dachshunds. J Vet Intern Med 1999;13:448–56.
4. Swenson L, Haggstrom J, Kvart C, et al. Relationship between parental cardiac status in Cavalier King Charles spaniels and prevalence and severity of chronic valvular disease in offspring. J Am Vet Med Assoc 1996;208:2009–12.

5. Meurs KM, Fox PR, Norgard MM, et al. A prospective genetic evaluation of familial dilated cardiomyopathy in the Doberman pinscher. J Vet Intern Med 2007;21:1016–21.

6. Meurs KM, Miller MW, Wright NA. Clinical features of dilated cardiomyopathy in Great Danes and results of a pedigree analysis: 17 cases (1990–2000). J Am Vet Med Assoc 1998;218:729–32.

7. Distl O, Vollmar AC, Broschk C, et al. Complex segregation analysis of dilated cardiomyopathy (DCM) in Irish wolfhounds. Heredity 2007;99:460–5.

8. Dukes-McEwan J, Jackson IJ. The promises and problems of linkage analysis by using the current canine genome map. Mamm Genome 2002;13:667–72.

9. Werner P, Raducha MG, Prociuk U, et al. A novel locus for dilated cardiomyopathy maps to canine chromosome 8. Genomics 2008;91:517–21.

10. Kittleson MD, Meurs KM, Munroe M, et al. Familial hypertrophic cardiomyopathy in Maine Coon cats: an animal model of human disease. Circulation 1999;99: 3172–6.

11. Meurs KM, Norgard MM, Ederer MM, et al. A substitution mutation in the myosin binding protein C gene in Ragdoll hypertrophic cardiomyopathy. Genomics 2007; 90:261–4.

12. Patterson DF, Pyle RL, Buchanan JW, et al. Hereditary patent ductus arteriosus and its sequelae in the dog. Circ Res 1971;29:1–13.

13. Patterson DF, Haskins ME, Schnarr WR. Hereditary dysplasia of the pulmonary valve in beagle dogs. Pathologic and genetic studies. Am J Cardiol 1981;47:631–41.

14. Patterson DF, Pyle RL, Van Meirop L, et al. Hereditary defects of the conotruncal septum in Keeshond dogs: pathologic and genetic studies. Am J Cardiol 1974; 34:187–205.

15. Andelfinger G, Wright KN, Lee HS, et al. Canine tricuspid valve malformation, a model of human Ebstein anomaly, maps to dog chromosome 9. J Med Genet 2003;40:320–4.

16. Pyle RL, Patterson DF, Chacko S. The genetics and pathology of discrete sub-aortic stenosis in the Newfoundland dog. Am Heart J 1976;92:324–34.

17. Diez-Prieto I, García-Rodríguez B, Ríos-Granja A, et al. Cardiac conotruncal malformations in a family of beagle dogs. J Small Anim Pract 2009;50:597–603.

18. Brown W. Ventricular septal defects in the English springer spaniel. In: Kirk RW, editor. Current veterinary therapy XII. Philadelphia: W.B. Saunders; 1995. p. 827–9.

19. Patterson DF. Companion animal medicine in the age of medical genetics. J Vet Intern Med 2000;14:1–9.

20. Zook BC, Paasch LH. Endocardial fibroelastosis in Burmese cats. Am J Pathol 1982;106:435–8.

21. Fox PR. Feline cardiomyopathies. In: Fox PR, Sisson D, Moise NS, editors. Textbook of canine and feline cardiology. Philadelphia: W.B. Saunders; 1999. p. 621–78.

22. Bonagura JD, Lehmkuhl LB. Congenital heart disease. In: Fox PR, Sisson D, Moise NS, editors. Textbook of canine and feline cardiology. Philadelphia: W.B. Saunders; 1999. p. 471–536.

23. Buchanan JW. Prevalence of cardiovascular disorders. In: Fox PR, Sisson D, Moise NS, editors. Textbook of canine and feline cardiology. Philadelphia: W.B. Saunders; 1999. p. 457–70.

24. Lee SA, Lee SG, Moon HS. Isolation, characterization and genetic analysis of canine GATA4 gene in a family of Doberman Pinschers with an atrial septal defect. J Genet 2007;86:241–7.

25. Sarkozy A, Conti E, Neri C, et al. Spectrum of atrial septal defects associated with mutations of NKX2.5 and GATA4 transcription factors. J Med Genet 2005;42:e16.
26. Werner P, Raducha MG, Prociuk U, et al. The keeshond defect in cardiac cono-truncal development is oligogenic. Hum Genet 2005;116:368–77.
27. Lee JS, Hyun C. Genetic screening of the canine zinc finger protein multitype 2 (cZFPM2) gene in dogs with tetralogy of Fallot (TOF). J Anim Breed Genet 2009;126:304–10.
28. Famula TR, Siemens LM, Davidson AP, et al. Evaluation of the genetic basis of tricuspid valve dysplasia in Labrador retrievers. Am J Vet Res 2002;63:816–20.
29. Kraus MS, Calvert CA, Jacobs GJ. Hypertrophic cardiomyopathy in a litter of five mixed-breed cats. J Am Anim Hosp Assoc 1999;35:293–6.
30. Meurs KM, Sanchez X, David RM, et al. Identification of a missense mutation in the cardiac myosin binding protein C gene in a family of Maine Coon cats with hypertrophic cardiomyopathy. Hum Mol Genet 2005;14:3587–93.
31. Keren A, Syrris P, McKenna WJ. Hypertrophic cardiomyopathy: the genetic deter-minants of clinical disease expression. Nat Clin Pract Cardiovasc Med 2008;5: 158–68.
32. Sampedrano CC, Chetboul V, Mary J, et al. Prospective echocardiographic and tissue Doppler imaging screening of a population of Maine Coon cats tested for the A31P mutation in the myosin-binding protein C gene: a specific analysis of the heterozygous status. J Vet Intern Med 2008;23:91–9.
33. Meurs KM, Mauceli E, Acland GM, et al. Genome-wide association identified a candidate mutation for ARVC in the Boxer dog. J Vet Intern Med 2009;23:687–8.
34. Osterziel K-J, Habfeld S, Geier C, et al. Familiare dilatative kardiomyopathie. Herz 2005;30:529–34.
35. Stabej P, Imholz S, Versteeg SA, et al. Characterization of the canine desmin gene and evaluation as a candidate gene for dilated cardiomyopathy in the Doberman. Gene 2004;340:241–9.
36. Stabej P, Leegwater PA, Imholz S, et al. The canine sarcoglycan delta gene: BAC clone contig assembly, chromosome assignment and interrogation as a candidate gene for dilated cardiomyopathy in Doberman dogs. Cytogenet Genome Res 2005;111:140–6.
37. Stabej P, Leegwater PA, Stokhof AA, et al. Evaluation of the phospholamban gene in purebred large-breed dogs with dilated cardiomyopathy. Am J Vet Res 2005; 66:432–6.
38. Meurs KM, Magnon AL, Spier AW, et al. Evaluation of the cardiac actin gene in Doberman pinschers with dilated cardiomyopathy. Am J Vet Res 2001;62:33–6.
39. Meurs KM, Hendrix KP, Norgard MM. Molecular evaluation of five cardiac genes in Doberman pinschers with dilated cardiomyopathy. Am J Vet Res 2008;68: 1050–3.
40. O'Grady MR, Horne R. Occult dilated cardiomyopathy: an echocardiographic and electrocardiographic study of 193 asymptomatic Doberman pinschers. In: 15th Annual Veterinary Medical Forum 1995. p. 298–99.
41. Calvert CA, Jacobs G, Smith D. Long -term ambulatory electrocardiographic (Holter) recordings in overtly healthy Doberman pinschers with normal echocar-diograms. J Am Vet Med Assoc 2000;216:34–9.
42. Oyama MA, Chittur S, Reynolds CA. Decreased triadin and increased calsatbin2 expression in Great Danes with dilated cardiomyopathy. J Vet Intern Med 2009; 23:1014–9.
43. Philipp U, Broschk C, Vollmar A, et al. Evaluation of tafazzin as candidate for dilated cardiomyopathy in Irish wolfhounds. J Hered 2007;98:506–9.

44. Phillip U, Vollmar A, Distl O. Evaluation of six genes for dilated cardiomyopathy in Irish wolfhounds. Anim Genet 2007;39:84–92.

45. Phillip U, Vollmar A, Distl O. Evaluation of the titin-cap (TCAP) as candidate for dilated cardiomyopathy in Irish wolfhounds. Anim Biotechnol 2008;19:231–6.

46. Brownlie SE, Cobb MA. Observations on the development of congestive heart failure in Irish wolfhounds with dilated cardiomyopathy. J Small Anim Pract 1999;40:371–7.

47. Vollmar AC. The prevalence of cardiomyopathy in the Irish wolfhound: a clinical study of 500 dogs. J Am Anim Hosp Assoc 2000;36:125–32.

48. Tidholm A, Jonsson L. Dilated cardiomyopathy in the Newfoundland: a study of 37 cases. J Am Anim Hosp Assoc 1996;32:465–70.

49. Dambach DM, Lannon A, Sleeper MM, et al. Familial dilated cardiomyopathy of young Portuguese water dogs. J Vet Intern Med 1999;13:65–71.

50. Swift S. The problems of inherited diseases: valvular disease in Cavalier King Charles spaniels. J Small Anim Pract 1996;37:505–6.

Status of Therapeutic Gene Transfer to Treat Canine Dilated Cardiomyopathy in Dogs

Meg M. Sleeper, VMD[a],*, Lawrence T. Bish, PhD[b],
H. Lee Sweeney, PhD[b]

KEYWORDS

- Cardiomyopathy • Animal model • Heart disease
- Gene transfer • Heart failure

Idiopathic dilated cardiomyopathy (DCM) is one of the most common acquired heart diseases in the dog, most often affecting large dog breeds.[1] DCM is a cardiac muscle disease characterized by enlargement of the cardiac chambers and a reduction in systolic function.[2] Etiologic mutations have not yet been identified but familial forms of canine DCM are recognized, suggesting the possibility that the disorder has a genetic basis. Large breeds of dog such as Dobermans, boxers, and Great Danes are over-represented, with most dogs presenting between 6 and 8 years of age.[3] Although there may be a long asymptomatic period, the disease eventually progresses into congestive heart failure if the dog does not succumb to a fatal arrhythmia.[4] Although various surgical options are available in human medicine, including the use of left ventricular assist devices and cardiac transplantation, medical management Is the only option available for dilated cardiomyopathic veterinary patients, with therapy based only on symptomatic relief. The median survival time in a recent large retrospective study that included 369 cases was 19 weeks, with a range of 4 to 60 weeks.[3] Novel therapeutic strategies are needed to augment the current treatment arsenal for canine DCM.

New approaches that target the underlying molecular defects of ventricular dysfunction are currently being studied. Therapeutic gene transfer is one molecular-based

[a] Section of Cardiology, Department of Clinical Studies, University of Pennsylvania Veterinary School, 3900 Delancey Street, Philadelphia, PA 19104, USA
[b] Department of Physiology, University of Pennsylvania School of Medicine, Philadelphia, 3700 Hamilton Walk, PA 19104, USA
* Corresponding author.
E-mail address: sleeper@vet.upenn.edu

option for heart disease patients. Gene therapy has traditionally been used to transfer a gene that encodes a functional protein into a diseased patient, resulting in long-term expression of the protein that was deficient.[5,6] This strategy is often referred to as gene replacement therapy, and it requires that the mutated gene be previously identified. This approach has been used effectively to treat canine hemophilia, lysosomal storage diseases, and inherited retinal diseases.[7–13] However, gene transfer can also be performed when the causative mutation is unknown or in acquired diseases, with the goal of increasing the concentration of a therapeutic gene product in a tissue or organ. When used in this manner, gene transfer results in a drug effect, and multiple therapeutic gene products can be considered.

When naked DNA is injected directly into cells, it is largely degraded. Therefore, most gene transfer techniques package the genetic material so that it can be more efficiently introduced into the cells of interest. Most commonly, viruses are used for this packaging purpose. Viruses bind to their host cells and introduce their genetic material (and directions for producing more copies of the virus) into the host cell as part of their replication process. Therapeutic gene transfer using viral vectors for gene delivery reengineers the virus to replace the viral disease-causing genes with the gene of interest (the therapeutic gene). Multiple viruses have been used for this packaging purpose, including retroviruses, adenoviruses, and adeno-associated viruses (AAV). All viral vectors have positive and negative aspects to their use in gene transfer. Retroviruses are efficient at transferring genetic material to the host cell (transduction), particularly dividing cells, and they can carry large genes. However, the genetic material is inserted into the host genome, and if this insertion occurs in the middle of one of the original genes, the gene can be disrupted. This process is termed insertional mutagenesis. If the disrupted gene happens to be one that regulates cell division, uncontrolled cell division (neoplasia) can result. Adenoviruses are also capable of packaging large genes, but the genetic material they carry is not incorporated into the host cell's genetic code, but remains free in the nucleus. It is believed that this characteristic will reduce the risk of cancer; however, adenoviral infection frequently results in an immune response. AAV are small viruses from the parvovirus family. The engineered vector (recombinant AAV [rAAV]) does not insert the viral gene into the host genome, therefore the risk of development of cancer seems to be lower. Also, the virus is nonpathogenic, so an inflammatory response should not occur after the therapy, which allows long-term production of the gene product. However, because of the small viral size, AAV can only carry small therapeutic transgenes. Nonviral methods of packaging DNA are also used because of low host immunogenicity and easy large-scale production; however, every method of gene transfer has shortcomings and the optimal carrier is dependent on the goal of therapy. For treatment of DCM, an ideal vector would result in long-term production of the gene product (months to years) with minimal immune response or risk of insertional mutagenesis.

There is substantial evidence that Ca^{2+} handling in the failing heart is impaired, and that abnormalities of calcium cycling represent a final common pathway in the pathogenesis of heart disease and failure.[14,15] The reduced rate at which cytosolic Ca^{2+} is returned to the sarcoplasmic reticulum results in impaired myocardial relaxation and a decrease in the amount of Ca^{2+} released via the ryanodine receptor. As understanding of the molecular Ca^{2+}-handling pathways has improved, various target proteins for gene transfer–based therapeutics have become possible. The intracellular calcium gradient is partially maintained by the cardiac sarcoplasmic reticulum Ca^{2+} ATPase (SERCA2a), an energy-dependent molecular pump that transports Ca^{2+} from the cytosol across the membrane of the sarcoplasmic reticulum. The activity of SERCA2a is modulated by several proteins, including phospholamban (PLB).[16] By altering expression of the proteins that move calcium between the cytosol and the sarcoplasmic reticulum, Ca^{2+} handling can be normalized in diseased myocardial cells, resulting in improved cardiac function regardless of the underlying disease. Dephosphorylated PLB inhibits the SERCA2a pump; however, once PLB is phosphorylated, inhibition is reversed so that SERCA2a activity and the rate of sarcoplasmic reticulum calcium uptake is increased. This improved Ca^{2+} uptake leads to increased velocity of relaxation and myocardial contractility.[16] Thus, PLB is a potential molecular target in attempts to improve calcium cycling in the cardiomyocyte. Specific strategies that have been used in experimental models include the introduction of gene products that behave similarly to phosphorylated PLB, therefore increasing calcium reuptake, as well as genetic ablation of PLB.

The principle of altering levels of calcium-handling proteins has been studied in many rodent experiments in which levels of various Ca^{2+} regulators were altered, including PLB, β-adrenergic receptor (βAR) kinase, and S100A1. Dieterle and colleagues[17] used adenovirus to over-express a recombinant, intracellularly expressed, antibody-derived protein targeting the cytoplasmic domain of PLB in a cardiomyopathic hamster model and showed that short-term expression improved left ventricular function and myocardial contractility in the failing heart. Another group used a recombinant AAV (rAAV) vector expressing a pseudophosphorylated mutant of PLB. The resultant gene product, which mimicked the conformation of the phosphorylated form of PLB, acted as a dominant negative mutant, suppressing progressive impairment of left ventricular function and contractility for up to 30 weeks in the BIO 14.6 cardiomyopathic hamster, a model of limb-girdle muscular dystrophy type F, and the muscle-specific LIM domain protein (MLP)-deficient cardiomyopathic mouse.[18] Adenovirus-mediated delivery of this pseudophosphorylated PLB mutant was also effective in reversing heart failure progression in a sheep model of pacing-induced failure.[19] However, uncertainty persists regarding the effect of PLB manipulations. Interventions that augment PLB activity, as well as those that suppress it, have been effective in experimental models of myocardial dysfunction. However, despite the results of some experimental studies, lack of PLB in humans is associated with DCM. Other groups have altered calcium cycling via targeting the βAR or its regulating kinase. For example, one group used a transgenic mouse model to show that acute βAR kinase inhibition can restore lost myocardial βAR responsiveness and adrenergic reserve.[14] S100A1, a Ca^{2+}-sensing protein that increases myocardial SERCA activity, diminishes diastolic sarcoplasmic Ca^{2+} leakage and results in an overall gain in sarcoplasmic reticulum Ca^{2+} cycling, has also proven to have great potential as a therapeutic myocardial transgene. It has been shown to improve myocardial function and reduce cardiac remodeling in a rat model of heart failure.[15,20]

Increased rates of apoptosis, or programmed cell death, have also been reported in diseased human and animal hearts.[21] Gene therapy using an antiapoptotic factor (Bcl-2) was protective in a rabbit model of ischemic heart disease.[22] Bcl-2 conferred protection from apoptosis during the entire 6-week period of the study and resulted in preserved left ventricular geometry and prevention of dilation.[22] Gene transfer of the apoptosis repressor with a caspase recruiting domain (ARC) had similar efficacy in the same rabbit model of heart failure.[23] A list of potential transgene targets to treat DCM is given in **Box 1**.

As suggested earlier, cardiac gene therapy has proven to be simple in rodents, with multiple studies showing stable and efficient global myocardial transgene expression using an rAAV vector.[24–27] However, myocardial transduction has proven more difficult in large animal models because myocardial volume is a determinant of the

Box 1
Target transgenes
PLB (S16E mutant)
S100a1
SERCA2a
βAR kinase
Bcl-2
ARC

proportion of the myocardial mass that is transduced by systemic administration of vector.[28,29] Groups have addressed the difficulty in achieving global cardiac transduction in large animals in variable ways. Although it is unclear what percentage of the myocardium will need to be successfully transduced for effective therapy, and the required number of transduced cells may vary depending on the underlying cause of cardiomyopathy, it is likely that at least 50% of the myocardial cells should be transduced. Several delivery methods have been investigated with varying degrees of success using AAV, adenovirus, or plasmid DNA as vectors. Pericardial instillation of vector results in gene transfer that is restricted to the epicardium.[30,31] Direct, transepicardial injection of vector following left thoracotomy allows delivery throughout the left ventricular free wall, but is highly invasive and cannot target the interventricular septum.[32–35] In addition, the gene transfer vectors used in these studies have been associated with inflammation and unstable expression in the case of adenovirus and low-efficiency, unstable expression in the case of plasmid DNA.[36] **Table 1** provides a summary of vector characteristics in rabbit myocardium.

Bridges and colleagues[29] showed efficient (approximately 50%) global cardiac expression of a transferred gene in a small group of dogs using β-galactosidase as a reporter transgene with a technique in which the heart was completely isolated in situ. While on cardiopulmonary bypass, the heart was isolated, and 10^{13} particles of adenovirus encoding the reporter transgene in addition to 15 μg of vascular endothelial growth factor were infused retrograde into the coronary sinus and recirculated for 30 minutes at pressures ranging from 60 to 80 mm Hg. Although this technique resulted in efficient expression, 1/6 normal dogs did not survive the procedure, and results have not been reported in cardiomyopathic dogs. Another group showed that infusion of adenovirus simultaneously through the left anterior descending artery and the great cardiac vein resulted in gene transfer to 78% of the perfused target area

Table 1			
Properties of gene transfer vectors in the rabbit heart[a]			
	Positive Cells/Field	**Stability of Expression**	**Immune Response[b]**
Naked plasmid DNA	0	N/A	No
Adenovirus	357	<21 d	Robust
Herpes simplex virus	16	<21 d	Robust
AAV	31	>21 d	No

[a] Following direct intramyocardial injection.
[b] Compared with control (direct injection of vehicle only).
Data from Wright MJ, Wightman LM, Lilley C, et al. In vivo myocardial gene transfer: optimization, evaluation and direct comparison of gene transfer vectors. Basic Res Cardiol 2001;96:227–36.

in the swine.[37] Both of these studies used the highly immunogenic and unstable adenovirus vector. More recently, a group has shown cardiac transduction in juvenile dogs using intravenous rAAV delivery in conjunction with immunosuppression.[38] rAAV is likely to be a better vector to treat cardiomyopathy because it results in long-term transduction with less of an immune response than is seen with adenovirus. However, because the virus packaging capacity is small, the size of the transgene is limited with rAAV.

The authors have developed a system in which intramyocardial injections (40–60) of rAAV are delivered throughout the left ventricle using a cardiac injection catheter and a carotid artery approach. The authors believe this technique will be better tolerated by patients with heart disease than direct injections via thoracotomy or other more invasive techniques such as the procedure described earlier.[35,36] Moreover, it eliminates the requirement for costly and potentially dangerous vascular endothelial growth factor. The authors have also shown that self-complementary rAAV results in superior expression compared with single-stranded rAAV.[39] Self-complementary AAV2/6 results in transduction of approximately 60% of the myocardium using this approach, which is in the order of 1 log superior to the expression obtained using self-complementary rAAV2/8 or rAAV2/9.[39] The authors are currently using this technique to alter intracellular Ca^{2+} cycling in dogs with a juvenile form of DCM.[40–42]

The authors have treated 3 dogs affected with juvenile DCM using the dominant negative mutant of PLB. When cells are transduced and produce the gene product, this mutant form of PLB will compete with the native PLB, thereby reducing its activity. In the 3 affected dogs treated with this approach, the disease process was slower than the typical progression in untreated dogs (Sleeper, unpublished data, 2009). The authors have also treated 3 normal mongrels with this transgene. All 3 of these dogs are currently more than 1 year posttreatment with normal cardiac function, showing that the approach should be safe in the long-term. Moreover, a cross of the PLB knockout mouse with the muscle lim protein knockout mouse (model of DCM) led to complete correction of the cardiac phenotype, suggesting that global reduction in PLB levels should be well tolerated.[43] The authors are currently evaluating the efficacy of a combined PLB inhibitor/s100a1 transgene to determine whether therapeutic efficacy will improve.

SUMMARY

Therapeutic gene transfer holds promise as a way to treat DCM from any underlying cause because the approach attempts to address metabolic disturbances that occur at the molecular level of the failing heart. Calcium-handling abnormalities[44] and increased rates of apoptosis[21,22] are abnormalities that occur in many types of heart disease, and gene therapies that target these metabolic defects have proven to be beneficial in numerous rodent models of heart disease. The authors are currently evaluating this approach to treat canine idiopathic DCM.

REFERENCES

1. Tidholm Λ, Jonooon L. A retrospective study of canine dilated cardiomyopathy (189 cases). J Am Anim Hosp Assoc 1997;33:544–50.
2. Richardson P, McKenna W, Bristow M, et al. Report of the 1995 World Health Organization/International Society and Federation of Cardiology Task Force on the Definition and Classification of Cardiomyopathies. Circulation 1996;93(5): 841–2.

3. Martin MW, Stafford Johnson MJ, Celona B. Canine dilated cardiomyopathy: a retrospective study of signalment, presentation and clinical findings in 369 cases. J Small Anim Pract 2009;50(1):23–9.

4. Borgarelli M, Santilli RA, Chiavegato D, et al. Prognostic indicators for dogs with dilated cardiomyopathy. J Vet Intern Med 2006;20:104–10.

5. Lyon AR, Sato M, Hajjar RJ, et al. Harding SE gene therapy: targeting the myocardium. Heart 2008;94:89–99.

6. Vinge LE, Raake PW, Koch WJ. Gene therapy in heart failure. Circ Res 2008;102: 1458–70.

7. Haskins M. Gene therapy for lysosomal storage diseases (LSDs) in large animal models. ILAR J 2009;50:112–21.

8. Tessitore A, Faella A, O'Malley T, et al. Biochemical, pathological and skeletal improvement of mucopolysaccharidosis VI after gene transfer to liver but not to muscle. Mol Ther 2008;16:30–7.

9. Margaritis P, Roy E, Aljamali MN, et al. Successful treatment of canine hemophilia by continuous expression of canine FVIIa. Blood 2009;113:3682–9.

10. Niemeyer GP, Herzog RW, Mount J, et al. Long term correction of inhibitor-prone hemophilia B dogs treated with liver-directed AAV2-mediated factor IX gene therapy. Blood 2008;113:797–806.

11. Acland GM, Aguirre GD, Bennet J, et al. Long term restoration of rod and cone vision by single dose rAAV-mediated gene transfer to the retina in a canine model of childhood blindness. Mol Ther 2005;12:1072–82.

12. Manno CS, Pierce GF, Arruda VR, et al. Successful transduction of liver in hemophilia by AAV-factor IX and limitations imposed by the host immune response. Nat Med 2006;12(3):342–7.

13. Ponder KP, Melniczek JR, Xu L, et al. Therapeutic neonatal gene therapy in mucopolysaccharidosis VII dogs. Proc Natl Acad Sci U S A 2002;99(20): 13102–7.

14. Manning BS, Shotwell K, Mao L, et al. Physiological induction of a beta-adrenergic receptor kinase inhibitor transgene preserves ss-adrenergic responsiveness in pressure-overload cardiac hypertrophy. Circulation 2000;102(22): 2751–7.

15. Most P, Pleger ST, Volkers M, et al. Cardiac adenoviral S100A1 gene delivery rescues failing myocardium. J Clin Invest 2004;114(11):1550–63.

16. Mattiazzi A, Mundina-Weilenmann C, Guoxiang C, et al. Role of phospholamban phosphorylation on Thr17 in cardiac physiological and pathological conditions. Cardiovasc Res 2005;68(3):366–75.

17. Dieterle T, Meyer M, Gu Y, et al. Gene transfer of a phospholamban-targeted antibody improves calcium handling and cardiac function in heart failure. Cardiovasc Res 2005;67(4):678–88.

18. Hoshijima M, Ikeda Y, Iwanaga Y, et al. Chronic suppression of heart-failure progression by a pseudophosphorylated mutant of phospholamban via in vivo cardiac rAAV gene delivery. Nat Med 2002;8(8):864–71.

19. Kaye DM, Preovolos A, Marshall T, et al. Percutaneous cardiac recirculation-mediated gene transfer of an inhibitory phospholamban peptide reverses advanced heart failure in large animals. J Am Coll Cardiol 2007;50(3):253–60.

20. Pleger ST, Most P, Boucher M, et al. Stable myocardial-specific AAV6-S100A1 gene therapy results in chronic functional heart failure rescue. Circulation 2007; 115(19):2506–15.

21. Olivetti G, Abbi R, Quaini F, et al. Apoptosis in the failing human heart. N Engl J Med 1997;336(16):1131–41.

22. Chatterjee S, Stewart AS, Bish LT, et al. Viral gene transfer of the antiapoptotic factor bcl-2 protects against chronic postischemic heart failure. Circulation 2002;106(12 Suppl. 1):212–7.

23. Chatterjee S, Bish LT, Jayasankar V, et al. Blocking the development of postischemic cardiomyopathy with viral gene transfer of the apoptosis repressor with caspase recruitment domain. J Thorac Cardiovasc Surg 2003;125(6):1461–9.

24. Gregorevic P, Blankinship MJ, Allen JM, et al. Systemic delivery of genes to striated muscles using adeno-associated viral vectors. Nat Med 2004;10(8):828–34.

25. Inagaki K, Fuess S, Storm TA, et al. Robust systemic transduction with AAV9 vectors in mice: efficient global cardiac gene transfer superior to that of AAV8. Mol Ther 2006;14(1):45–53.

26. Woo YJ, Zhang JC, Taylor MD, et al. One year transgene expression with adeno-associated virus cardiac gene transfer. Int J Cardiol 2005;100(3):421–6.

27. Bish LT, Morine K, Sleeper MM, et al. AAV9 provides global cardiac gene transfer superior to AAV1, AAV6, AAV7 and AAV8 in the mouse and rat. Hum Gene Ther 2008;19:1359–68.

28. Bridges CR, Burkman JM, Malekan R, et al. Global cardiac-specific transgene expression using cardiopulmonary bypass with cardiac isolation. Ann Thorac Surg 2002;73(6):1939–46.

29. Bridges CR, Gopal K, Holt DE, et al. Efficient myocyte gene delivery with complete cardiac surgical isolation in situ. J Thorac Cardiovasc Surg 2005; 130(5):1364.

30. Lamping KG, Rios CD, Chun JA, et al. Intrapericardial administration of adenovirus for gene transfer. Am J Physiol 1997;272:H310–7.

31. Lazarous DF, Shou M, Stiber JA, et al. Adenoviral-mediated gene transfer induces sustained pericardial VEGF expression in dogs: effect on myocardial angiogenesis. Cardiovasc Res 1999;44:294–302.

32. Ferrarini M, Arsic N, Recchia FA, et al. Adeno-associated virus-mediated transduction of VEGF165 improves cardiac tissue viability and functional recovery after permanent coronary occlusion in conscious dogs. Circ Res 2006;98: 954–61.

33. Laguens R, Cabeza MP, Vera JG, et al. Cardiomyocyte hyperplasia after plasmid-mediated vascular endothelial growth factor gene transfer in pigs with chronic myocardial ischemia. J Gene Med 2004;6:222–7.

34. McTiernan CF, Mathier MA, Zhu X, et al. Myocarditis following adeno-associated viral gene expression of human soluble TNF receptor (TNFRII-Fc) in baboon hearts. Gene Ther 2007;14:1613–22.

35. Vera Janavel G, Crottogini A, Cabexa Meckert P, et al. Plasmid-mediated VEGF gene transfer induces cardiomyogenesis and reduces myocardial infarct size in sheep. Gene Ther 2006;13:1133–42.

36. Li JJ, Ueno H, Pan Y, et al. Percutaneous transluminal gene transfer into canine myocardium in vivo by replication-defective adenovirus. Cardiovasc Res 1995; 30:97–105.

37. Sasano T, Kikuchi K, McDonald AD, et al. Targeted high-efficiency, homogeneous myocardial gene transfer. J Mol Cell Cardiol 2007;42(5):954–61.

38. Gregorevic P, Schultz BR, Allen JM, et al. Evaluation of vascular delivery methodologies to enhance rAAV6-mediated gene transfer to canine striated musculature. Mol Ther 2009;17(8):1427–33.

39. Bish LT, Sleeper MM, Brainard B, et al. Percutaneous transendocardial delivery of self-complementary adeno-associated virus 6 achieves global cardiac gene transfer in canines. Mol Ther 2008;16:1953–9.

40. Dambach D, Lannon A, Sleeper M, et al. Familial dilated cardiomyopathy of young Portuguese water dogs. J Vet Intern Med 1999;13:65–71.

41. Sleeper M, Henthorn P, Vijayasarathy C, et al. Characterization of juvenile dilated cardiomyopathy in Portuguese water dogs. J Vet Intern Med 2002;16:52–62.

42. Werner P, Raducha MG, Prociuk U, et al. A novel locus for dilated cardiomyopathy maps to canine chromosome 8. Genomics 2008;91:517–21.

43. Minamisawa S, Hoshijima M, Chu G, et al. Chronic phospholamban-sarcoplasmic reticulum calcium ATPase interaction is the critical calcium cycling defect in dilated cardiomyopathy. Cell 1999;19(3):313–22.

44. Diedrichs H, Hagemeister J, Chi M, et al. Activation of the calcineurin/NFAT signalling cascade starts early in human hypertrophic myocardium. J Int Med Res 2007;35:803–18.

Index

Note: Page numbers of article titles are in **boldface** type.

A

Acquired heart defects, in small animals, surgical procedures for, 616–618

Acquired heart disease, in small animals, genetics of, 707–709

Amplatz Canine Duct Occluder, for PDA, 591–593

Amplatzer Canine Duct Occluder, for PDA, 586–588

Amplatzer Vascular Plug, for PDA in dogs, 588–591

Arrhythmia(s), feline, **643–650**

  AV block, 646–648

  HCM, 648

  hyperkalemia, 643–645

  ventricular tachyarrhythmias, 645–646

Arrhythmogenic right ventricular cardiomyopathy (ARVC), in boxers, genetics of, 709–710

ARVC. See *Arrhythmogenic right ventricular cardiomyopathy (ARVC)*.

ASD. See *Atrial septal defect (ASD)*.

Atrial septal defect (ASD)

  canine, occlusion procedures for, 593–594

  in small animals

    genetics of, 704–705

    surgical procedures for, 615

Atrioventricular (AV) block, feline, 646–648

Atrioventricular (AV) valve stenosis, canine, occlusion procedures for, 599

Autosomal dominant genes, cardiac disease in small animals and, 702

Autosomal recessive genes, cardiac disease in small animals and, 701–702

AV. See *Atrioventricular (AV)*.

B

Balloon dilation, canine

  of pulmonic stenosis, 596–597

  of SAS, 598–599

Bartonella spp., infective endocarditis in dogs due to, 667–669

Biomarkers, in pulmonary hypertension in dogs diagnosis, 627–628

Blood pressure, natriuretic peptides in cats effects on, 564

BNP. See *B-type natriuretic peptide (BNP)*.

Boxer(s), ARVC in, genetics of, 709–710

B-type natriuretic peptide (BNP), testing of, in human medicine, 546–547

C

Calcium-sensitizing agents, for canine pulmonary hypertension, 635

Cardiac disease, in small animals

  genetics of, **701–715**. See also specific animals and diseases.

Vet Clin Small Anim 40 (2010) 725–732

doi:10.1016/S0195-5616(10)00075-6

0195-5616/10/$ – see front matter © 2010 Elsevier Inc. All rights reserved.

vetsmall.theclinics.com

Moving?

Make sure your subscription moves with you!

To notify us of your new address, find your **Clinics Account Number** (located on your mailing label above your name), and contact customer service at:

Email: journalscustomerservice-usa@elsevier.com

800-654-2452 (subscribers in the U.S. & Canada)
314-447-8871 (subscribers outside of the U.S. & Canada)

Fax number: 314-447-8029

Elsevier Health Sciences Division
Subscription Customer Service
3251 Riverport Lane
Maryland Heights, MO 63043

*To ensure uninterrupted delivery of your subscription, please notify us at least 4 weeks in advance of move.

Printed and bound by CPI Group (UK) Ltd, Croydon, CR0 4YY

03/10/2024

01040448-0001